Anti-Angiogenesis Drug Discovery and Development

(Volume 5)

Edited by

Atta-ur-Rahman, *FRS*
Kings College,
University of Cambridge, Cambridge,
UK

&

Muhammad Iqbal Choudhary
H.E.J. Research Institute of Chemistry,
International Center for Chemical and Biological Sciences,
University of Karachi, Karachi,
Pakistan

Anti-Angiogenesis Drug Discovery and Development

Volume # 5

Editors: Prof. Atta-ur-Rahman and Prof. M. Iqbal Choudhary

ISSN (Online): 2210-268X

ISSN (Print): 2452-3240

ISBN (Online): 978-981-14-3287-3

ISBN (Print): 978-981-14-3286-6

©2020, Bentham eBooks imprint.

Published by Bentham Science Publishers Pte. Ltd. Singapore. All Rights Reserved.

need for a court order if at any point you breach any terms of this License Agreement. In no event will any delay or failure by Bentham Science Publishers in enforcing your compliance with this License Agreement constitute a waiver of any of its rights.

3. You acknowledge that you have read this License Agreement, and agree to be bound by its terms and conditions. To the extent that any other terms and conditions presented on any website of Bentham Science Publishers conflict with, or are inconsistent with, the terms and conditions set out in this License Agreement, you acknowledge that the terms and conditions set out in this License Agreement shall prevail.

Bentham Science Publishers Pte. Ltd.
80 Robinson Road #02-00
Singapore 068898
Singapore
Email: subscriptions@benthamscience.net

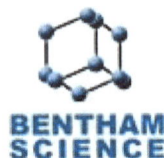

BENTHAM SCIENCE

CONTENTS

PREFACE

Angiogenesis, formation of new blood vessels, is one of the most vigorously studied processes due to its central place in normal physiology and in the on-set of diseases. Imbalance in tightly regulated angiogenesis leads to complex chronic disorders, especially solid tumors and other malignancies. A complex cascade of angiogenic signaling molecules, including vascular endothelial growth factors (VEGF), is involved that has attracted immense scientific interest as possible drug targets. Several inhibitors of angiogenesis have been developed and extensive preclinical and clinical studies are underway.

The book series *"Anti-angiogenesis Drug Discovery and Development"* covers a broad range of topics focusing on the development of anti-angiogenic agents and their mechanisms of actions. Volume 5 has five comprehensive reviews, contributed by leading experts in these fields. These reviews broadly cover various important drug targets, and new classes of anti-angiogenic therapies for the prevention or treatment of cancers.

The review by Mabeta *et al* focuses on complex molecular mechanisms of angiogenesis, and their role as drug targets. Therapeutic approaches that target multiple pathways and components of the microenvironment as well as those normalize the vasculature, are explored. In addition, applications of noninvasive imaging to monitor the effects of AIs on tumor vessels is discussed. The review of Khan *et al*. focuses on various types of antiangiogenic agents, biochemical, chemical, and recombinant, in clinical trials or those recently approved against breast and prostate cancers and their respective mechanisms of action.

Microorganisms have been rich sources of biologically active molecules since the discovery of penicillin. Khurshid *et al* have reviewed the recent literature on innovative approaches involving microbe-based anti-angiogenic anti-cancer therapeutics. These include DNA vaccination, bactofection, alternative gene therapy and RNA interferences, as well as genetically modified bacteria as antiangiogenic agents. Soleimanjahi and Ala Habibian have contributed a comprehensive review on various classes of antiangiogenic agents which target powerful regulators that play a crucial role in cell proliferation and tumor microenvironment. These agents include VEGF inhibition, mesenchymal stem cells (MSCs) as vehicles for antiangiogenic agents, use of oncolytic viruses which selectively replicate in tumor cells, *etc*. Last but not the least, the review of Costa *et al* covers recent progress on coumarin- and chromene-based anticancer agents. Chromenes and coumarins are naturally occurring polyphenolic compounds, which are known to regulate the expressions of VEGF, matric metalloproteinases (MMPs), and receptor tyrosine kinases (RTKs) signaling pathways. Many of them are in various stages of development.

We would to express our gratitude to all the authors of above cited review articles for their excellent scholarly works in this dynamic and exciting field of biomedical and pharmaceutical research. The efforts of the excellent team of Bentham Science Publishers for the timely production of the 5th volume are greatly appreciated particularly the efforts of Ms. Mariam Mehdi (Assistant Manager Publications), and Mr. Mahmood Alam (Director Publications). We hope that the efforts of the contributing authors, and the production team will help readers in gaining a better understanding of this important area of biomedical research.

Prof. Dr. Atta-ur-Rahman *FRS*
Kings College
University of Cambridge
Cambridge
UK

&

Prof. Dr. M. Iqbal Choudhary
H.E.J. Research Institute of Chemistry
International Center for Chemical and Biological Sciences
University of Karachi
Karachi
Pakistan

LIST OF CONTRIBUTORS

Ala Habibian	Department of Virology, Faculty of Medical Sciences, Tarbiat Modares University, Tehran, Iran
Alexandre Bridoux	Integral University, Lucknow, India Laboratoire Centre Atlantique, Zone Industrielle Chef de Baie, 1 rue Samuel de Champlain, Cs 41074, 17000la Rochelle, France
Ana Raquel-Cunha	Life and Health Sciences Research Institute (ICVS), University of Minho, Campus of Gualtar, Braga, Portugal ICVS/3Bs-PT Government Associate Laboratory, Braga/Guimarães, Portugal
Asad Ali Shah	Department of Bioinformatics & Biotechnology, Government College University Faisalabad, Pakistan
Fátima Baltazar	Life and Health Sciences Research Institute (ICVS), University of Minho, Campus of Gualtar, Braga, Portugal ICVS/3Bs-PT Government Associate Laboratory, Braga/Guimarães, Portugal
Hoorieh Soleimanjahi	Department of Virology, Faculty of Medical Sciences, Tarbiat Modares University, Tehran, Iran
Marta Costa	Life and Health Sciences Research Institute (ICVS), University of Minho, Campus of Gualtar, Braga, Portugal ICVS/3Bs-PT Government Associate Laboratory, Braga/Guimarães, Portugal
Mike Sathekge	Department of Nuclear Medicine, University of Pretoria, Pretoria, South Africa
Mohammad Yusuf	College of Pharmacy, Taif University, Al-Haweiah, Taif, KSA
Mohsin Khurshid	Department of Microbiology, Government College University Faisalabad, Pakistan
Muhammad Shahid	Department of Bioinformatics & Biotechnology, Government College University Faisalabad, Pakistan
Muhammad Sajid Hamid Akash	Department of Pharmaceutical Chemistry, Government College University Faisalabad, Pakistan
Naseem Akhtar	College of Pharmacy, Buraydah Colleges, Qassim, KSA
Olga Martinho	Life and Health Sciences Research Institute (ICVS), University of Minho, Campus of Gualtar, Braga, Portugal ICVS/3Bs-PT Government Associate Laboratory, Braga/Guimarães, Braga, Portugal Molecular Oncology Research Center, Barretos Cancer Hospital, Barretos, São Paulo, Brazil
Olívia Pontes	Life and Health Sciences Research Institute (ICVS), University of Minho, Campus of Gualtar, Braga, Portugal ICVS/3Bs-PT Government Associate Laboratory, Braga/Guimarães, Portugal

Peace Mabeta	Department of Physiology, University of Pretoria, Pretoria, South Africa
Riaz A. Khan	Manav Rachna International Institute of Research & Study (MRIIRS)-Manav Rachna International University (MRIU), Faridabad, HR 121 001, India College of Pharmacy, Qassim University, Qassim, KSA
Samman Munir	Department of Bioinformatics & Biotechnology, Government College University Faisalabad, Pakistan
Salman A. A. Mohammed	College of Pharmacy, Qassim University, Qassim, KSA
Shilpa J. Newati	Manav Rachna International Institute of Research & Study (MRIIRS)-Manav Rachna International University (MRIU), Faridabad, India
Sofia Oliveira-Pinto	Life and Health Sciences Research Institute (ICVS), University of Minho, Campus of Gualtar, Braga, Portugal ICVS/3Bs-PT Government Associate Laboratory, Braga/Guimarães, Portugal
Usman Ali Ashfaq	Department of Bioinformatics & Biotechnology, Government College University Faisalabad, Pakistan
Vanessa Steenkamp	Department of Pharmacology, Faculty of Health Sciences, University of Pretoria, Pretoria, SouthAfrica
Varsha M. Singh	Manav Rachna International Institute of Research & Study (MRIIRS)-Manav Rachna International University (MRIU), Faridabad, HR 121 001, India

CHAPTER 1

Therapeutic Targeting of the Tumor Vasculature: Past, Present and Future

Peace Mabeta[1,*], Mike Sathekge[2] and **Vanessa Steenkamp[3]**

[1]*Department of Physiology, University of Pretoria, Pretoria, South Africa*
[2]*Department of Nuclear Medicine, University of Pretoria, Pretoria, South Africa*
[3]*Department of Pharmacology, Faculty of Health Sciences, University of Pretoria, Pretoria, South Africa*

Abstract: Tumor progression relies on a constant supply of oxygen and nutrients. Angiogenesis, the formation of neovessel from existing microvessels, is a prerequisite for the growth of many tumors. Significant advances have been made in delineating the interplay between pro- and anti-angiogenic factors that foster an environment that promotes the angiogenic phenotype in tumors. Of these angiogenic regulators, vascular endothelial growth factor-A (VEGF-A) and its cognate receptor, vascular endothelial growth factor receptor-2 (VEGFR-2) have been the most studied.

Various angiogenesis inhibitors (AIs) that target VEGF-A and VEGFR-2 have been developed for use as monotherapy or as part of combination therapies with standard chemotherapy. However, these AIs have thus far produced modest results, in part owing to compensatory pathways that have led to disease refractory.

To overcome refractory to disease, normalization of the tumor vasculature and broadening of the scope of therapeutic targeting are necessary. Furthermore, predictive biomarkers can enhance efficacy by enabling the early detection of resistance as well as the determination of clinical benefit. Herein, the therapeutic approaches that target multiple pathways and components of the tumor microenvironment, as well as those that normalize the vasculature are explored. In addition, the future application of non-invasive imaging to monitor the effects of AIs on the tumor vessels is discussed.

Keywords: Angiogenesis, Bevacizumab, Cancer, Imaging, Immunotherapy, Hypoxia, Vascular endothelial growth factor.

INTRODUCTION

The functions of the blood vasculature include the transport of nutrients and gasses, transcapillary filtration, vascular tone, hemostasis, and hormone traffic-

---

* **Corresponding author Peace Mabeta**: Department of Physiology, University of Pretoria, Pretoria, South Africa;
E-mail: peace.mabeta@up.ac.za

Atta-ur-Rahman & M. Iqbal Choudhary (Eds.)

king [1]. Endothelial cells provide a non-thrombogenic environment which facilitates the transit of plasma and cellular constituents of blood throughout the vasculature [1, 2]. The functions of blood vessels are mainly effected through various ligands including growth factors and their receptors, cytokines, as well as transcription factors such as hypoxia inducible factor-1α (HIF-1α) [2, 3]. Some of these molecules also modulate vascular homeostasis by regulating the process of angiogenesis.

Angiogenesis is the formation of blood vessels from an existing microvasculature [4, 5]. During embryonic development, angiogenesis is necessary for the remodeling of the primordial vasculature, while in postnatal development, the process of angiogenesis is important for tissue growth [5]. However, in the adult, the endothelium is in a relatively quiescent state, which is maintained by a balance between anti-angiogenic and pro-angiogenic factors [6]. Under such conditions, angiogenesis is observed only in a few instances such as during wound healing. In the female, vascular homeostasis is also periodically interrupted during the reproductive cycle [7].

The process of angiogenesis also occurs during pathological conditions such as cancer [2, 8]. Indeed, sustained angiogenesis is a hallmark of various malignancies [9, 10].

ANGIOGENESIS IN TUMOR PROGRESSION

For tumors to grow beyond 1-2mm in diameter, they need to elaborate a vascular supply [2]. Angiogenesis enables tumor neovascularization, thus providing a route for nutrient delivery [2, 8]. The steps involved in angiogenesis include the disruption of the basement membrane and remodeling of the extracellular matrix (ECM) [8].

In addition, endothelial cells (ECs) migrate and proliferate in the direction of the stimulus, and coalesce to form capillary channels through which blood flow can be established [6, 8]. The maturation of the newly formed is the recruitment of supporting cells such as pericytes [4, 9]. Unlike blood vessels formed through physiological angiogenesis, the tumor vessels are structurally and functionally abnormal.

The Tumor Vasculature

Tumor blood vessels are chaotic and lack the normal architecture observed in normal vessels. These blood vessels are also tortuous, and they have few pericytes, making them immature and unstable [2, 6]. Furthermore, due to the loss of VE-Cadherin, cell-cell contacts are compromised, resulting in a loss of vessel integrity [6].

Some of the vessels are susceptible to collapse, thus leading to erratic blood flow and poor perfusion [2]. This in turn hampers proper delivery of drugs. Also, the vessels are leaky, which supports tumor cell extravazation into the circulation [5, 6]. It is for this reason that vascular normalization has been recognized as important for effective tumor antiangiogenesis therapies.

The trigger for tumor angiogenesis is a local imbalance between pro-angiogenic factors and anti-angiogenic factors, which is tilted towards angiogenesis stimulators [2, 6]. In response to hypoxia, tumor cells secrete proteins that stimulate angiogenesis (Fig. **1**). Of the secreted proteins, the vascular endothelial growth factor-A (VEGF-A) is the best characterized [11].

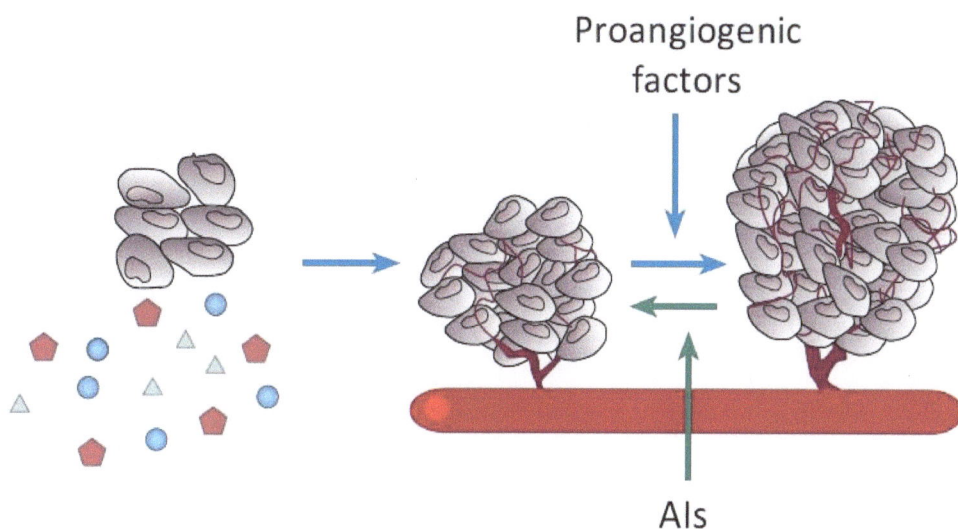

Fig. (1). Schematic representation of the induction of angiogenesis by angiogenic growth factors secreted by tumor cells. Proangiogenic factors such as VEGF stimulate the vasculature to sprout new vessels. The newly formed vessels enable further tumor growth. Angiogenesis inhibitors limit tumor neovascularization and sometimes normalize the tumor vasculature.
AIs – angiogenesis inhibitors

    - vascular endothelial growth factor (VEGF),   - basic fibroblast growth factor (bFGF),   - platelet derived growth factor (PDGF)

Importance of Vascular Endothelial Growth Factor Signaling in Cancer

In humans, the vascular endothelial growth factor (VEGF) family consists of VEGF -A, -B, -C, -D, and placental growth factor (PlGF) [12]. The most studied angiogenic growth factor in this family is VEGF-A (referred to herein as VEGF). It is an important mediator of angiogenesis both in physiological and pathological settings [12]. The principal receptors for VEGF are VEGFR-1 and VEGFR-2, although VEGFR-2 presents greater signaling activity [13]. As such, the mitogenic actions of VEGF in endothelial cells are mediated mainly *via* VEGFR-2 [12, 13]. In addition, VEGFR-2 plays a key role in modulating cell migration and vascular permeability in response to VEGF, whereas VEGFR-1 has a weak or undetectable response [12].

Upon binding of VEGF to VEGFR-2, phosphatidylinositol-4,5-bisphosphate 3-kinase (PI3k) is recruited to the internal side of the cell membrane and activated through phosphorylation (Fig. **2**) [14, 15]. Activated PI3k phosphorylates phosphatidylinositol 4,5-bisphosphate (PIP2) to form phosphatidylinositol 3,4,5-trisphosphate (PIP3) [14].

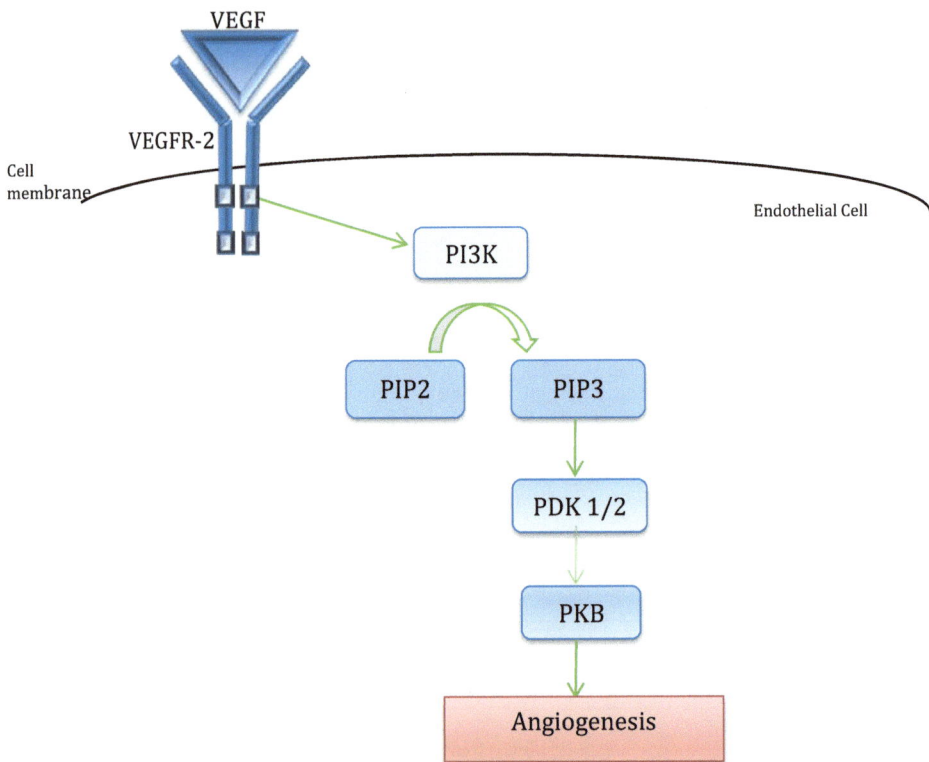

Fig. (2). A schematic diagram showing the activation of PI3K/PKB signaling which occurs following the binding of VEGF to VEGFR-2. The pathway promotes angiogenesis.

Phosphatidylinositol 3,4,5-trisphosphate initiates a cascade of events that lead to the phosphorylation of 3-phosphoinositide-dependent protein kinase-1 and -2 (PDK1/2), which in turn activate protein kinase B (PKB), a key downstream effector of PI3k, ultimately leading to angiogenesis (Fig. **2**) [14, 15].

Investigations have shown unequivocally that angiogenesis promotes tumor progression and in some cancers, metastasis. Accordingly, the targeting of the tumor vasculature has become an important approach in anti-cancer therapy [8, 10, 11]. In particular, the development of drugs that target vascular endothelial growth factor signaling has received considerable attention over the past two decades.

Studies on human and murine tumors have shown that VEGFR-2 is upregulated in tumors [8, 16]. Also, high levels of VEGF have also been measured in blood and urine samples of patients with different neoplasms [17 - 19]. Additionally, in some cancers, high levels of VEGF correlate with a poor prognosis [19]. The clinical development of angiogenesis inhibitors (AIs) has also focused on the cognate receptor for vascular endothelial growth factor, namely, VEGFR-2 [18, 19].

Therapeutic Targeting of Vascular Endothelial Growth Factor

The discovery that VEGF is over-expressed in many neoplasms, and that it is a key mediator of tumor angiogenesis, made it an important target in anti-cancer therapy. Preclinical studies in xenograft models of various cancers found that the inhibition of VEGF resulted in a decrease in microvascular density (MVD) and in the suppression of tumor growth [20].

The inhibition of VEGF with a neutralizing antibody led to reduced metastasis in preclinical models of colorectal cancer [20]. Based on these observations, the targeting of VEGF was further tested in patients.

It is worth noting that the clinical testing of a VEGF targeting antibody was preceded by the development of TNP-470, an analogue of Fumagillin. TNP-470 was one of the first drugs to undergo clinical testing for angiogenesis inhibition in cancer patients [21]. Unfortunately negative results such as a short half-life and severe side-effects hampered its further clinical development. Nonetheless, efforts to develop anti-angiogenic drugs continued and by 2004, Ferrara and colleagues had designed a humanized VEGF antibody (Ab) to target the tumor vasculature [16].

Although the neutralization of VEGF with a VEGF antibody was successful in preclinical studies, the humanized Ab was much weaker than the murine Ab in terms of binding affinity to the growth factor [22]. The humanized Ab was thus further engineered by replacing 7 residues in the variable heavy domain [22]. The newly engineered human VEGF monoclonal antibody, which was named bevacizumab, underwent testing in patients with diseases characterized by excessive angiogenesis such as macular degeneration and cancer.

In initial studies, bevacizumab did not improve the overall survival of breast cancer patients when compared to chemotherapy [22]. However, in further clinical studies the drug was shown to improve both overall survival (OS) and progression free survival (PFS) in metastatic colorectal cancer as either first line or second line treatment [16, 23]. In 2003 a positive outcome was obtained in phase III trials when bevacizumab was used in combination with chemotherapy. The study showed that patients receiving a combination of bevacizumab plus chemotherapy had a 50% increased chance of survival compared to patients who received chemotherapy alone [23].

In February 2004 bevacizumab became the first AI to be granted approval by the United States Food and Drug Administration (FDA) for the treatment of metastatic colorectal cancer [16].

Bevacizumab has had response rates of up to 10% as monotherapy, with higher response rates of 55% being observed in glioblastoma multiforme [24]. Promising results were also observed in lung, ovarian, endometrial, mesothelioma and cervical cancers as indicated by increased progression-free survival [22]. Bevacizumab is approved for metastatic colorectal cancer, non-squamous non-small cell lung cancer, glioblastoma and metastatic renal cell carcinoma [23]. Bevacizumab, in combination with interferon alpha (IFNα), has become standard therapy for metastatic renal cell carcinoma (mRCC) [25].

However, the observation in cancer patients treated with bevacizumab was that following the discontinuation of therapy, the vasculature is re-established [26]. This necessitated prolonged use of the drug in order to improve therapeutic effect, thus increasing the risk of exposure to toxicity or undesirable effects [26]. In addition, in other neoplastic diseases such as breast, melanoma, pancreatic and prostate cancers, bevacizumab failed to significantly increase patient survival, even when combined with chemotherapy.

BEYOND BEVACIZUMAB

Given the limitations of targeting VEGF with bevacizumab, other angiogenesis inhibitors were developed to target its key receptor, VEGFR-2 [27, 28].

Ramucirumab

Ramucirumab is a humanized IgG monoclonal antibody that targets the extracellular domain of VEGFR-2, thereby inhibiting angiogenesis by blocking VEGF binding to the receptor [27]. From preclinical studies it is evident that ramucirumab inhibits cell proliferation *in vitro*, as well as tumor progression in mouse xenograft models of human cancer [27]. The effects of the drug have also been studied in patients [28, 29].

In phase I clinical trials in patients with advanced neoplastic diseases such as NSCLC, gastric and colorectal cancers. Results showed that weekly and fortnightly schedules of ramucirumab were well tolerated, with the most common adverse effect being hypertension [29]. Another study was undertaken to evaluate ramucirumab as a second-line treatment in advanced gastric cancer.

The drug decreased the risk of disease progression by 37–52% and death by 19–22% [28]. Studies using dynamic contrast enhanced magnetic resonance imaging (DCE-MRI) revealed that ramucirumab decreased tumor vascularity in 69% of treated patients, including those with multiple tumors [29].

Ramucirumab has also been shown to improve overall survival by an average of 5.2 months in a phase III clinical trial in patients with advanced gastric cancer [30]. In another Phase III trial ramucirumab was evaluated as single therapy and in combination with paclitaxel in patients with advanced gastric cancer or gastro-esophageal adenocarcinoma. The median OS was 5.2 months in the ramucirumab group, compared to 3.8 months in the placebo group [31].

Progression free survival was prolonged with a median of 2.1 months in the ramucirumab group *vs.* 1.3 months in the placebo group [31]. The overall survival with ramucirumab plus paclitaxel was 9.6 months *vs* 7.4 months with placebo plus ramucirumab [31].

Phase II trials evaluated ramucirumab in different combinations and in several neoplasms, with dacarbazine in melanoma, mitoxantrone/prednisone in prostate cancer, carboplatin/paclitaxel in NSCLC and with oxaliplatin/folinic acid/5-fluorouracil in colorectal cancer [28]. While ramucirumab has shown promising results, he outcome of these clinical trials will shed further light on the effectiveness of the drug when used in combination therapies.

Apatinib

Apatinib is another novel tyrosine kinase inhibitor that targets vascular endothelial growth factor receptor-2 [32]. *In vitro* apatinib was shown to decrease endothelial cell proliferation, migration and tube formation [32]. In preclinical studies using nude mice injected with lung or colon cancer cells, apatinib inhibited tumor progression [32]. A phase II clinical trial demonstrated the survival benefit of apatinib monotherapy in advanced NSCLC [33, 34]. The 12-month OS rate in the study was approximately 57% [32 - 34].

Another study revealed that apatinib monotherapy and apatinib plus docetaxel have potential as therapeutic options for heavily pretreated patients with advanced non-squamous NSCLC [35]. The study showed that both apatinib monotherapy and apatinib plus docetaxel treatment had a positive response, with progression-free survival durations of 5 months and 6 months respectively being attained [35]. In a different study Apatinib was well tolerated when administered as third-line or beyond therapy in patients with chemotherapy-refractory advanced or metastatic adenocarcinoma of the stomach or gastroesophageal junction. The main side-effect was hypertension [33].

Of interest is whether VEGFR-2 inhibitors are more effective than anti-VEGF therapy in inhibiting tumor angiogenesis and suppressing tumor progression. Very few studies have been conducted to compare these two approaches. It appears that different approaches have therapeutic benefits in different disease settings.

Effectiveness of Anti-VEGF *Versus* Anti-VEGFR Therapy

A study was undertaken to compare the efficacy of bevacizumab with cediranib, a VEGFR inhibitor, in a phase III study of advanced colorectal cancer [22]. The drugs were combined with oxaliplatin-based chemotherapy [22]. No significant difference in PFS was observed between the two regimens [22]. Although there were therapeutic benefits observed with the use of both VEGF and VEGFR-2 targeting therapies, such benefits have been modest.

DEVELOPMENT OF RESISTANCE TO VEGF/VEGFR-2 TARGETING DRUGS

The limitations of anti-VEGF therapy have been partly attributed to the triggering of alternative proangiogenic pathways [22, 26]. Although VEGF is a specific endothelial cell mitogen associated with angiogenesis, several other proangiogenic molecules can contribute to tumor angiogenesis, albeit not with the same potency [26].

Clinical trials have revealed that in some tumors blocking VEGF/VEGFR signaling can aggravate tumor hypoxia, which results in the tumor cells secreting proteins such as placental growth factor (PlGF), basic fibroblast growth factor (bFGF) and platelet derived growth factors (PDGFs) [26]. The latter were shown to stimulate angiogenesis and thus improve the supply of oxygen and nutrients to the tumor [26]. Other proangiogenic proteins that promote tumor angiogenesis and that seem to promote resistance to anti-VEGF therapy include basic fibroblast growth factor and angiopoietins [26]. These factors have also been linked to tumor aggressive growth in various neoplastic diseases such as melanoma, NSCLC and breast cancer [11, 36].

Platelet-Derived Growth Factor Pathway

Platelet-derived growth factors (PDGFs) are a family of peptides made up of PDGF-A, -B, -C, and -D that interact with trans-membrane tyrosine kinase receptors, PDGFR-α and -β [37]. The activation of PDGFs promotes angiogenesis by activating MEK/ Extracellular Signal-Regulated Kinase

(ERK), which leads to EC proliferation and migration (Fig. **3**) [36]. Signaling through PDGFs also promotes the recruitment of pericytes and supports vessel maturation [36].

Genes associated with PDGF receptors are mutated in a number of malignancies. For instance, point mutations in PDGFR-α were found in 5% of gastrointestinal stromal tumors [37]. In addition, 5-10% of glioblastoma multiforme patients had an amplified PDGFR-α gene [37]. As a result of this gene amplification, the ECs in the tumor stroma become susceptible to stimulation by low levels of PDGF [37]. Such stimulation promotes tumor angiogenesis.

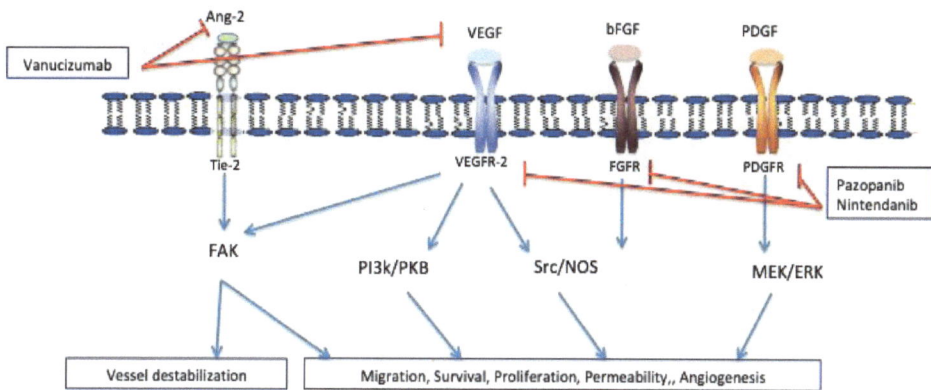

Fig. (3). A diagram showing ligands that promote tumor angiogenesis and the pathways they elicit. Angiopoietin-2 (Ang-2) binds to the Tie-2 receptor and activates focal adhesion kinase (FAK), leading to vessel destabilization, while bFGF and VEGF bind FGFR and VEGFR-2 respectively to activate signaling through Src and nitric oxide synthase (NOS), which in turn promotes vessel permeability, EC proliferation and migration, and tube formation. Binding of VEGF to VEGFR-2 also promotes EC survival, through the PI3k, VEGF also promotes EC migration *via* FAK. Platelet-derived growth factor (PDGF) binds PDGFR and promotes angiogenesis through the MEK/ERK pathway. The AIs Pazopanib and Nintendab inhibit VEGFR-2, FGFR and PDGFR, while vanucizumab inhibits Ang-2 and VEGF.

Due to the role of PDGFs and their receptors in human malignancies, a number of therapeutic molecules have been developed to target the PDGFRs [37]. The drugs include sorafenib and sunitinib, which do not only inhibit PDGFRs but also target other receptors involved in angiogenesis, such as fibroblast growth factor receptors [37].

Fibroblast Growth Factor Signaling in Anti-Cancer Therapy

Fibroblast growth factors (FGFs) are a family of pleiotropic ligands comprising of approximately 22 members that vary in size ranging from 17 kDa to 34 kDa [38]. The ligands bind to specific tyrosine kinase receptors known as fibroblast growth factor receptors (FGFRs) [39].

The overexpression, co-activation or mutation of these receptors contributes to cancer [39, 40]. For instance, the amplification of FGFR-1 is approximately 17% of non-squamous lung carcinoma patients, and approximately 15% of estrogen receptor positive breast cancer patients [40]. As a result, drugs that target FGFR-1 were developed [40]. However, the efficacy of FGFR-1 inhibition has yielded poor results and some of these inhibitors have not progressed beyond phase II trials [40].

Genetic alterations in FGFR-1 and FGFR-2, as well as in FGFR-3, -4 and -19, have been linked to cancer progression in preclinical models [41]. In addition, FGFR-2 is mutated in endometrial, lung and gastric cancers [42].

Drugs that target additional fibroblast growth factor receptors have been developed as tyrosine kinase receptor inhibitors and monoclonal antibodies [42]. The drugs exert their action by inhibiting FGFR dimerization or by preventing receptor phosphorylation [40]. Several of these drugs that target the FGF receptors, such as ponatinib and AZD4547, have progressed to clinical trials. The drugs may hold promise in the inhibition of tumor angiogenesis, especially in combination with other anti-cancer drugs.

Angiopoietin-Tie Pathway in Therapeutic Anti-Angiogenesis

Angiopoietins are a family of growth factors made up of angiopoietin (Ang)-1, Ang-2, Ang-3 and Ang-4. These growth factors bind to tyrosine kinase receptors Tie-1 and Tie-2, which are mainly expressed on endothelial cells (ECs) [12, 43]. Whereas Ang-1 is important for vessel maturation, Ang-2 induces vessel regression and is required during the early stages of angiogenesis [43]. The binding of Ang-1 to the Tie-2 receptor leads to the recruitment of pericytes to premature segments of newly formed vessels, thus promoting the re-enforcement of these vessels and their maturation [44, 45]. However, it is Ang-2 and the Tie-2 receptor that appear to play an important role in tumor angiogenesis. Indeed, some tumor cells express Ang-2 and the Tie-2 receptor [44].

The interaction of angiopoietin-2 with the Tie-2 receptor promotes tumor cell plasticity as well as the remodeling of the tumor vasculature [44]. Furthermore, the overexpression of Ang-2 has been linked to poor clinical prognosis in various cancers [46]. As a result, the design of drugs that target the tumor vasculature has also focused on targeting this pathway.

Vanucizumab was developed to target Ang-2/Tie-2 signaling. The drug is a bi-specific monoclonal antibody against Ang-2 and VEGF. A phase I study evaluating the safety, pharmacokinetics, pharmacodynamics and antitumor activity of vanucizumab in adults with advanced solid tumors (including renal cell and colon cancers) refractory to standard therapies was published recently [46].

The study found that bi-weekly doses of vanucizumab had an acceptable safety and tolerability profile consistent with single-agent use of selective inhibitors of the VEGF pathway [46].

Another study, a double-blind, randomized phase II study of vanucizumab (VAN) plus FOLFOX *vs.* bevacizumab (BEV) plus FOLFOX in patients with previously untreated metastatic colorectal carcinoma (mCRC) showed that VAN plus FOLFOX did not improve PFS compared to BEV plus FOLFOX [47]. Furthermore, the VAN-FOLFOX combination increased the risk of hypertension [47]. More studies are needed to identify effective doses and combination approaches using VAN with other drugs.

Various other AIs target receptors such as the epidermal growth factor receptor (EGFR) as well as adhesion molecules such as integrins (Table **1**) may have potential in combination strategies and thus warrant further investigation.

The limitations of single molecule targeting AIs (Table **1**) have necessitated a radical shift in the rationale for drug targeting. Indeed, the development of AIs that target more than one molecule or pathway simultaneously has become the focus in the quest to design more effective therapeutics.

THERAPEUTIC TARGETING OF MULTIPLE ANGIOGENIC PATHWAYS

Angiogenesis inhibitors that target several angiogenic pathways have been demonstrated to increase progression free survival in various tumors [28, 48 - 51]. These include multi-targeting tyrosine kinase inhibitors and monoclonal antibodies (Fig. **4**) [28]. Some of the approved drugs that target multiple pathways in therapeutic angiogenesis are listed in Table **2**.

Table 1. Selected angiogenesis inhibitors that have undergone clinical testing [71, 72].

Antibodies			
Target	**Drug**	**Status**	**Indications**
EGFR	Cetuximab	FDA approved	Colorectal cancer, head and neck carcinoma
EGFR	Panitumumab	FDA approved	Colorectal cancer
VEGF	Bevacizumab	FDA approved	NSCLC, Colorectal cancer
Her2	Trastuzumab	FDA approved	Her2 positive breast cancer
Integrin $\alpha v\beta_3$	Vitaxin	Phase II	Metastatic cancers, bone cancer
Integrin $\alpha v\beta_5$	Celengitide	Phase II	Glioblastoma
VEGF	Pegatinib	FDA approved	Age-related macular degeneration
Tyrosine kinase inhibitors			
Target	**Drug**	**Status**	**Indications**
EGFR	Gefitinib	FDA approved	NSCLC
EGFR	Erlotinib	FDA approved	NSCLC, pancreatic cancer
EGFR	Lapatinib	FDA approved	Her2 positive breast cancer

Table 2. Selected multi-targeting angiogenesis inhibitors that have been approved for the treatment of various malignancies.

Target	Drug	Indications
VEGFR-1,-2,-3, EGFR, PDGFRβ	Sorafenib	Renal cell cancer, hepatocellular carcinoma
VEGFR-1,-2,-3, PDGFRβ, FLT3, c-KIT	Sunitinib	Renal cell cancer, gastrointestinal stromal tumor
VEGFR-1,-2,-3, FGFR -1,-3, KIT, PDGFR-β	Pazopanib	Ovarian carcinoma, soft tissue sarcoma, Advanced Renal cell carcinoma
VEGFR-1,-2,-3, PDGFRs, FGFRs	Nintedanib	Lung cancer

Multi-Targeting Tyrosine Kinase Inhibitors

Tyrosine kinase inhibitors (TKIs) are small molecules that inhibit tyrosine kinases, a group of transmembrane receptors involved in various signaling pathways [16]. The kinases exert their effects through different mechanisms: i. they can compete with adenosine triphosphate (ATP), ii. they can catalyze the phosphorylation of other signaling molecules, iii. they can bind to a molecule allosterically at a site different from the active site, and thus alter the activity of that molecule [16, 52]. Anti-angiogenic TKIs have been employed in cancer treatment as single agents and in combination with other drugs [52]. The receptors targeted by these TKIs include VEGFRs, PDGFRs, EGFRs, c-KIT, fms-like tyrosine kinase 3 (FLT3) and FGFRs (Table **3**) [52 - 54].

Some multi-targeting TKIs such as sorafenib and Sunitinib have been approved for the treatment of various neoplasms.

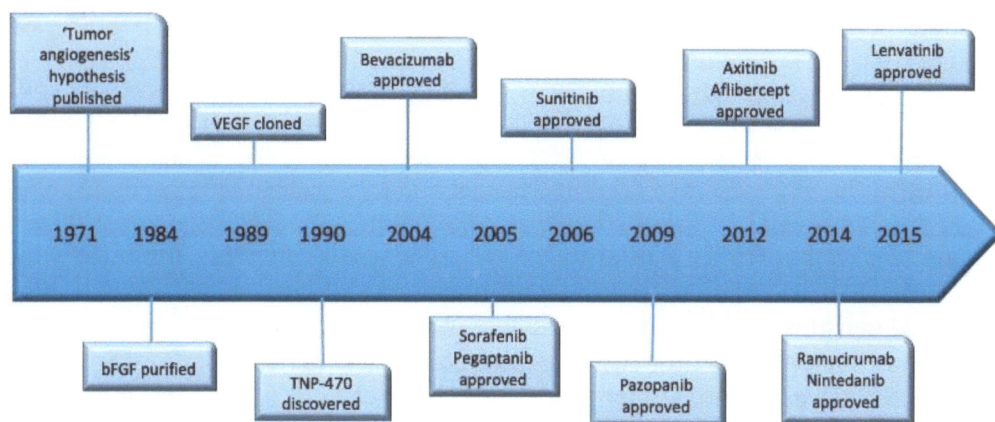

Fig. (4). A diagram representing some of the key milestones in the development of angiogenesis inhibitors.

Table 3. Clinical trials involving combined regimens of angiogenesis inhibitors and immunotherapy [100].

Treatment	Type of cancer	Clinical trial
Sorafenib + Pexa Vec	Hepatocellular carcinoma	NCT02562755
Bevacizumab + atezolizumab + liposomal doxorubicin	Ovarian, fallopian tube peritoneal cancer	NCT02839707
Bevacizumab + atezolizumab	Advanced renal cell carcinoma	NCT02420821
Axitinib + avelumab	Advanced renal cell carcinoma	NCT02684006

Sorafenib

Sorafenib is a multi-kinase inhibitor that targets VEGFR-2, VEGFR-3, PDGFR and Raf [55, 56]. *In vitro* studies have revealed that sorafenib inhibits the proliferation of human hepatocellular carcinoma cells [56, 57]. In preclinical xenograft models of human hepatocellular carcinoma, the drug was shown to inhibit angiogenesis and tumor growth [57, 58].

Sorafenib has been employed in the treatment of various cancers as monotherapy and in combination with chemotherapy to improve patient outcome [59 - 61]. Hwang and colleagues (2017) observed complete remission following the administration of a combination of sorafenib and tegafur, an orally administered fluoro-uracil based chemotherapeutic, in a hepatocellular carcinoma (HCC) patient with progressed disease [61]. Sorafenib was also shown to improve OS in

RCC patients [61 - 63].

In a multi-center phase III trial using sorafenib in advanced renal cell carcinoma (RCC), the 1-year PFS and OS were 58.4% and 64.6% respectively [63].

In some countries including those in the European Union and the USA, oral sorafenib is the approved treatment for patients with advanced HCC [64]. The various clinical trials have shown that sorafenib improves OS, especially when administered as part of combination therapies.

Sunitinib

Sunitinib, also known as Sunitinib malate, is a small-molecule inhibitor which targets vascular endothelial growth factor receptors (VEGFR-1, -2, -3), PDGFR-β, Flt3, glial cell-line derived neurotropic factor receptor (RET), macrophage colony stimulating factor 1 receptor (CSF-1R) and stem cell factor receptor (KIT) [65 - 68]. Sunitinib has demonstrated anti-angiogenic effects in *in vitro* models and anti-tumor effects in cancer cell lines that express its target receptors [66, 67].

The drug is approved in various countries for the treatment of advanced renal cell carcinoma as well as for imatinib resistant gastrointestinal stromal tumor (GIST) [68]. The mechanism of sunitinib in RCC has been attributed to its anti-angiogenic effects. Indeed, decreased levels of soluble VEGFR-2 were measured in plasma samples of RCC patients that were on sunitinib treatment [68]. In addition, in RCC and GIST patients, sunitinib induced a decrease in soluble KIT, a stem cell factor receptor that is involved in the promotion of angiogenesis [68 - 70].

Sunitinib has since become the reference standard of care for first line mRCC treatment [70]. In a global expanded clinical trial undertaken in 50 countries, sunitinib increased OS by 18.7 months, and clinical benefit was observed in naïve and previously treated patients [70]. Furthermore, clinical benefit was observed across age and even in patients with poor prognosis, including those with brain metastasis [70].

In treatment combinations employing sunitinib plus the chemotherapeutic drug gemcitabine in patients with sarcomatoid mRCC, and with sunitinib plus the immunotherapy drug AGS-003, there was improved survival in both instances and the therapies were well tolerated [69, 70]. It is anticipated that these treatments will improve the standard of care for RCC patients [70].

Axitinib

Other multi-targeting TKIs that have received approval for the treatment of various cancers (Table **2**) include axitinib and pazopanib [55]. Axitinib is a second-generation inhibitor of VEGFR-1, VEGFR-2, and VEGFR-3. Axitinib inhibited tumor growth in a pre-clinical model of breast cancer. The drug also induced partial response in clinical trials involving patients with various cancers [55]. Axitinib is currently approved for the treatment of advanced renal-cell carcinoma [55].

Pazopanib

Pazopanib is another second generation TKI which inhibits VEGF receptors [73]. It inhibits the VEGF signaling pathway *via* ATP-competitive inhibition of VEGFRs, with IC_{50} values of approximately 10 nm, 30 nm, and 47 nm for VEGFR-1, VEGFR-2, and VEGFR-3, respectively [74]. The drug also inhibits PDGFR-α, PDGFR-β, fibroblast growth factor receptor (FGFR)-1, FGFR-3, and c-KIT [74]. Pazopanib has been shown to be effective in the treatment of patients with metastatic renal cell cancer [75].

Nintedanib

A recently developed TKI, nintedanib, was approved for the treatment of pulmonary fibrosis in 2014. The drug was later tested in a phase III clinical trial in non-small-cell lung carcinoma patients [76]. Nintedanib was evaluated in combination with docetaxel as second-line treatment, and the combination reduced tumor size by approximately 9 mm after 6 months [76].

Multi-Targeting Versus Mono-Targeting AIs

Few studies have been conducted to compare the efficacy of mono- and multi-targeting AIs in cancer treatment. A phase III study compared bevacizumab and sunitinib in breast cancer patients where both drugs were combined with paclitaxel [77].

Bevacizumab showed superior results as the median PFS was 7.4 months with sunitinib-paclitaxel *vs.* 9.2 months with bevacizumab-paclitaxel [77]. However, a systematic review of several clinical trials compared the clinical effectiveness of the two drugs in RCC. Evidence revealed that Sunitinib was statistically superior to bevacizumab plus interferon [78].

In addition to TKIs other molecules that target angiogenesis have been explored in various studies, especially for use in combination approaches [79].

FUSION PEPTIDES AND DECOY RECEPTORS

Other AIs that do not target RTKs, such as fusion peptides (aflibercept) and decoy receptors (abexinostat) have also been developed to target multiple proangiogenic pathways simultaneously.

Aflibercept

Aflibercept is a fusion protein that consists of portions of VEGFR-1 and -2 fused with the Fc portion of human IgG [80]. Aflibercept binds multiple proangiogenic factors (VEGF, VEGF-B and PlGF) and leads to their neutralization [80].

Preclinical studies in a xenograft model of colon cancer showed that aflibercept inhibits angiogenesis [80]. In clinical studies aflibercept was shown to improve PFS and OS in advanced colorectal cancer [80]. Furthermore, the drug was found to improve PFS in advanced non- small cell lung cancer, although it did not improve OS [81].

Phase III clinical studies in mCRC revealed that a combination of the drug with folinic acid, fluorouracil, and irinotecan (FOLFIRI), improved overall survival by 13.5 months [82]. Noteworthy is that the adverse effects with aflibercept, although similar to those observed with bevacizumab, were less severe.

Abexinostat and Panobinostat Attenuate Hypoxia

Abexinostat is a non-selective pan-histone deacetylase (HDAC) inhibitor that is in the experimental stage [83]. Of note is that HDAC has been associated with HIF-dependent gene expression and the promotion of hypoxia [83, 84]. Abexinostat thus suppresses hypoxia by inhibiting HDAC [83]. In pre-clinical studies the drug was found to be effective in inhibiting the growth of different types of tumors by inhibiting angiogenesis [85].

Previous studies have shown that hypoxia-induced alterations in the tumor microenvironment can promote resistance to AIs [86]. These alterations include the increased secretion of proangiogenic growth factors, mobilization of bone marrow-derived endothelial cells, the induction of epithelial-to-mesenchymal transition (EMT) and vessel co-option [87, 88].

Phase I clinical studies have revealed that abexinostat enhances the effects of the AI pazopanib [84]. In another study, the effect of a combination of pazopanib and abexinostat in cancer treatment was evaluated. Both drugs target hypoxia-inducible factor and VEGF-A respectively. With the inclusion of abexinostat, prolonged exposure of patients to pazopanib was possible and resistance was overcome [84]. Indeed, resistance is known to develop when pazopanib is used alone [89].

Another HDAC inhibitor, panobinostat, was tested in a phase II study in combination with rituximab, a monoclonal antibody against the B-lymphocyte antigen CD20 in 18 patients with relapsed diffuse large B-cell lymphoma [90]. The results of the study showed that the combination of panobinostat with rituximab induced a response in 11% of the patients [90]. Currently panobinostat is undergoing Phase II clinical trials for the treatment of B-cell lymphoma. It is anticipated that these hypoxia-suppressing drugs will contribute to the reduction of resistance to most AIs.

IMMUNE CELLS AND THE EFFECTIVENESS OF ANGIOGENESIS INHIBITORS

In addition to hypoxia, there are factors within the tumor microenvironment that promote the development of resistance to AIs [26]. Studies have revealed that tumor stromal tissue uniquely expresses proteins that promote endothelial cell migration and proliferation and could thus promote resistance to anti-angiogenic therapy [26, 91]. The tumor stroma consists of tumor infiltrating and resident immune cells, which secrete cytokines that can promote negatively, affect the effectiveness of AIs [92].

Immune cell types found within this microenvironment include macrophages, neutrophils, natural killer cells and B-cells [93]. Growth factors and cytokines secreted by these immune cells have been associated with the stimulation of angiogenesis and the development of resistance to AIs [94, 95].

The presence of immune cells further promotes tumor resistance to therapy and is linked to the chronic inflammation associated with tumors [95].

OVERCOMING INFLAMMATION - ANGIOGENESIS INHIBITORS AND IMMUNOTHERAPY

Inflammation is a physiological response to tissue damage or infection. It is a beneficial process that restores homeostasis and is self-limiting under physiological conditions [96]. When factors that initiate inflammation persist or the mechanisms that resolve inflammation fail, chronic inflammation results [97, 98]. Indeed, neoplastic cells produce cytokines that attract diverse leukocyte populations. These leukocytes, which include neutrophils, eosinophils, macrophages, mast cells and lymphocytes can promote chronic inflammation and thus create a permissive environment for continued tumor growth [96].

A prominent component of the inflammatory infiltrate is tumor-associated macrophages (TAMs) [93]. Upon recruitment to the tumor site, the macrophages are transformed by factors in the tumor stroma into TAMs [47]. Tumor-associated macrophages produce molecules such as VEGF, PDGF and FGFs, which have been implicated in the activation of the angiogenic switch [99].

Tumor cells also secrete cytokines that bind to receptors on the surface of infiltrating lymphocytes. Such binding enables the tumor to escape immune check-points [100]. Cancer immunotherapy has thus emerged as an important anti-cancer strategy over the past two decades.

A number of therapies such as Pembrolizumab, an immune-check-point inhibitor, have been tested in clinical trials on patients with neoplasms such as melanoma, prostate, advanced squamous-cell NSCLC, metastatic urothelial carcinoma and advanced renal cell carcinoma [100, 101].

Unfortunately, immunotherapy was only found to be effective in approximately 20% of these cancers. Moreover, in cases where there was efficacy, pre-existing immunity already existed. Furthermore, these patients who had showed response rapidly developed resistance to immunotherapy [100].

The abnormal architecture of the tumor vasculature has been regarded as an obstacle to the effective delivery of immunotherapy [92]. Therefore, AIs that normalize the tumor vasculature have been considered in order to enhance drug delivery.

In addition, the contribution of the cross-talk between ECs and immune cells within the tumor stroma to disease progression is well-documented [102]. As such a number of AIs have been evaluated for efficacy in combination with immunotherapy in pre-clinical and clinical studies [102 - 105].

In preclinical studies, Lenvatinib (Fig. **3**), a multi-targeting tyrosine kinase inhibitor of VEGFR 1-3, FGFR 1-4, PDGFR β, RET and KIT induced significant tumor regression when administered in a combination approach incorporating cellular immunotherapy [105].

Given the role played by interactions between endothelial and immune cells in promoting tumor progression, there is rationale for the combination of drugs that target these components of the TME. The combination of immunotherapy and AIs has been tested in various clinical trials and these are listed in Table **3**.

Normalization of the Tumor Vasculature

Vascular normalization is the restoration of a defective vascular phenotype to a near 'normal' architecture that allows for improved perfusion [106]. Vascular normalization improves the delivery of oxygen, thus reducing the chances of developing hypoxia. In addition, it enables the improved delivery of therapies to the tumor. Vascular normalization was first proposed following observation of the effectiveness of combination approaches utilizing anti-VEGF plus chemotherapy [106, 107]. Normalization of the tumor vasculature has improved drug delivery in various tumor types and enhanced treatment efficacy.

In hepatocellular carcinoma, FGFRs are overexpressed and impaired FGF signaling is considered a critical contributor to neoplastic progression [107]. The FGFR inhibitor infigratinib normalized the tumor vasculature in a xenograft model of hepatocellular carcinoma and reduced tumor growth [107]. In breast cancer patients, bevacizumab administered preoperatively, followed with a combination of bevacizumab plus chemotherapy normalized the tumor vasculature [108].

There is an urgent need for predictive biomarkers that will enable the monitoring of AIs as well as AI-immunotherapy combination approaches in order to minimize toxicity.

FUTURE PERSPECTIVE - IMAGING BIOMARKERS IN ANGIOGENESIS

As demonstrated above, many promising new antiangiogenic therapies targeting the VEGF-VEGFR axis with different mechanisms of action have been evaluated in recent years [109]. However, not all patients respond to antiangiogenic therapy [110, 111]. Surprisingly, since the elucidation of the angiogenic switch in the 1970's, there is still no validated predictive biomarker for the selection of antiangiogenic therapy [112].

While angiogenesis is an important component in the progression of a number of diseases, it is clear that all angiogenic processes are not regulated by the same signals and are often distinct to different pathologies [113]. Hence it is increasingly evident that the successful implementation of antiangiogenic therapies requires improved diagnostic tools that can identify the patient population that is most likely to respond and match it with the optimal treatment [114].

In addition, a noninvasive imaging technique for monitoring the status of tumor angiogenesis that could provide a prompt readout of post-treatment response is highly desirable [115].

Encouraging imaging results have been obtained with two VEGF isoforms, namely, VEGF165 and VEGF121, which have been labeled with various radionuclides such as iodine-123 and -125, copper-64, gallium-68 and technetium-99m. [116-120]. Prostate-specific membrane antigen (PSMA) labeled to gallium 68 has also been suggested as another potential measure in imaging tumor vessels. [116-120].

CONCLUSION

The recognition that tumors require a vascular supply in order to grow beyond 1-2mm heralded a new era in the treatment of cancer. Since the pioneering work of Folkman and colleagues in unraveling the mechanisms by which tumors recruit blood vessels, the complex molecular pathways that govern tumor angiogenesis have been elucidated. As well, multiple molecules have been identified for pharmacological manipulation of the tumor vasculature.

Key in the identification of potential therapeutic targets was the discovery of the potent angiogenic factor, VEGF. Accordingly, preclinical and clinical research mostly focused on the design of drugs targeting VEGF or its cognate receptor VEGFR-2. The various VEGF and VEGFR-2 inhibitors showed promise, however, the improvement in OS was offset by the development of resistance.

The emerging question is what mediates the resistance that has limited the effectiveness of these treatment approaches. A number of obstacles have emerged from literature: i. the existence of different angiogenesis regulators that are tumor specific, ii. the activation of alternative pathways that promote angiogenesis, iii. the development of hypoxia, iv. the tortuous nature of tumor blood vessels, v. the presence of immune cells which further support angiogenesis and enable tumor escape from immune surveillance, vi. a lack of predictive biomarkers.

To address the first two obstacles, drugs that target multiple receptors and downstream molecules in pathways that regulate angiogenesis have been designed. These multi-targeting drugs mainly inhibit tyrosine kinases. While there are few studies that compare single-targeting and multi-targeting AIs, *in vivo* and *in vitro* data support the use of multi-targeting drugs as a sound therapeutic approach. However, the matching of appropriate multi-targeting AIs with the tumors that overexpress specific molecules relies on an ability to effectively identify tumor specific biomarkers.

With regard to hypoxia, drugs such as abexinostat, which have been designed to target HIF-1α in order to reduce hypoxia within the tumor microenvironment, are being used to further enhance the efficacy of AIs.

To overcome the limitations posed by the chaotic architecture of tumor vessels, angiogenesis inhibitors have been employed to normalize the tumor vasculature and thus improve the delivery of chemotherapy, immune check-point inhibitors as well as other forms of immunotherapy.

The combination of AIs with chemotherapy and other drugs that target different components of the TME has shown potential in improving OS and PFS.

There is undoubtedly a futuristic need to develop advanced techniques for the noninvasive visualization of tumor blood vessels to guide therapeutic design. For this purpose, imaging agents for single photon emission computed tomography (SPECT) and positron emission tomography (PET) targeting VEGFRs and their ligands could enable a detailed characterization of the molecular status of the endothelium in the tumor and thus enhance therapeutic monitoring.

CONSENT FOR PUBLICATION

Not applicable.

CONFLICT OF INTEREST

The author confirms that this chapter contents have no conflict of interest.

ACKNOWLEDGEMENTS

The authors thank the National Research Foundation (project 114403) and the NRF-University of Pretoria mentorship program for funding.

REFERENCES

[1]   Pries AR, Secomb TW. Blood Flow in Microvascular Networks. Microcirculation. 2nd ed. San Diego: Academic Press 2008; pp. 1-36.
[http://dx.doi.org/10.1016/B978-0-12-374530-9.00001-2]

[2]   Ronca R, Benkheil M, Mitola S, Struyf S, Liekens S. Tumor angiogenesis revisited: Regulators and clinical implications. Med Res Rev 2017; 37(6): 1231-74.
[http://dx.doi.org/10.1002/med.21452] [PMID: 28643862]

[3]   Janmohamed SR, Brinkhuizen T, den Hollander JC, *et al.* Support for the hypoxia theory in the pathogenesis of infantile haemangioma. Clin Exp Dermatol 2015; 40(4): 431-7.
[http://dx.doi.org/10.1111/ced.12557] [PMID: 25511669]

[4]   Folkman J. Angiogenesis and apoptosis. Semin Cancer Biol 2003; 13(2): 159-67.
[http://dx.doi.org/10.1016/S1044-579X(02)00133-5] [PMID: 12654259]

[5]   Folkman J. Antiangiogenesis in cancer therapy--endostatin and its mechanisms of action. Exp Cell Res 2006; 312(5): 594-607.
[http://dx.doi.org/10.1016/j.yexcr.2005.11.015] [PMID: 16376330]

[6]   Pepper MS. Manipulating angiogenesis. From basic science to the bedside. Arterioscler Thromb Vasc Biol 1997; 17(4): 605-19.
[http://dx.doi.org/10.1161/01.ATV.17.4.605] [PMID: 9108772]

[7]   De Sanctis F, Ugel S, Facciponte J, Facciabene A. The dark side of tumor-associated endothelial cells. Semin Immunol 2018; 35: 35-47.
[http://dx.doi.org/10.1016/j.smim.2018.02.002] [PMID: 29490888]

[8]   Mabeta P, Pepper MS. A comparative study on the anti-angiogenic effects of DNA-damaging and cytoskeletal-disrupting agents. Angiogenesis 2009; 12(1): 81-90.

[http://dx.doi.org/10.1007/s10456-009-9134-8] [PMID: 19214765]

[9] Potente M, Gerhardt H, Carmeliet P. Basic and therapeutic aspects of angiogenesis. Cell 2011; 146(6): 873-87.
[http://dx.doi.org/10.1016/j.cell.2011.08.039] [PMID: 21925313]

[10] Xu JX, Maher VE, Zhang L, *et al.* FDA approval summary: Nivolumab in advanced renal cell carcinoma after anti-angiogenic therapy and exploratory predictive biomarker analysis. Oncologist 2017; 22(3): 311-7.
[http://dx.doi.org/10.1634/theoncologist.2016-0476] [PMID: 28232599]

[11] Lopes-Bastos BM, Jiang WG, Cai J. Tumour-endothelial cell communications: Important and indispensable mediators of tumour angiogenesis. Anticancer Res 2016; 36(3): 1119-26.
[PMID: 26977007]

[12] Ribatti D. The Discovery of Angiogenesis Factors. Judah Folkman. Springer 2018; pp. 37-45.
[http://dx.doi.org/10.1007/978-3-319-92633-9_4]

[13] Sakao S, Taraseviciene-Stewart L, Cool CD, *et al.* VEGF-R blockade causes endothelial cell apoptosis, expansion of surviving CD34+ precursor cells and transdifferentiation to smooth muscle-like and neuronal-like cells. FASEB J 2007; 21(13): 3640-52.
[http://dx.doi.org/10.1096/fj.07-8432com] [PMID: 17567571]

[14] Graupera M, Potente M. Regulation of angiogenesis by PI3K signaling networks. Exp Cell Res 2013; 319(9): 1348-55.
[http://dx.doi.org/10.1016/j.yexcr.2013.02.021] [PMID: 23500680]

[15] Mabeta P. Inhibition of phosphoinositide 3-kinase is associated with reduced angiogenesis and an altered expression of angiogenic markers in endothelioma cells. Biomed Pharmacother 2014; 68(5): 611-7.
[http://dx.doi.org/10.1016/j.biopha.2014.03.017] [PMID: 24773755]

[16] Ferrara N, Hillan KJ, Gerber HP, Novotny W. Discovery and development of bevacizumab, an anti-VEGF antibody for treating cancer. Nat Rev Drug Discov 2004; 3(5): 391-400.
[http://dx.doi.org/10.1038/nrd1381] [PMID: 15136787]

[17] Chan LW, Moses MA, Goley E, *et al.* Urinary VEGF and MMP levels as predictive markers of 1-year progression-free survival in cancer patients treated with radiation therapy: A longitudinal study of protein kinetics throughout tumor progression and therapy. J Clin Oncol 2004; 22(3): 499-506.
[http://dx.doi.org/10.1200/JCO.2004.07.022] [PMID: 14752073]

[18] Li L, Wang L, Zhang W, *et al.* Correlation of serum VEGF levels with clinical stage, therapy efficacy, tumor metastasis and patient survival in ovarian cancer. Anticancer Res 2004; 24(3b): 1973-9.
[PMID: 15274387]

[19] Duque JLF, Loughlin KR, Adam RM, Kantoff PW, Zurakowski D, Freeman MR. Plasma levels of vascular endothelial growth factor are increased in patients with metastatic prostate cancer. Urology 1999; 54(3): 523-7.
[http://dx.doi.org/10.1016/S0090-4295(99)00167-3] [PMID: 10475365]

[20] Vasudev NS, Reynolds AR. Anti-angiogenic therapy for cancer: Current progress, unresolved questions and future directions. Angiogenesis 2014; 17(3): 471-94.
[http://dx.doi.org/10.1007/s10456-014-9420-y] [PMID: 24482243]

[21] Bhargava P, Marshall JL, Rizvi N, *et al.* A Phase I and pharmacokinetic study of TNP-470 administered weekly to patients with advanced cancer. Clin Cancer Res 1999; 5(8): 1989-95.
[PMID: 10473076]

[22] Limaverde-Sousa G, Sternberg C, Ferreira CG. Antiangiogenesis beyond VEGF inhibition: A journey from antiangiogenic single-target to broad-spectrum agents. Cancer Treat Rev 2014; 40(4): 548-57.
[http://dx.doi.org/10.1016/j.ctrv.2013.11.009] [PMID: 24360358]

[23] Ferrara N, Adamis AP. Ten years of anti-vascular endothelial growth factor therapy. Nat Rev Drug

Discov 2016; 15(6): 385-403.
[http://dx.doi.org/10.1038/nrd.2015.17] [PMID: 26775688]

[24]   Wong ET, Gautam S, Malchow C, Lun M, Pan E, Brem S. Bevacizumab for recurrent glioblastoma multiforme: A meta-analysis. J Natl Compr Canc Netw 2011; 9(4): 403-7.
[http://dx.doi.org/10.6004/jnccn.2011.0037] [PMID: 21464145]

[25]   Rini BI, Bellmunt J, Clancy J, *et al.* Randomized phase III trial of temsirolimus and bevacizumab versus interferon alfa and bevacizumab in metastatic renal cell carcinoma: INTORACT trial. J Clin Oncol 2014; 32(8): 752-9.
[http://dx.doi.org/10.1200/JCO.2013.50.5305] [PMID: 24297945]

[26]   Ribatti D. Tumor refractoriness to anti-VEGF therapy. Oncotarget 2016; 7(29): 46668-77.
[http://dx.doi.org/10.18632/oncotarget.8694]

[27]   Krupitskaya Y, Wakelee HA. Ramucirumab, a fully human mAb to the transmembrane signaling tyrosine kinase VEGFR-2 for the potential treatment of cancer. Curr Opin Investig Drugs 2009; 10(6): 597-605.
[PMID: 19513949]

[28]   Vlachostergios PJ, Lee A, Thomas C, Walsh R, Tagawa ST. A critical review on ramucirumab in the treatment of advanced urothelial cancer. Future Oncol 2018; 14(11): 1049-61.
[http://dx.doi.org/10.2217/fon-2017-0473] [PMID: 29231057]

[29]   Vennepureddy A, Singh P, Rastogi R, Atallah JP, Terjanian T. Evolution of ramucirumab in the treatment of cancer - A review of literature. J Oncol Pharm Pract 2017; 23(7): 525-39.
[http://dx.doi.org/10.1177/1078155216655474] [PMID: 27306885]

[30]   Mawalla B, Yuan X, Luo X, Chalya PL. Treatment outcome of anti-angiogenesis through VEGF-pathway in the management of gastric cancer: A systematic review of phase II and III clinical trials. BMC Res Notes 2018; 11(1): 21.
[http://dx.doi.org/10.1186/s13104-018-3137-8] [PMID: 29329598]

[31]   Shimodaira Y, Elimova E, Wadhwa R, *et al.* Ramucirumab for the treatment of gastroesophageal cancers. Expert Opin Orphan Drugs 2015; 3(6): 737-46.
[http://dx.doi.org/10.1517/21678707.2015.1040390] [PMID: 27570714]

[32]   Xiang Y, Zhang W, Wu Z, Qian Z, Zhou J, Wang X, *et al.* Enhanced antitumor and anti-angiogenic effects of Apatinib combined with chemotherapy in a zebrafish model of non-small cell lung cancer. Am J Respir Crit Care Med 2017; 77(13): 1818.

[33]   Qin S, Deng W, Wen L, Wang J, Zhang G, Zhong H, *et al.* Apatinib as third-line or beyond therapy in patients with chemotherapy-refractory advanced or metastatic adenocarcinoma of stomach or gastroesophageal junction: An open-label, multicenter, post-marketing phase IV study (Ahead-G201). J Clin Oncol 2018; 36(4_suppl): 103.

[34]   Gou M, Si H, Zhang Y, *et al.* Efficacy and safety of apatinib in patients with previously treated metastatic colorectal cancer: A real-world retrospective study. Sci Rep 2018; 8(1): 4602.
[http://dx.doi.org/10.1038/s41598-018-22302-z] [PMID: 29545575]

[35]   Wu F, Zhang S, Gao G, Zhao J, Ren S, Zhou C. Successful treatment using apatinib with or without docetaxel in heavily pretreated advanced non-squamous non-small cell lung cancer: A case report and literature review. Cancer Biol Ther 2018; 19(3): 141-4.
[http://dx.doi.org/10.1080/15384047.2017.1414757] [PMID: 29261000]

[36]   de Castro G Junior, Puglisi F, de Azambuja E, El Saghir NS, Awada A. Angiogenesis and cancer: A cross-talk between basic science and clinical trials (the "do ut des" paradigm). Crit Rev Oncol 2006; 59(1): 40-50.

[37]   Bartoschek M, Pietras K. PDGF family function and prognostic value in tumor biology. Biochem Biophys Res Commun 2018; 503(2): 984-90.
[http://dx.doi.org/10.1016/j.bbrc.2018.06.106] [PMID: 29932922]

[38] Naito H, Kidoya H, Sato Y, Takakura N. Induction and expression of anti-angiogenic vasohibins in the hematopoietic stem/progenitor cell population. J Biochem 2009; 145(5): 653-9.
[http://dx.doi.org/10.1093/jb/mvp021] [PMID: 19179360]

[39] Eswarakumar VP, Lax I, Schlessinger J. Cellular signaling by fibroblast growth factor receptors. Cytokine Growth Factor Rev 2005; 16(2): 139-49.
[http://dx.doi.org/10.1016/j.cytogfr.2005.01.001] [PMID: 15863030]

[40] Liang G, Liu Z, Wu J, Cai Y, Li X. Anticancer molecules targeting fibroblast growth factor receptors. Trends Pharmacol Sci 2012; 33(10): 531-41.
[http://dx.doi.org/10.1016/j.tips.2012.07.001] [PMID: 22884522]

[41] Gerwins P, Sköldenberg E, Claesson-Welsh L. Function of fibroblast growth factors and vascular endothelial growth factors and their receptors in angiogenesis. Crit Rev Oncol Hematol 2000; 34(3): 185-94.
[http://dx.doi.org/10.1016/S1040-8428(00)00062-7] [PMID: 10838264]

[42] Fearon AE, Gould CR, Grose RP. FGFR signalling in women's cancers. Int J Biochem Cell Biol 2013; 45(12): 2832-42.
[http://dx.doi.org/10.1016/j.biocel.2013.09.017] [PMID: 24148254]

[43] Bach F, Uddin FJ, Burke D. Angiopoietins in malignancy. Eur J Surg Oncol 2007; 33(1): 7-15.
[http://dx.doi.org/10.1016/j.ejso.2006.07.015] [PMID: 16962282]

[44] Papetti M, Herman IM. Mechanisms of normal and tumor-derived angiogenesis. Am J Physiol Cell Physiol 2002; 282(5): C947-70.
[http://dx.doi.org/10.1152/ajpcell.00389.2001] [PMID: 11940508]

[45] Otrock ZK, Mahfouz RAR, Makarem JA, Shamseddine AI. Understanding the biology of angiogenesis: Review of the most important molecular mechanisms. Blood Cells Mol Dis 2007; 39(2): 212-20.
[http://dx.doi.org/10.1016/j.bcmd.2007.04.001] [PMID: 17553709]

[46] Hidalgo M, Martinez-Garcia M, Le Tourneau C, *et al.* First-in-Human phase I study of single-agent Vanucizumab, a first-in-class bispecific anti-angiopoietin-2/Anti-VEGF-A antibody, in adult patients with advanced solid tumors. Clin Cancer Res 2018; 24(7): 1536-45.
[http://dx.doi.org/10.1158/1078-0432.CCR-17-1588] [PMID: 29217526]

[47] Bendell JC, Sauri T, Cubillo A, López-López C, Garcia Alfonso P, Hussein MA, *et al.* Final results of the McCAVE trial: A double-blind, randomized phase 2 study of vanucizumab (VAN) plus FOLFOX *vs.*bevacizumab (BEV) plus FOLFOX in patients (pts) with previously untreated metastatic colorectal carcinoma (mCRC). J Clin Oncol 2017; 35(15): 3539.
[http://dx.doi.org/10.1200/JCO.2017.35.15_suppl.3539]

[48] Rajkumar SV, Witzig TE. A review of angiogenesis and antiangiogenic therapy with thalidomide in multiple myeloma. Cancer Treat Rev 2000; 26(5): 351-62.
[http://dx.doi.org/10.1053/ctrv.2000.0188] [PMID: 11006136]

[49] Dong X, Han ZC, Yang R. Angiogenesis and antiangiogenic therapy in hematologic malignancies. Crit Rev Oncol Hematol 2007; 62(2): 105-18.
[http://dx.doi.org/10.1016/j.critrevonc.2006.11.006] [PMID: 17188504]

[50] Teicher BA. Angiogenesis and cancer metastases: Therapeutic approaches. Crit Rev Oncol Hematol 1995; 20(1-2): 9-39.
[http://dx.doi.org/10.1016/1040-8428(94)00142-G] [PMID: 7576200]

[51] Allen J, Bergsland EK. Angiogenesis in colorectal cancer: Therapeutic implications and future directions. Hematol Oncol Clin North Am 2004; 18(5): 1087-1119, ix.
[http://dx.doi.org/10.1016/j.hoc.2004.05.002] [PMID: 15474337]

[52] Landuyt W, Ahmed B, Nuyts S, *et al.* In vivo antitumor effect of vascular targeting combined with either ionizing radiation or anti-angiogenesis treatment. Int J Radiat Oncol Biol Phys 2001; 49(2):

443-50.
[http://dx.doi.org/10.1016/S0360-3016(00)01470-X] [PMID: 11173139]

[53]   El Alaoui-Lasmaili K, Faivre B. Antiangiogenic therapy: Markers of response, "normalization" and resistance. Crit Rev Oncol Hematol 2018; 128: 118-29.
[http://dx.doi.org/10.1016/j.critrevonc.2018.06.001] [PMID: 29958627]

[54]   Lai Y, Zhao Z, Zeng T, *et al.* Crosstalk between VEGFR and other receptor tyrosine kinases for TKI therapy of metastatic renal cell carcinoma. Cancer Cell Int 2018; 18(1): 31.
[http://dx.doi.org/10.1186/s12935-018-0530-2] [PMID: 29527128]

[55]   Kyriakopoulos CE, Rini BI. Tyrosine kinase inhibitors: Sorafenib, Sunitinib, Axitinib, and Pazopanib.Renal Cell Carcinoma. Springer Japan 2017; pp. 253-72.
[http://dx.doi.org/10.1007/978-4-431-55531-5_10]

[56]   Zhang M, Liu T, Xia B, Yang C, Hou S, Xie W, *et al.* Platelet-derived growth factor D is a prognostic biomarker and is associated withplatinum resistance in epithelial ovarian cancer. Int J Gynaecol Obstet 2018; 28(2): 323-31.

[57]   Keating GM. Bevacizumab: A review of its use in advanced cancer. Drugs 2014; 74(16): 1891-925.
[http://dx.doi.org/10.1007/s40265-014-0302-9] [PMID: 25315029]

[58]   Liu Z, Battinelli E, Sparger KA, Ross A, Johnson KE, Laforest T, *et al.* Noval insights into the role of platelet angiogenic growth factors on the regulation of normal vascular development. Blood 2017; 130(1): 2299.

[59]   Dal Lago L, D'Hondt V, Awada A. Selected combination therapy with sorafenib: A review of clinical data and perspectives in advanced solid tumors. Oncologist 2008; 13(8): 845-58.
[http://dx.doi.org/10.1634/theoncologist.2007-0233] [PMID: 18695262]

[60]   Chen SC, Chao Y, Yang MH. Complete response to the combination of pembrolizumab and sorafenib for metastatic hepatocellular carcinoma: A case report. Am J Gastroenterol 2017; 112(4): 659-60.
[http://dx.doi.org/10.1038/ajg.2017.1] [PMID: 28381841]

[61]   Hwang SY, Lee SM, Im JW, Jeon KJ, Ahn SB, Park JY, *et al.* A case of achieving complete remission with a combination of Sorafenib and Tegafur in patients with hepatocellular carcinoma with progression of disease after Sorafenib therapy. J Liver Cancer 2017; 17(1): 88-93.
[http://dx.doi.org/10.17998/jlc.17.1.88]

[62]   Cheng AL, Kang YK, Chen Z, *et al.* Efficacy and safety of sorafenib in patients in the Asia-Pacific region with advanced hepatocellular carcinoma: A phase III randomised, double-blind, placebo-controlled trial. Lancet Oncol 2009; 10(1): 25-34.
[http://dx.doi.org/10.1016/S1470-2045(08)70285-7] [PMID: 19095497]

[63]   Zhang H, Dong B, Lu JJ, *et al.* Efficacy of sorafenib on metastatic renal cell carcinoma in Asian patients: Results from a multicenter study. BMC Cancer 2009; 9(1): 249.
[http://dx.doi.org/10.1186/1471-2407-9-249] [PMID: 19622166]

[64]   Zhang XP, Wang K, Guo WX, Chen ZH, Cheng SQ. Is sorafenib an optimal treatment for hepatocellular carcinoma with macrovascular invasion or metastatic disease? Hepatology 2018; 68(2): 786.
[http://dx.doi.org/10.1002/hep.29862] [PMID: 29500904]

[65]   Griffioen AW, Mans LA, de Graaf AMA, *et al.* Rapid angiogenesis onset after discontinuation of sunitinib treatment of renal cell carcinoma patients. Clin Cancer Res 2012; 18(14): 3961-71.
[http://dx.doi.org/10.1158/1078-0432.CCR-12-0002] [PMID: 22573349]

[66]   Mankal P, O'Reilly E. Sunitinib malate for the treatment of pancreas malignancies--where does it fit? Expert Opin Pharmacother 2013; 14(6): 783-92.
[http://dx.doi.org/10.1517/14656566.2013.776540] [PMID: 23458511]

[67]   Nör JE, Christensen J, Liu J, *et al.* Up-Regulation of Bcl-2 in microvascular endothelial cells enhances intratumoral angiogenesis and accelerates tumor growth. Cancer Res 2001; 61(5): 2183-8.

[PMID: 11280784]

[68]   Christensen JG. A preclinical review of sunitinib, a multitargeted receptor tyrosine kinase inhibitor with anti-angiogenic and antitumour activities. Ann Oncol 2007; 18(10) (Suppl. 10): x3-x10.
[http://dx.doi.org/10.1093/annonc/mdm408] [PMID: 17761721]

[69]   Deprimo S, Friece C, Huang X, Smeraglia J, Sherman L, Collier M, *et al.* Effect of treatment with sunitinib malate, a multitargeted tyrosine kinase inhibitor, on circulating plasma levels of VEGF, soluble VEGF receptors 2 and 3, and soluble KIT in patients with metastatic breast cancer. J Clin Oncol 2006; 24(18): 578.

[70]   Motzer RJ, Escudier B, Gannon A, Figlin RA. Sunitinib: Ten years of successful clinical use and study in advanced renal cell carcinoma. Oncologist 2017; 22(1): 41-52.
[http://dx.doi.org/10.1634/theoncologist.2016-0197] [PMID: 27807302]

[71]   Burotto M, Manasanch EE, Wilkerson J, Fojo T. Gefitinib and erlotinib in metastatic non-small cell lung cancer: A meta-analysis of toxicity and efficacy of randomized clinical trials. Oncologist 2015; 20(4): 400-10.
[http://dx.doi.org/10.1634/theoncologist.2014-0154] [PMID: 25795635]

[72]   van Cruijsen H, Voest EE, Punt CJ, *et al.* Phase I evaluation of cediranib, a selective VEGFR signalling inhibitor, in combination with gefitinib in patients with advanced tumours. Eur J Cancer 2010; 46(5): 901-11.
[http://dx.doi.org/10.1016/j.ejca.2009.12.023] [PMID: 20061136]

[73]   Climent MA, Muñoz-Langa J, Basterretxea-Badiola L, Santander-Lobera C. Systematic review and survival meta-analysis of real world evidence on first-line pazopanib for metastatic renal cell carcinoma. Crit Rev Oncol Hematol 2018; 121: 45-50.
[http://dx.doi.org/10.1016/j.critrevonc.2017.11.009] [PMID: 29279098]

[74]   van Geel RM, Beijnen JH, Schellens JH. Concise drug review: Pazopanib and axitinib. Oncologist 2012; 17(8): 1081-9.
[http://dx.doi.org/10.1634/theoncologist.2012-0055] [PMID: 22733795]

[75]   McCormack PL. Pazopanib: A review of its use in the management of advanced renal cell carcinoma. Drugs 2014; 74(10): 1111-25.
[http://dx.doi.org/10.1007/s40265-014-0243-3] [PMID: 24935162]

[76]   Reck M, Mellemgaard A, Novello S, *et al.* Change in non-small-cell lung cancer tumor size in patients treated with nintedanib plus docetaxel: Analyses from the Phase III LUME-Lung 1 study. OncoTargets Ther 2018; 11: 4573-82.
[http://dx.doi.org/10.2147/OTT.S170722] [PMID: 30122949]

[77]   Robert NJ, Saleh MN, Paul D, *et al.* Sunitinib plus paclitaxel versus bevacizumab plus paclitaxel for first-line treatment of patients with advanced breast cancer: A phase III, randomized, open-label trial. Clin Breast Cancer 2011; 11(2): 82-92.
[http://dx.doi.org/10.1016/j.clbc.2011.03.005] [PMID: 21569994]

[78]   Thompson Coon JS, Liu Z, Hoyle M, *et al.* Sunitinib and bevacizumab for first-line treatment of metastatic renal cell carcinoma: A systematic review and indirect comparison of clinical effectiveness. Br J Cancer 2009; 101(2): 238-43.
[http://dx.doi.org/10.1038/sj.bjc.6605167] [PMID: 19568242]

[79]   Touyz RM, Herrmann J. Cardiotoxicity with vascular endothelial growth factor inhibitor therapy. NPJ Precis Oncol 2018; 2(1): 13.
[http://dx.doi.org/10.1038/s41698-018-0056-z] [PMID: 30202791]

[80]   Van Cutsem E, Tabernero J, Lakomy R, *et al.* Addition of aflibercept to fluorouracil, leucovorin, and irinotecan improves survival in a phase III randomized trial in patients with metastatic colorectal cancer previously treated with an oxaliplatin-based regimen. J Clin Oncol 2012; 30(28): 3499-506.
[http://dx.doi.org/10.1200/JCO.2012.42.8201] [PMID: 22949147]

[81]   Ramlau R, Gorbunova V, Ciuleanu TE, *et al.* Aflibercept and Docetaxel versus Docetaxel alone after platinum failure in patients with advanced or metastatic non-small-cell lung cancer: A randomized, controlled phase III trial. J Clin Oncol 2012; 30(29): 3640-7.
[http://dx.doi.org/10.1200/JCO.2012.42.6932] [PMID: 22965962]

[82]   Zhao L, Li W, Zhang H, Hou N, Guo L, Gao Q. Angiogenesis inhibitors rechallenge in patients with advanced non-small-cell lung cancer: A pooled analysis of randomized controlled trials. OncoTargets Ther 2015; 8: 2775-81.
[PMID: 26491352]

[83]   Rivera S, Leteur C, Mégnin F, *et al.* Time dependent modulation of tumor radiosensitivity by a pan HDAC inhibitor: Abexinostat. Oncotarget 2017; 8(34): 56210-27.
[http://dx.doi.org/10.18632/oncotarget.14813] [PMID: 28915585]

[84]   Ma S, Pradeep S, Hu W, Zhang D, Coleman R, Sood A. The role of tumor microenvironment in resistance to anti-angiogenic therapy. F1000 Res 2018; 7: 326.
[http://dx.doi.org/10.12688/f1000research.11771.1] [PMID: 29560266]

[85]   Zang J, Liang X, Huang Y, *et al.* Discovery of novel Pazopanib-based HDAC and VEGFR dual inhibitors targeting cancer epigenetics and angiogenesis simultaneously. J Med Chem 2018; 61(12): 5304-22.
[http://dx.doi.org/10.1021/acs.jmedchem.8b00384] [PMID: 29787262]

[86]   Blagosklonny MV. Antiangiogenic therapy and tumor progression. Cancer Cell 2004; 5(1): 13-7.
[http://dx.doi.org/10.1016/S1535-6108(03)00336-2] [PMID: 14749122]

[87]   Jain RK. Antiangiogenesis strategies revisited: From starving tumors to alleviating hypoxia. Cancer Cell 2014; 26(5): 605-22.
[http://dx.doi.org/10.1016/j.ccell.2014.10.006] [PMID: 25517747]

[88]   Li Q, Xia S, Fang H, Pan J, Jia Y, Deng G. VEGF treatment promotes bone marrow-derived CXCR4$^+$ mesenchymal stromal stem cell differentiation into vessel endothelial cells. Exp Ther Med 2017; 13(2): 449-54.
[http://dx.doi.org/10.3892/etm.2017.4019] [PMID: 28352314]

[89]   Aggarwal R, Thomas S, Pawlowska N, *et al.* Inhibiting histone deacetylase as a means to reverse resistance to angiogenesis inhibitors: Phase I study of Abexinostat plus Pazopanib in advanced solid tumor malignancies. J Clin Oncol 2017; 35(11): 1231-9.
[http://dx.doi.org/10.1200/JCO.2016.70.5350] [PMID: 28221861]

[90]   Barnes JA, Redd R, Fisher DC, *et al.* Panobinostat in combination with rituximab in heavily pretreated diffuse large B-cell lymphoma: Results of a phase II study. Hematol Oncol 2018; 36(4): 633-7.
[http://dx.doi.org/10.1002/hon.2515] [PMID: 29956350]

[91]   Ribatti D. Endogenous inhibitors of angiogenesis: A historical review. Leuk Res 2009; 33(5): 638-44.
[http://dx.doi.org/10.1016/j.leukres.2008.11.019] [PMID: 19117606]

[92]   Torok S, Rezeli M, Kelemen O, *et al.* Limited tumor tissue drug penetration contributes to primary resistance against angiogenesis inhibitors. Theranostics 2017; 7(2): 400-12.
[http://dx.doi.org/10.7150/thno.16767] [PMID: 28042343]

[93]   Hanahan D, Coussens LM. Accessories to the crime: Functions of cells recruited to the tumor microenvironment. Cancer Cell 2012; 21(3): 309-22.
[http://dx.doi.org/10.1016/j.ccr.2012.02.022] [PMID: 22439926]

[94]   Coffelt SB, Hughes R, Lewis CE. Tumor-associated macrophages: Effectors of angiogenesis and tumor progression. Biochim Biophys Acta 2009; 1796(1): 11-8.
[PMID: 19269310]

[95]   Ye W. The Complexity of translating anti-angiogenesis therapy from basic science to the clinic. Dev Cell 2016; 37(2): 114-25.
[http://dx.doi.org/10.1016/j.devcel.2016.03.015] [PMID: 27093081]

[96] Colotta F, Allavena P, Sica A, Garlanda C, Mantovani A. Cancer-related inflammation, the seventh hallmark of cancer: Links to genetic instability. Carcinogenesis 2009; 30(7): 1073-81.
[http://dx.doi.org/10.1093/carcin/bgp127] [PMID: 19468060]

[97] Williams BH, Weiss CA. Neoplasia.Ferrets, rabbits, and rodents Clinical Medicine and Surgery. 2nd ed. Saint Louis: W.B. Saunders 2004; pp. 91-106.
[http://dx.doi.org/10.1016/B0-72-169377-6/50011-3]

[98] Xiao X, Liu J, Sheng M. Synergistic effect of estrogen and VEGF on the proliferation of hemangioma vascular endothelial cells. J Pediatr Surg 2004; 39(7): 1107-10.
[http://dx.doi.org/10.1016/j.jpedsurg.2004.03.067] [PMID: 15213909]

[99] Pradel LP, Ooi CH, Romagnoli S, *et al.* Macrophage susceptibility to emactuzumab (RG7155) treatment. Mol Cancer Ther 2016; 15(12): 3077-86.
[http://dx.doi.org/10.1158/1535-7163.MCT-16-0157] [PMID: 27582524]

[100] Ramjiawan RR, Griffioen AW, Duda DG. Anti-angiogenesis for cancer revisited: Is there a role for combinations with immunotherapy? Angiogenesis 2017; 20(2): 185-204.
[http://dx.doi.org/10.1007/s10456-017-9552-y] [PMID: 28361267]

[101] Russo M, Giavazzi R. Anti-angiogenesis for cancer: Current status and prospects. Thromb Res 2018; 164 (Suppl. 1): S3-6.
[http://dx.doi.org/10.1016/j.thromres.2018.01.030] [PMID: 29703482]

[102] Huang Y, Yuan J, Righi E, *et al.* Vascular normalizing doses of antiangiogenic treatment reprogram the immunosuppressive tumor microenvironment and enhance immunotherapy. Proc Natl Acad Sci USA 2012; 109(43): 17561-6.
[http://dx.doi.org/10.1073/pnas.1215397109] [PMID: 23045683]

[103] Stylianopoulos T, Munn LL, Jain RK. Reengineering the tumor vasculature: Improving drug delivery and efficacy. Trends Cancer 2018; 4(4): 258-9.
[http://dx.doi.org/10.1016/j.trecan.2018.02.010] [PMID: 29606306]

[104] Khan KA, Kerbel RS. Improving immunotherapy outcomes with anti-angiogenic treatments and vice versa. Nat Rev Clin Oncol 2018; 15(5): 310-24.
[http://dx.doi.org/10.1038/nrclinonc.2018.9] [PMID: 29434333]

[105] Cai C, Tang J, Shen B, *et al.* Preclinical trial of the multi-targeted lenvatinib in combination with cellular immunotherapy for treatment of renal cell carcinoma. Exp Ther Med 2017; 14(4): 3221-8.
[http://dx.doi.org/10.3892/etm.2017.4858] [PMID: 28912872]

[106] Jain RK. Normalization of tumor vasculature: An emerging concept in antiangiogenic therapy. Science 2005; 307(5706): 58-62.
[http://dx.doi.org/10.1126/science.1104819] [PMID: 15637262]

[107] Huynh H, Lee LY, Goh KY, *et al.* Infigratinib Mediates Vascular Normalization, Impairs Metastasis, and Improves Chemotherapy in Hepatocellular Carcinoma. Hepatology 2019; 69(3): 943-58.
[http://dx.doi.org/10.1002/hep.30481] [PMID: 30575985]

[108] Tolaney SM, Boucher Y, Duda DG, *et al.* Role of vascular density and normalization in response to neoadjuvant bevacizumab and chemotherapy in breast cancer patients. Proc Natl Acad Sci USA 2015; 112(46): 14325-30.
[http://dx.doi.org/10.1073/pnas.1518808112] [PMID: 26578779]

[109] Dvorak HF. Vascular permeability factor/vascular endothelial growth factor: A critical cytokine in tumor angiogenesis and a potential target for diagnosis and therapy. J Clin Oncol 2002; 20(21): 4368-80.
[http://dx.doi.org/10.1200/JCO.2002.10.088] [PMID: 12409337]

[110] Diaz RJ, Ali S, Qadir MG, De La Fuente MI, Ivan ME, Komotar RJ. The role of bevacizumab in the treatment of glioblastoma. J Neurooncol 2017; 133(3): 455-67.
[http://dx.doi.org/10.1007/s11060-017-2477-x] [PMID: 28527008]

[111] Castro BA, Flanigan P, Jahangiri A, *et al.* Macrophage migration inhibitory factor downregulation: A novel mechanism of resistance to anti-angiogenic therapy. Oncogene 2017; 36(26): 3749-59.
[http://dx.doi.org/10.1038/onc.2017.1] [PMID: 28218903]

[112] Wilson PM, LaBonte MJ, Lenz HJ. Assessing the *in vivo* efficacy of biologic antiangiogenic therapies. Cancer Chemother Pharmacol 2013; 71(1): 1-12.
[http://dx.doi.org/10.1007/s00280-012-1978-8] [PMID: 23053262]

[113] Friedlander M, Theesfeld CL, Sugita M, *et al.* Involvement of integrins alpha $_v$ beta $_3$ and alpha $_v$ beta $_5$ in ocular neovascular diseases. Proc Natl Acad Sci USA 1996; 93(18): 9764-9.
[http://dx.doi.org/10.1073/pnas.93.18.9764] [PMID: 8790405]

[114] Murukesh N, Dive C, Jayson GC. Biomarkers of angiogenesis and their role in the development of VEGF inhibitors. Br J Cancer 2010; 102(1): 8-18.
[http://dx.doi.org/10.1038/sj.bjc.6605483] [PMID: 20010945]

[115] Tolmachev V, Stone-Elander S, Orlova A. Radiolabelled receptor-tyrosine-kinase targeting drugs for patient stratification and monitoring of therapy response: Prospects and pitfalls. Lancet Oncol 2010; 11(10): 992-1000.
[http://dx.doi.org/10.1016/S1470-2045(10)70088-7] [PMID: 20667780]

[116] Li S, Peck-Radosavljevic M, Koller E, *et al.* Characterization of (123)I-vascular endothelial growth factor-binding sites expressed on human tumour cells: Possible implication for tumour scintigraphy. Int J Cancer 2001; 91(6): 789-96.
[http://dx.doi.org/10.1002/1097-0215(200002)9999:9999<::AID-IJC1126>3.0.CO;2-K]   [PMID: 11275981]

[117] Yoshimoto M, Kinuya S, Kawashima A, Nishii R, Yokoyama K, Kawai K. Radioiodinated VEGF to image tumor angiogenesis in a LS180 tumor xenograft model. Nucl Med Biol 2006; 33(8): 963-9.
[http://dx.doi.org/10.1016/j.nucmedbio.2006.08.006] [PMID: 17127168]

[118] Cai W, Chen K, Mohamedali KA, *et al.* PET of vascular endothelial growth factor receptor expression. J Nucl Med 2006; 47(12): 2048-56.
[PMID: 17138749]

[119] Kang CM, Kim SM, Koo HJ, *et al. In vivo* characterization of 68Ga-NOTA-VEGF 121 for the imaging of VEGF receptor expression in U87MG tumor xenograft models. Eur J Nucl Med Mol Imaging 2013; 40(2): 198-206.
[http://dx.doi.org/10.1007/s00259-012-2266-x] [PMID: 23096079]

CHAPTER 2

Anti-angiogenic Mechanism, Biochemical Factors' Roles, Therapeutic Agents, and Under Clinical Trial Drugs for Breast and Prostate Cancers

Varsha M. Singh[1], Shilpa J. Newati[1], Mohammad Yusuf[2], Alexandre Bridoux[3,4], Salman A. A. Mohammed[5], Naseem Akhtar[6] and Riaz A. Khan[1,5,*]

[1] *Manav Rachna International Institute of Research & Study (MRIIRS)-Manav Rachna International University (MRIU), Faridabad, HR 121 001, India*

[2] *College of Pharmacy, Taif University, Al-Haweiah, Taif, KSA*

[3] *Integral University, Lucknow, India*

[4] *Laboratoire Centre Atlantique, Zone Industrielle Chef de Baie, 1 rue Samuel de Champlain, Cs 41074, 17000la Rochelle, France*

[5] *College of Pharmacy, Qassim University, Qassim, KSA*

[6] *College of Pharmacy, Buraydah Colleges, Qassim, KSA*

Abstract: The genesis of new blood vessels is the culmination of angiogenic activity which is responsible for the spreading of the tumors and other malignant masses. The blood supply also provides nourishment to non-malignant tissues and helps in their maintenance, growth, and proliferation. The major biological factors that significantly favor the angiogenic processes includes vascular endothelial growth factors (VEGFs), tumor necrosis factors (TNFs), and fibroblast growth factors (FGFs). The disruption and inhibition of angiogenic growth factors and their biochemical pathways during the cancer cycle are among the obvious choices to control the growth and proliferation of cancers. The current work deals in details about the growth factors, their roles, contextual biomechanics, and approaches to control angiogenesis through different inhibitory mechanisms involving biochemical pathways, growth factors, and structural motifs, playing part in the angiogenesis. The approaches to find novel molecular templates, new chemical entities, bio-macromolecular substrates, and probable drug leads for anti-angiogenic pharmacology are discussed. The chapter enlists various anti-angiogenesis drugs, under clinical trials, new chemical entities, and other biochemical and recombinant therapeutic agents, used either as mono or as combination therapy in treatment of various forms of cancers, especially breast and prostate cancers.

** **Corresponding author Professor Riaz A. Khan, (MRSC, UK):** Manav Rachna International Institute of Research & Study (MRIIRS)-Manav Rachna International University (MRIU), Faridabad, HR 121 001, India, and College of Pharmacy, Qassim University, KSA; E-mail: kahnriaz@gmail.com*

Atta-ur-Rahman & M. Iqbal Choudhary (Eds.)

Keywords: Angiogenesis, Angiogenin, Angiostatin, Antiangiogensis, Bevacizumab, Decorin, FGF, Ephrin, Endostatin, Interferon, Interleukin, Integrin, Matrix Metallo-Proteinases (MMP), TNFα, Thrombospondin, US-FDA Approved Anti-Cancer Drugs, Vitaxin.

INTRODUCTION: THE ANGIOGENESIS AND CANCERS

Angiogenesis, a natural and crucial process in the living systems through the modes of sprouting and splitting of existing vasculature, results in the formation of new blood vessels. It initiates during embryonic growth through various phases of development and is principally involved in injury remediation and wound recovery during life-cycle. The process is a balance of activators and inhibitors, forming the on-off trigger-based switch mechanism. The process is also mandatory for nourishing tumor for its maintenance, growth, multiplication, and lastly, relocations. The tumor, which can grow up to 50-100 cells or 1-2 mm^3 in blood-deprived conditions because of multiple biochemical factors, may become necrotic. The tumor-induced vascularization controlled by the release of various growth factors is crucial for angiogenesis, but their inhibitions curtail the tumor maintenance, growth, and its relocation. The anti-angiogenesis is currently the new area of interest in designing newer molecular templates, finding drugs lead, developing new chemical entities, and drug candidates as anti-cancer and anti-tumor agents [1].

The angiogenesis switch is governed by its activators and inhibitors to make it functional and inactivate, respectively. During tumor development and consequent growth, the endothelium gets operative according to the physiological and pathological needs of the tumor and activators promote endothelial cells growth while the inhibitors check on the endothelial cell proliferation and not let it grow beyond requirements (Fig. **1** and Table **1**).

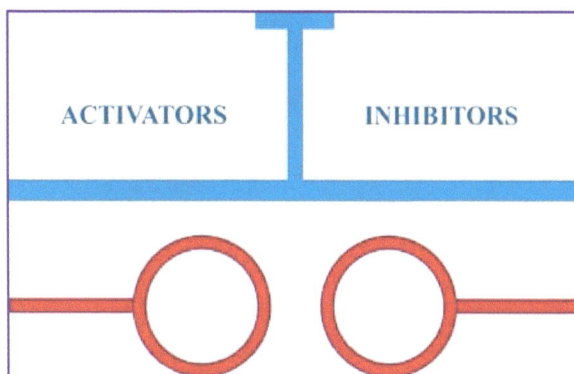

Fig. (1). Angiogenesis: The Switch.

Table 1. Major process regulators of angiogenesis.

Serial	Activator
1.	Vascular Endothelial Growth Factors (VEGF) family
2.	Fibroblast Growth Factors (FGF)
3.	Tumor Necrosis Factor-α (TNF-α)
4.	Plated-delivered Endothelial Growth Factor
5.	Interleukin-1, 6, and 8
6.	Endogenous Modulators (αVβ-3 integrin), Hypoxia, Nitric Oxide Synthase
7.	Matrix Metalloproteinases (MMP)

ANGIOGENIC BIOMECHANISMS: NORMAL *VERSUS* TUMOR-INDUCED

The angiogenesis is a vital process responsible for the healthy development, growth, wound healing, and formation of granulation tissues. It plays an essential part in tumor growth and transition to malignancy from the benign tumor. The first identified angiogenesis type, the sprouting angiogenesis, is manifested in various stages, and the angiogenic growth factors involved in biological signaling help to activate the endothelial based receptors present on the blood vessels to release proteases for detachment of basement membrane of the endothelial cells on the vessels. The detached endothelial cells reach into the nearby matrices and generate sprouts to connect other vessels through adhesion molecules, *i.e.*, integrins. The migrating endothelial cells and sprouts form the initial lumen for the vessel. Sprouting occurs at a faster pace, and gaps are initiated in the newly formed vasculature. The splitting form of angiogenesis, intussusceptive angiogenesis, generates new vessels by splitting the existing vessels into two vessels [2].

The tumors through secretions of various growth factors and necessary proteins induce the angiogenesis to produce new blood vessels and its further growth into the expanding tumor (Fig. **2**). The self-directed and irregular tumor cells divisions give rise to expanding tumor mass which releases angiogenic stimulators. These stimulators activate the endothelial cell receptors on the existing blood vessel to let them secrete proteolytic enzymes, which in turn works at a particular location on the vessel to form pores for generating the new blood vessels for the blood supply to the tumor area [3, 4]. The metastatic cancer also follows the angiogenesis, and a single cancer cell leaves the solid tumor and travels through the blood to another location where it implants itself to produce the secondary tumor and follows the same cycle to produce new blood vessels [5].

Herein, certain signaling entities help in stimulating the development of new blood vessels, and these processes help tumors in growth and migration to different locations. The stimulation for angiogenesis is controlled by several factors, which also includes integrin and prostaglandin molecules. A list of stimulators and their roles in angiogenesis are presented in Table **2**.

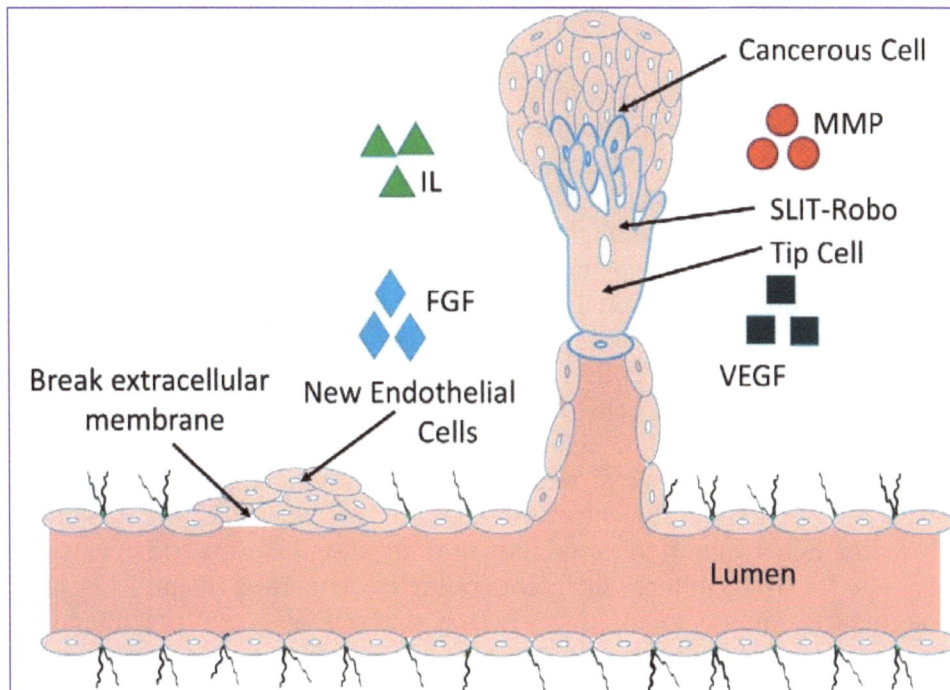

Fig. (2). Representative sketch for the tumor-induced angiogenesis.

Table 2. Angiogenesis Stimulators*.

Stimulator	Roles
Ang1, 2	Stabilizes the vessels
Ephrin	Determines the formation of arteries or veins
FGF	Proliferation, differentiation of fibroblast, endothelial and smooth muscle cells
Integrins αVβ3, αVβ5, α5β1	Binds matrix macromolecules and proteinases
ID1/ID3	Regulates endothelial trans-differentiation
PDGF (BB-Homodimer), PDGFR	Recruits smooth muscle cells
Plasminogen Activators	Remodels extracellular matrix releases and activates growth factors
Plasminogen Activator Inhibitor-1	Stabilizes nearby vessels

(Table 2) cont.....

Stimulator	Roles
Semaphorins (class III)	Modulates endothelial cells adhesion, migration, proliferation and apoptosis, alters vascular permeability
TGF-β, Endoglin, TGF-β Receptors	Increases extracellular matrix production
VE-Cadherin, CD31	Endothelial junctional molecules
VEGF	Affects permeability
VEGFR, NRP-1 (Neuropilin-1)	Integrate survival signals

sourced from https://en.wikipedia.org/wiki/Angiogenesis

The angiogenesis nourishes the tumor by providing the blood supply which contains oxygen and required nutrients. The cancerous cells grow to certain genetically-predefined size and specifications, and eventually their migration to other places takes place with the blood supply. The signaling entities including growth factors, *i.e.*, vascular endothelial growth factor (VEGF), and several other requisite signaling processes combine to initiate the angiogenesis process while some of the anti-angiogenic signaling entities restrict the angiogenic process and play their role to restrict the growth of the cancerous mass. The normal angiogenesis is a highly controlled process based on signaling phenomenon. As the blood supply reaches the cells, it helps to pave the way for migration of cells and various other signaling molecules. The migrating and multiplying tumor cells require nourishment for survival and consequently switches on the angiogenic process. The VEGF is responsible for vascular permeability [6, 7], and this growth factor helps tumor to enter into normal vascular-web and metastasize feasibly. The VEGF have three different coding regions-189, 165 and 121 amino acids segments. Among them, the $VEGF_{165}$ and $VEGF_{121}$ are the abundantly secreted isoforms, and with the latest known class of receptors on tumor and endothelial cells, the neuropilin (Npn)-1, and Npn-2 which have the affinity to bind with $VEGF_{165}$ [8, 9], results in uncontrolled growth of cells in the tumor. The nutrients requirement for tumor and cancers' survival makes these cells mimic the angiogenesis process in the pre-existing vasculature (Fig. 3).

Tumor Vasculature

The tumor cells get their nourishment through the angiogenesis processes, and the new blood vessels called, 'mother vessels' arise from the healthy blood vessels. The tumor cells can also suckle on the local vessels and avoid angiogenesis for a certain period. Anatomically, the tumor vasculatures are atypical, and may be deficient in specific functional cells and base membrane's presence [10]. They are not porous to the outsized macromolecules and are unable to discard the left-overs. Their cell wall consists of transcellular dumps, and small apertures are responsible for making vessels drippy. These small apertures let water and plasma proteins to leak [11].

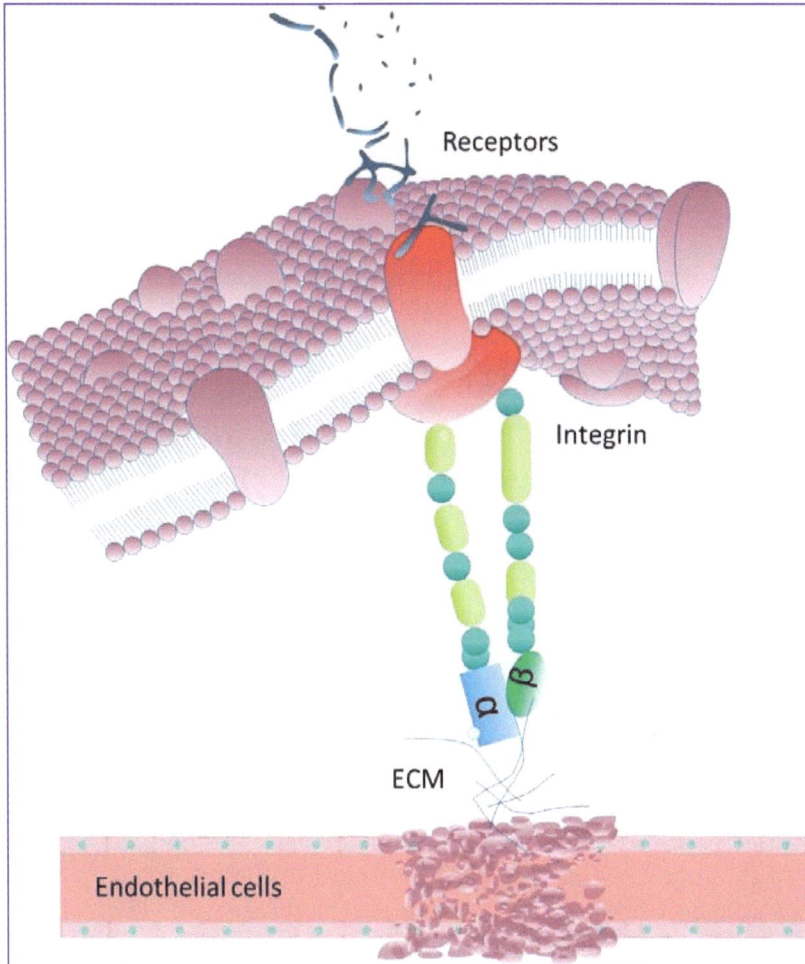

Fig. (3). Cells proliferation, migration, and survival.

Operational Signaling Pathways in Tumor

Although the growth factors of tumor cells are indeed the same as in the case of normal angiogenesis processes [12, 13], the lack of cross-regulation control factors, and downstream signaling leads to abnormal vascular synthesis. This process results in an abnormal vascular system with the irregular flow and improper nutrients supply [14, 15]. A variety of signaling molecules play essential roles in tumor angiogenesis: VEGF with VEGFR-1,-2 as receptors, and the NRP-

1 protein. Furthermore, the angiogenic remodeling requires angiopoietins, the ligands of Tie receptors, while another two important notch receptors for tumor angiogenesis are Delta-like 4 (DLL4) Jagged-1; the ephrins, and Eph receptors including the slits glycoproteins/roundabout receptors pathways (ROBO). These growth factors, signaling, and receptors help in growth, organization, and metastasis of the vascular system for the tumor cells [16]. These operational signals help to grow and to spread the tumor cells with two most necessary conditions of nutrients and oxygen supplies through blood for cancer to grow in the body. For cancer to stop flourishing, these growth factors-cum-receptors need to be suppressed [17, 18].

Angiogenic Promoters and their Involvement in Breast Cancer

The cancer survival depends on two requirements. First, the nourishment, and second is to relocate from place to place, even in the vicinity. The angiogenic process fulfills both of these basic requirements, promoted by many factors, *i.e.*, vascular endothelial growth factors (VEGF), Fibroblast growth factors (FGF), Interleukins (IL), and Matrix Metalloproteinases (MMP). These factors, or signals when interacting with their respective receptors, aid to the basic requirement for any cancer to flourish.

Angiogenin

Angiogenin (ANG) is a 14-kDa single chain extracellular protein, initially isolated in the tumor cells conditioned medium [19 - 21]. The ANG was identified because of its ability to induce neovascularization. The ANG has shown structural similarly of 35% sequence homology to pancreatic RNAse.

In addition to the increased levels of ANG found in the plasma, the ANG is also present in its vascular endothelial and smooth muscle cells. The ANG has also been detected in the fetus as well as in adult's heart, spleen, lung, and liver [22]. No preclinical studies on knockout mice exist in rodents due to the complexity in knocking out the genes. In comparison to humans having single ANG gene, the mouse has five genes (ANG 1-5) in addition to 3 pseudogenes but only one gene, in mice, has shown to possess angiogenic activity with an identical structure as to that of the human gene. Another vertebrate's *viz.* rat, pig, and turtle have been reported to possess two genes each while cattle have three ANG genes. The absence of the angiogenin gene in douc langur monkeys indicated that angiogenin might not be an essential gene for survival [23]. Recently, the angiogenin gene-deficiency were reported in other animals, *i.e.*, dog, guinea pig, and the giant panda. The CRISPR/CAS9 is a gene editing technique which also failed to report , till date, any success of generating transgenic mice from ANG-1.

The activated signal transduction is achieved through cell migration and invasion. Under stress, the endocytosis of ANG starts from the cells surface to the inner side of the cells followed by its accumulation in the nucleoli leading to the activation of signal transduction pathways thereby promoting the cell migration and invasion. The angiogenin also contributes to ubiquitination of p53by inhibiting the serine-15 phosphorylation of p53. Under hypoxic stress condition, the ANG levels increase malignant melanoma and instance of cervical cancers [24, 25].

The molecular function of angiogenin includes signal transduction. Nuclear translocation has the potential to stimulate endothelial proliferation, migration, invasion, and tubular structure formation [26, 27]. Some protein factors that include angiogenin in addition to other factors influence vascularization and angiogenesis. The ANG also participates in the immune defense of intestine [28] and acts as an antimicrobial peptide on the surface of the eyes [29, 30]. The ANG possesses anti-fungal activities by suppressing the replication of X4 HIV strains. The overexpressed ANG levels influence all steps of tumor growth and progression and evaluated by serum ANG levels [18]. For example, a high serum level of ANG is found in the solid tumor [31 - 33]. The ANG serum levels in non-malignant diseases like inflammatory bowel disease [34], diabetes [35, 36], and endometriosis [37] are reported to be an indicator/biomarker. In neurodegenerative disease, ANG correlates with the pathogenesis of the amyotrophic lateral sclerosis (ALS) [38].

The promising findings reported various animal models inhibition of tumor growth using various ANG inhibitors like neomycin, neamine, siRNA, antisense, and enzymatic inhibitors [33, 39 - 41]. However, the high levels of ANG in human serum makes it a challenging task to neutralize it by inhibitors. Even though blocking of ANG is a daunting task due to its high incidence in the plasma, cancer, and various inflammatory disease treatment approach could be achieved by blocking the attaching of ANG to its receptor. Furthermore, recombinant ANG could be another approach in neuroprotective therapies. The multi-function protein, like ANG with its varied mechanisms of action, has potential not only as a diagnostic marker but also for the treatment of cancers and other diseases. Further research might unravel new roles of ANG towards developing new therapies.

Vascular Endothelial Growth Factors (VEGFs)

The VEGFs, a sub-family of growth factors, are considered potent stimulator and prime contributor in angiogenesis. Together with bFGF (basic fibroblast growth factor), it is responsible for an increase in several capillaries formed as a consequence of plated endothelial cells migration and proliferation. The VEGF starts the process of tyrosine kinase signaling and series of signaling events in the endothelial cells. These events lead to production of responsible factors for stimulating vessel permeability by eNOS (endothelial nitric oxide synthase), production of NO, the survival and proliferation by the bFGF during the migration by matrix metalloproteinase, intercellular (CD54) and vascular adhesion molecules, and finally maturation to the blood vessel. The increased blood flow causes an increase in mRNA production of VEGF receptors 1 and 2, which consequently causes massive signaling related to angiogenesis. As part of the angiogenic signaling cascade, the NO works as a significant participant to angiogenic response [42].

Again, the VEGF play essential roles in many vital processes, *e.g.*, osteogenesis, wound healing, and other developmental processes. In mammals, there are five main VEGF molecules with three different VEGF receptors [43 - 45]. The interaction between these VEGF ligands and receptors expression levels is very high, and they are within the ambit of responsibility for any cancerous material to proliferate and migrate. In case of breast cancer, the VEGF types, VEGF-A, and VEGFR-1 and VEGFR-2 are responsible for cell division/proliferation and migration [46 - 53]. The PIGF (placental growth factor, a member of the VEGF family) is also accountable in pro-inflammatory and pro-angiogenic activities that support cancer cells relocation. A brief role of these factors is presented in Table 3.

Table 3. Growth factors and their roles.

Serial	VEGF	VEGFR	Roles
1.	A	2	Stimulates angiogenesis
2.	B	1	Stimulates plasminogen, and metastasis
3.	C	2,3	Stimulates angiogenesis, and lymph-angiogenesis
4.	D	Lymph-angiogenesis	Stimulates lymphatic vessels
5.	PIGF (Placental Growth Factor)	1	Embryogenesis

Interleukins

The interleukins are neutrophilic, chemotactic, and inflammatory cytokines, and act as a critical mediator of the immune system. The neutrophils can degrade the base membrane and extracellular matrix to influence the affected site on getting signal from the immune system. It is also present in storage vesicles of endothelial cells. One of the interleukins, IL-8, produced by endothelial cells, can bind with many receptors, but it has more affinity to G protein-coupled serpentine receptors CXCR-1 and CXCR-2. However, the IL-8 is more expressed in CXCR-1, and its expression levels are very high in case of breast cancer. The IL-8 in breast cancer progression is related to its interaction with the Estrogen Receptor (ER), and Human Epidermal Growth Factor Receptor-2 (HER-2). The IL-8 is exclusively expressed highly in the ER- and HER+ breast cancers [54].

Fibroblast Growth Factors (FGF)

The fibroblast growth factors (FGF) family comprises acidic FGF-1 (aFGF) and basic FGF-2 (bFGF) along with 22 other members [55]. The FGFs stimulate different cellular functions by binding to cell surface FGF-receptor proteins, which are single-chain receptor tyrosine kinase activated by autophosphorylation. This activation produces signals cascade leading to proliferation, cell differentiation, and matrix dissolution to initiate mitogenic activity essential for endothelial cells, fibroblasts, and smooth muscle cells growth. The FGF-1 binds to all seven receptor-subtypes, and is a potent mitogen capable of starting angiogenesis in hypoxic masses. It also stimulates the proliferation and cell differentiation for building up of smooth muscle, endothelial cells and arterial vessels [56]. The FGF-2, participating in endothelial cells proliferation organizes tubular structures of the endothelial cells towards angiogenesis. It is more potent than vascular and platelet-derived growth factors, but less potent than the FGF-1. The FGF-2, responsible for division and relocation of endothelial cells, consequently enhances the breast cancer occurrences [57]. The protein appears in five different forms having different molecular weights wherein the 18-kDa bFGF is the most common FGF, which communicates with all other seven FGF-Receptors. The bFGF initiates the angiogenesis process when heparin sulfate enters the extracellular matrix [58 - 63].

Matrix MetalloProteinases (MMPs) and Matrix Remodeling

The matrix metalloproteinases, or matrixins are the highly regulated proteolytic enzymes controlling protein degradation of the vessel walls to let the endothelial cells move into the interstitial matrix for taking part in the sprouting angiogenesis. The MMPs are of endopeptidase class wherein Zn ion works as a cofactor. The MMPs favor cell expressions, development and cell divisions along with the cellular movement to specific directions and locations, when needed, during various immune responses as well as wound healing processes. They also prepare cells to differentiate for angiogenesis. They allow the normal preexisting blood vessels destabilized by ruining of the matrix proteins, and specific evolutionary DNA sequences to participate in the process. This process helps in relocating endothelial cells [64 - 73].

The metalloproteinases (MMPs) are generally of 5 types. They are secreted as inactive zymogens in the beginning and becomes active when in communication with other proteolytic enzymes in the extracellular matrix. The MMPs are governed differently in breast cancer cells. They are essential in tumor raid, spread, and angiogenesis. Thus, the MMPs have great potential as a drug target and potential to develop as biomarkers for diagnosis purposes [74]. The MMPs, *i.e.*, MMP-2, and MMP-9, synthesized by stromal cells, supports the growth of breast cancer [75]. The MMP-7 synthesized by tumor cells have high expressions and helps in the propagation of the tumor. These MMPs act as a diagnostic marker not only in the revealing but also in observing of malignant lesions status [76]. The MMP-9 is a pivotal candidate in tumor angiogenesis because it takes care of the bioavailability of VEGF. It is an effective inducer of angiogenesis. The MMP-9 and MMP-2 triggers are transforming growth factor-β (TGF-β) signaling to endorse tumor raid, angiogenesis, and tumor distribution, *i.e.*, metastasis [74]. Thus, the formation of new capillaries is controlled by inhibiting the MMPs [77].

Angiopoietins

Angiopoietin, a family of vascular growth factors, play essential roles in postnatal and embryonic angiogenesis and are responsible for assembling/disassembling endothelial linings of the blood vessels. The related cytokines control the microvascular permeation, dilation, and vasoconstrictions. Out of the four angiopoietins, ANGPT1, 2, 3, and 4, the ANGPT1 and 2, take part in the maturation of blood vessels as being part of the crucial growth factors responsible for angiogenesis through binding with their receptors, Tie-1, and Tie-2 wherein it is thought that cells signals are mostly transmitted by Tie-2, the tyrosine kinases type receptors. The phosphorylation on tyrosine during dimerization compel to initiate cell signaling by activation of downstream intracellular enzymes termed as cell signaling [78]. The ANGPT1 have multiple roles in adhesion, migration, survival, and vessel maturation while the ANGPT2 causes apoptosis together with vascularization disruptions; nonetheless, together with VEGF, the ANGPT2 promotes neovascularization [79].

Roles of Integrins in Tumorigenesis

These proteinases adhesive bodies are heterodimers of subunits alpha (α) and beta (β) which helps in the transduction of biochemical signals from the extracellular matrix to cytoskeleton. The integrins αvβ3 and αvβ5 play significant roles in angiogenesis. These transmembrane linkers transfer signals from the extracellular matrix to the cytoskeleton and help in relocation and survival of the endothelial cells. In a typical unchanged environment, αvβ3 is inactive and comes in action mode with the help of cytokines present on both endothelial and vascular cells of the tumor environment [80, 81].

ANGIOGENIC INHIBITORS

Interferons

The interferons are signal proteins released for defending against pathogens and tumor cells. Along with chemotherapy and radiation, the interferons are used as a treatment tool against cancers. They have growth inhibition effects on tumor cells, and in general, there are two types of interferons; type I that includes α and β and they bind with similar kinds of receptor whereas type II interferon, Υ is activated by Interleukin-12, and released by T-helper cells, which binds with the receptors on the cell surface. The interferons have shown anti-proliferative effects on breast cancer cell lines in different concentrations of estradiol. At 1000 IU/ml concentrations, the effect is maximum, and β type has significant effects among α and Υ irrespective of the receptors on the cell surface [82]. Similarly, on the MCF-7 cell lines, α and Υ interferons have cells inhibition effects [83]. Some of the inhibitors are listed in Table **4**.

Table 4. Natural angiogenic inhibitors.

Serial	Inhibitor	Role
1.	Interferons	Hinder angiogenesis promoters; prevent cell migration of endothelial cells.
2.	Endostatin	Prevent relocation of the cell, cell multiplying, and sustained existence of endothelial cells.
3.	Angiostatin	Hinder cell multiplying, and encourage endothelial cells death.
4.	Thrombospondin	Prevents relocation of the cell, cell multiplying, cell union, and sustained existence of endothelial cells.
5.	Decorin	Prevent relocation of the cell, cell multiplying, and encourage endothelial cells death.

Endostatin

Endostatin, a natural, all-purpose pro-angiogenic inhibitor, restricts the actions of VEGF, and bFGF/FGF-2 growth factors. It also inhibits tumor necrosis factor TNF-α, which activates the c-Jun N-terminal kinase (JNK) pathway opposite of the cell surface receptors, α_v- and α_5- integrins [84]. The Endostatin is also responsible for inhibition of endothelial cells progressions [85]. The JNK signaling pathways are initiated by cellular stress and help in tumor necrosis factor, TNF-α to provoke cell death [86].

Angiostatin

A natural anti-angiogentic agent to inhibit tumor growth and proliferation [87 - 90], it binds with adenosine triphosphate (ATP) synthase, and integrin $\alpha_v\beta_3$ to inhibit cell multiplications. It is also involved in activating the MAPK (Mitogen-Activated Protein Kinase), extracellular-signal-regulated kinases-1(ERK1), and ERK2, which are required for cell proliferation, and differentiation. Also, it suppresses the FGF-2 and VEGF activities in h-SVC (human skin vascular cells) [91, 92].

Thrombospondin

The thrombospondins (TSPs) family consists of five members. They are calcium-binding extracellular glycoproteins. The TSP family members (TSP-1 and 2) are effective in angiogenesis inhibition as well as in endothelial cell migration induced by VEGF or, the basic-fibroblast growth factor (bFGF) [93]. The TSPs also helps in inducing endothelial cells apoptosis [94]. Both, the TSP-1 and TSP-2, hinders the cell cycle, initiated by many mitogen proteins, and stops cells in the G_0/G_1 phase. The TSP-1 has antiangiogenic effects. It also blocks the nitric oxide (NO) by CD36 and CD47 [95] driven proangiogenic responses, and inhibits the endothelial cell multiplications [96].

Decorin

The leucine-rich proteoglycan, decorin [97, 98], has been studied as a potential anticancer agent. It contributes crucially in tumor-induced angiogenesis, and is the first proteoglycan expressed in the stroma of colon cancers [99, 100]. The systemic delivery of decorin reduces not only the breast tumor size but also it's metabolism and relocation to other body parts, especially lungs [101] by downregulating the multiple receptor tyrosine kinases (RTKs) [102 - 104], and the receptor tyrosine-protein kinase (ErbB2) [105, 106]. Decorin help in controlling, tumor growth [107]. The cyclin-dependent kinase inhibitor p21^{WAF1} (p21) which is a physiological controller of breast cancer [108, 109], as well as regulation of intracellular Ca^{2+} which, in turn, helps in working of anticancer agents [110], is this way taken care by the decorin. The decorin provokes the Met proto-oncogene

[111] *via* caveolae-mediated endocytosis [112], and discontinues the signals similar to EGFR [113]. This process helps Met to activate downstream signals [114, 115] to inhibit tumor-induced angiogenesis.

Commercially Aailable Angiogenic Inhibitors

The United States Food and Drug Administration (USFDA) approved several angiogenesis inhibitors for treating various cancers (https://www.cancer.gov/about-cancer/treatment/types/immunotherapy/angiogenesis-inhibitors-fact-sheet). A single inhibitor works for multiple cancer types and is used as a monotherapy, or as part of combination therapy with drugs and adjuvants. These inhibitors are also substantiated through combination dosing with hormone, and other modes of cancer therapies wherein these work as targeted therapies or precision-medicine and specifically target the VEGF, its receptor, and other specific molecules involved in the process of angiogenesis. The approved and commercially registered angiogenesis inhibitors, along with their trade names, include:

Axitinib (Inlyta®)

Bevacizumab (Avastin®)

Cabozantinib (Cometriq®)

Everolimus (Afinitor®)

Lenalidomide (Revlimid®), Lenvatinib mesylate (Lenvima®)

Pazopanib (Votrient®)

Ramucirumab (Cyramza®), Regorafenib (Stivarga®)

Sorafenib (Nexavar®), Sunitinib (Sutent®)

Thalidomide (Synovir®, Thalomid®)

Vandetanib (Caprelsa®)

Ziv-aflibercept (Zaltrap®)

CLINICAL TRIALS TOWARDS ANTI-ANGIOGENIC DRUGS DEVELOPMENT

There have been distinct developments in the drug discovery and development processes for anti-angiogenic drugs. However, the majority of antiangiogenic drug candidates have failed to produce significant survival benefits for patients with metastatic breast cancer (MBC). Some drug candidates neutralize the VEGF ligand; the drugs are working on blocking of the respective receptors involved in the angiogenesis processes, and some of the drug candidates are capable of interrupting of the transduction of the signal, or disrupting the cellular signaling involved in the angiogenesis processes. The anti-angiogenic therapy for most of the trials have provided transitory improvements in the form of tumor status quo or its size-reduction, giving increased survival time for certain patients, but have often failed to produce long-term or permanent clinical benefits. The resistance is either intrinsic or acquired. The success of therapy is dependent upon proper timing window for tumor vascular normalization process, and the inhibitor therapy needs to target at this early stage to confront the progression of the tumor. The prolonged anti-angiogenic therapy may lead to low levels of oxygen availability in the tumor, which increases the VEGF production to sustain itself along with instability in the extracellular environment and it produces vascular permeability of the tumor. The subsequent reduction in blood flow reduces oxygen and nutrient concentrations at the tumor site, putting stress on the tumor growth. However, this process is less effective against the established tumor vessels, and the response of the therapy met with resistance [116]. Nonetheless, the anti-angiogenic drug developmental exercises have yielded some anti-angiogenic drugs which have passed the developmental stages and are commercially available. These drugs are protein and small molecule-based new chemical entities. With different specifications, these drugs interfere with the VEGF signaling pathway. However, monovalent antibiotic drugs are antigen-specific and inhibit the roles of factors involved in the angiogenesis. The ramucirumab communicates with VEGFR2 and does not allow communication with the VEGF-A-C-D. Some of the approved and underdevelopment anti-angiogenesis drugs/drug candidates, especially for breast cancers, are discussed and represented (Fig. **4**) here.

Bevacizumab

Bevacizumab works as VEGF-antagonist by hindering binding to its receptors VEGFR-1 and 2 for inhibiting the tumor growth without affecting other signaling pathways [117 - 121]. The US-FDA approved bevacizumab under the trade name Avastin in 2008. The drug belongs to biopharmaceutical class, and is structurally a humanized monovalent antibody, administered intravenously. It is considered as the first anti-angiogenetic drug against many cancers, *i.e.*, ovarian, colon, lung, breast, renal-cell carcinoma, and gliomas [122 - 142]. It was considered insignificant for prolonged use with *progression-free survival* (PFS) due to certain side-effects.

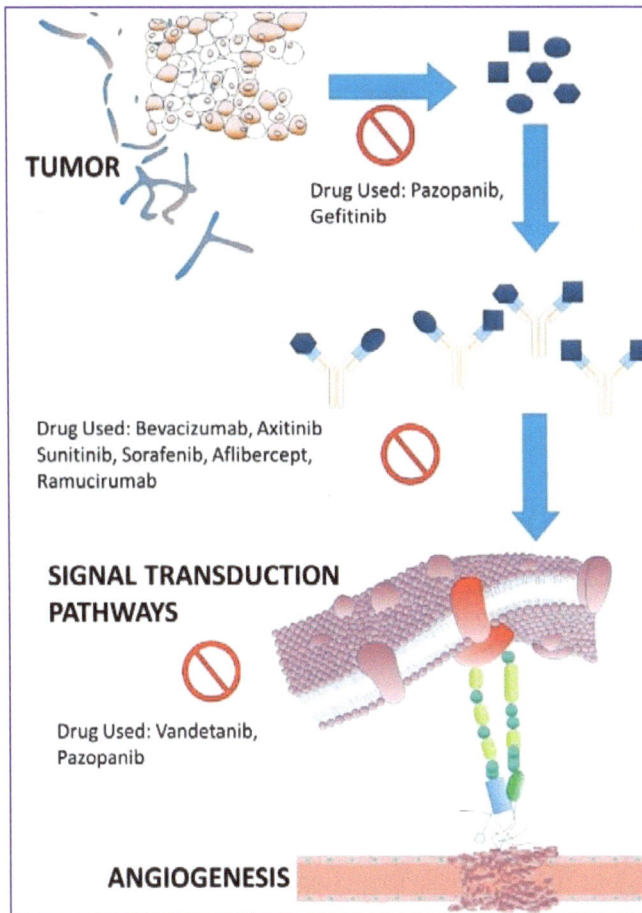

Fig. (4). Angiogenic inhibitors at different levels.

During the first phase of safety trial on 75 patients with metastatic breast cancer, when drug administered intravenously every 2 weeks at different dose concentrations, 4 patients at dose levels of 20 mg/kg felt headache with queasiness, unsettled stomach, and sudden elevation of cerebral arterial pressure, kidney problems and secretion of high volume of proteins in the urine. However, it was seen that at dose levels 10 mg/kg for two weeks, the drug was well tolerated.

In most of the trials, the PFS increased considerably on a combination of bevacizumab with a chemotherapy agent during first-line therapy of HER2-negative breast cancers. In AVF2119 study involving 462 MBC patients, the comparative study of capecitabine effect (with the two divided daily doses of 2500 mg/m^2 for two weeks with 1 week off in between) with capecitabine in combination with bevacizumab (dose of 15 mg/kg for 3 weeks) showed an increase in Objective Response Rate (ORR) from 9.1% to 19.8%. The PFS and the overall survival remained unchanged along with the side effects of proteinuria and hypertension [143]. In another trial, ECOG 2100, the effects of paclitaxel and paclitaxel with bevacizumab was studied on 722 patients with MBC. The patients were randomly administered paclitaxel as 90 mg/m^2 or a combination of paclitaxel with bevacizumab at dose levels of 10 mg/kg/week to show improved therapeutic action. These studies concluded that patients taking a combination of paclitaxel with bevacizumab showed an improvement in PFS, but somehow, the overall survival rate remained unchanged. It also resulted in various side effects, such as hypertension, headache, cerebrovascular ischemia, and proteinuria in the patients [144]. In another AVADO trial, a combination of bevacizumab with docetaxel did not significantly impacted the outcome. The bevacizumab, 15 mg/kg, in a combination with docetaxel for every other third week, increased the PFS period in first-line treatment for MBC patients as compared with the docetaxel and placebo groups [145]. In RIBBON 1 and 2 trials, the bevacizumab combined with capecitabine, taxanes or anthracycline antibiotics, the chemotherapeutic systems in both the PFS and ORR studies, increased slightly, whereas overall survival rate was not affected as compared with various other kinds of treatments. As a result, FDA disapproved bevacizumab as a drug for treating metastatic breast cancer on 28 November 2011.

Cilengitide

It is the first small molecule anti-angiogenic drug (Fig. **5**) and targets the integrins αvβ3, αvβ5, and α5β1. It works as an anti-proliferation entity and is useful in cell necrosis and in stopping the bone metastasis [146 - 149]. The drug is helpful in tumor-size reduction with negligible toxicity. However, there is no significant effect on the overall survival rate in comparison to other chemotherapeutic treatments [150 - 153].

The drug is in phase III clinical trial evaluation for the treatment of glioblastomas while second phase clinical trial concerns with several other tumors [154]. The drug is being investigated in clinical trial phase-I with paclitaxel for aggressive breast cancers [155].

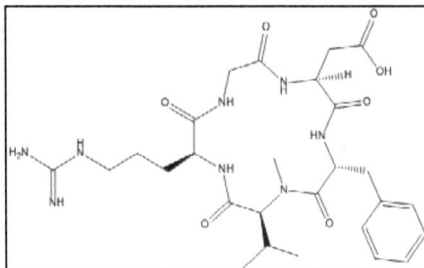

Fig. (5). Cilengitide chemical structure.

Aflibercept

It is an anti-VEGF drug that absorbs soluble VEGF-A, B, and PlGF-1, 2. The drug was tested in previously treated patients with anthracycline and a taxane class drug, *i.e.* paclitaxel and docitaxel. Also, MBC patients pretreated for metastatic breast cancer showed tumor shrinkage of about 5%, and a PFS rate of 10% after six months of trials (ClinicalTrials.gov, Identifier: NCT001843725). Aflibercept works as VEGF trap neutralizing VEGF-A, VEGF-B, and PlGF, and is considered as useful as an add-on drug to adjuvant and neoadjuvant chemotherapy, although it has only been tested at primary scale. The inhibition of Ang1 and Ang2 signaling is part of the mode of biochemical mechanistic action of the drug, and which is important, but the Ang1 inhibition was not found to be very pronounced [156].

The drug was approved by US-FDA for metastasized colorectal cancer in the US and according to Cancer Research, UK (canceresesarchuk.org) for advanced bowel cancer in the UK. Aflibercept was tested in combination with capecitabine for chemo-refractory digestive tumors, and breast tumors in phase I trials, including other tumors. Aflibercept has generally been more in use for ophthalmic purposes, and has been approved by USFDA for age-related neovascular macular degeneration, macular edema after retinal-vein occlusion, diabetic macular edema, and diabetic retinopathy according to American Academy of Ophthalmology (https://eyewiki.aao.org/Aflibercept).

Ramucirumab

This human monoclonal antibody, cyramza, or ramucirumab, inhibits VEGF ligands, VEGF-A,C,D, from binding extracellularly. It inhibits the proliferation and migration of human endothelial cells [157]. The drug has also not been very effective in combination with capecitabine (CAP) for previously treated unresectable, locally advanced, MBC patients. The phase-I study dose level showed anti-angiogenic and anti-tumor effects with maximum tolerant dose level at 13 mg/kg. The phase III clinical trials used docetaxel in combination with ramucirumab, or placebo in breast cancer patients (clinicalTrials.gov, Identifier: NCT00703326, 2017/11 update), and the PFS of the ramucirumab (IMC-1121B) and docetaxel combination was 8.3 to 9.8 with overall survival rates of 23.6 to 29.1%, while the placebo and docetaxel PFS showed 7.1 to 8.5% range with an overall survival rate from 24.3 to 32.2%.

Sorafenib

Sorafenib (Fig. 6), an oral multi-tyrosine inhibitor acts upon BRAF (human gene encoding B-Raf protein, also referred to as proto-oncogene B-Raf and v-Raf murine sarcoma viral oncogene homolog B), C-RAF (a human enzyme encoded by RAF1 gene which is also termed as proto-oncogene c-RAF, C-Raf is a member of the Raf kinase family of serine/threonine-specific protein kinases, from the TKL group of kinases, or simply proto-oncogene serine/threonine-protein kinase, a part of the ERK1/2 [Extracellular signal Regulated Kinases] pathway as a MAP3kinase functioning downstream of the Ras subfamily of membrane associated GTPases), VEGFR, PDGFR (platelet-derived growth factor receptor), RET, c-KIT, and FMS-like tyrosine kinase-3 ligands. It's anti-cancer action is manifested through inhibiting the growth and progression of the tumor, and inhibition of the metastasis and angiogenesis [158, 159].

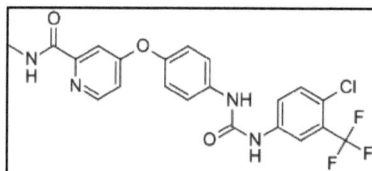

Fig. (6). Sorafenib chemical structure.

The sorafenib as a monotherapy trial for phase II, in a Mayo Clinic trial, showed insignificant anti-tumor action [160], while in Phase III randomized, double-blind study with combination of sorafenib or placebo with capecitabine in HER2-negative breast cancer also proved ineffective. Similarly, an arbitrarily II b study on paclitaxel with the combination of sorafenib (600 mg/d) versus paclitaxel with placebo performed on 537 females suffering from locally recurring or metastatic breast cancers showed remarkable enhancement in PFS and ORR. However, sorafenib, in combination with capecitabine, showed no improvement for HER2-negative advanced breast cancer patients in PFS, OS (overall survival), or ORR. However, the grade-3 toxicities were higher for sorafenib treated patients [161].

In another phase I/II study on 35 females after menopause with hormone receptor-positive MBC, the participants were unaffected to aromatase inhibitors except 23% patients whom benefitted. In SOLTI-0701 trial, the participating 229 patients suffering from locally advanced or MBC were observed. The study analyzed the worthiness and suitability of the sorafenib and capecitabine. Herein, the capecitabine was given either with placebo, or sorafenib and analysis revealed that improvement in PFS was obtained but with least or no changes in the overall survivals [162, 163]. More recent studies [164 - 168], and breast cancer trials (https://clinicaltrials.gov/ct2/show/NCT00096434) are undergoing.

Sunitinib

The Sunitinib, or Sutent (Fig. **7**) is an anti VEGF2, small molecule, oral, multi-targeted Receptor Tyrosine Kinase (RTK) inhibitor drug working through inhibitions of platelet-derived growth factor receptor (PDGFR), stem cell factor receptor (c-Kit), and FLT3 (a cytokine receptor belonging to receptor tyrosine kinase class-III, cytokine receptor involved in normal hematopoiesis) tyrosine kinase signaling pathways. During the interventional study on 23 cases pretreated with standard neoadjuvant, the sunitinib as a single agent in segment 1 for 3 weeks followed by sunitinib with paclitaxel in segment 2 for 16 weeks, further followed by segment 3 with doxorubicin and cyclophosphamide for 8 weeks, demonstrated that changes in IFP (Interstitial Fluid Pressure) in segment 1 was at 14 mmHg, in segment 2 the IFP shifted to 1.7 mmHg.

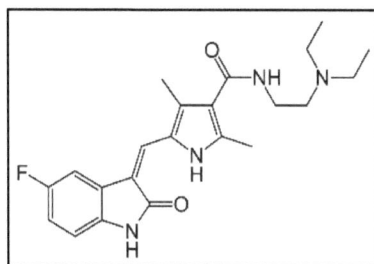

Fig. (7). Sunitinib chemical structure.

However, the Complete Response Rate (CRR) for patients treated in segment two, followed by segment three, 53.3%. In another clinical phase II trial on 13 patients, the effects of sunitinib on occult tumor cells in bone marrow with high early-stage breast cancer were observed. All cases were treated with sunitinib for six months with a dose of 37.5 mg daily, and the analysis revealed a 39% change from baseline in distributed tumor cells (DTC) in the bone marrow, but 84.61%, *i.e.*, 11 out of 13 patients were able to tolerate the drug for the selected period of trial lasting six months. Another phase II clinical trial consisting of 83 patients showing advanced levels of breast cancer pathology were put on an oral dose of 31.5 mg/day, only 1.08% patients benefitted from the drug with PFS observance at 2.4 to 3.9%, and an overall survival rate of 14 to 22.7% was observed. In another cluster of 64 patients treated with an anthracycline and a taxane class drug with sunitinib at dose level of 50 mg/day for 6-week cycle, the partial and overall positive responses included about 11% of cases whereas 5% of the subjects maintained stable conditions of the disease for approximately six more months. Also, the PFS and overall survival rates were satisfactory. As far as the adverse events were concerned, 56% of the total cases showed signs of fatigue, nausea, diarrhea, mucosal inflammation, and anorexia. In combination dosage with trastuzumab (Herceptin®) for treatment-naïve patients with HER2-positive ABC (Advanced Breast Cancer) that have not received any prior anthracycline therapy, the responses did not touch the median survivals. In overall summary, the drug showed the modest antitumor effect on patients with refractory multidrug-resistant MBC, and enhanced metastasis in tumors showing innate resistance towards therapy. The addition of sunitinib with capecitabine also did not improve the outcome for MBC patients whom were pretreated with anthracyclines and taxanes [169]. Studies on multi-drug resistant metastatic cancer [170] and sunitinib as mono and multi-drug therapy with unimpressive outcome is reported [171]. Moreover, metastasis enhancement of innately drug-resistant breast tumors is also [172].

Vandetanib

Vandetanib (Fig. **8**) a multikinase inhibitor for intracellularly involved signaling pathways contributing towards tumor growth, progression, proliferation, and angiogenesis through VEGFR-2, EGFR (epidermal growth factor receptor), and RET (REarranged during Transfection) tyrosine kinase receptors. It prevents the hormone-therapy resistant, and aromatase resistant breast cancer cells' growth. The drug has demonstrated little efficacy in patients with MBC. In phase-I trial to investigate anti-tumor activity, in cases of advanced solid tumors, the drug doses at 100-300 mg were given orally once daily [173], but its action remained limited in patients pretreated with various chemotherapeutic agents [174]. In case of phase II clinical trial on patients who have advanced breast cancers, the docetaxel (100 mg/meter square/21 days orally) with placebo, vandetanib was administered intravenously, and vandetanib with docetaxel was administered in another trial in which docetaxel was administered intravenously while vandetanib was given one oral dose daily, the numbers of patients with diseased progression events were 24 out of 35, and 18 out of 25 in case of vandetanib with docetaxel, and placebo with docetaxel, respectively. Vandetanib addition with docetaxel did not affect the risk of disease progression as compared with the placebo, and docetaxel, while both being monotherapy agents. However, adverse effects were recorded, which included 15 out of 35, and 11 out of 29 patients treated with vandetanib with docetaxel, and placebo with docetaxel administered cases. The blood and lymphatic, cardiac and gastrointestinal disorders, hypertension, ear and labyrinth, eye and skin conditions related adverse effects were observed [ClinicalTrials.gov Identifier: NCT00494481].

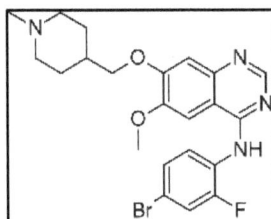

Fig. (8). Vandetanib chemical structure.

Fulvestrant is a selective estrogen receptor (ER) down-regulator, also used alone as part of hormone therapy to treat post-menopausal patients with hormone-receptor- positive advanced breast cancers as second-line of treatment, after progression of the tumor as shown by patients after aromatase inhibitors, *e.g.*, tamoxifen, has been proposed to be used in combination with vandetanib, and also with palbociclib (a Cyclin-D-dependent Kinase, CDK), for hormone therapy-resistant cases in pre/peri/post-menopausal patients showing breast cancer progression despite endocrine therapy. The results are awaited, nonetheless, the drug; Vandetanib was approved by US-FDA for advanced and metastatic medullary thyroid cancers patients [175-78; http://isrctn.com/ISRCTN13663157; https://clinicaltrials.gov/ct2/show/NCT01934335; https://accessdata.fda.gov/drugsatfda_docs/label/2014/022405s007lbl.pdf].

Axitinib

Axitinib, (Fig. 9), the small molecule tyrosine kinase inhibitor (TKI), developed by Pfizer, has shown significant growth inhibition in experimental breast cancer (xenograft) with partial responses in clinical trials conducted for renal cell carcinoma (RCC) along with different tumors. The phase I and II clinical trials on randomized 174 patients, whom have metastatic breast cancer without chemotherapy, were studied by administering axitinib with docetaxel. The patients were daily administered 5 mg axitinib, through the oral route-twice daily, starting from the third day of the first cycle, in total cycles of 3 weeks. A dose of 80 mg/m^2 was administered intravenously hourly on the first day of each cycle, in cycles of 3 weeks, wherein, only one patient showed positive clinical progression.

The axitinib with docetaxel in phase II was not encouraging, and the response was at 31.9% to 50.8% while the docetaxel and placebo combination in phase II double-blind clinical trial, the time taken for tumor progression was 215 days, and the objective response rate was at 13.2% to 37.0%. In the case of axitinib phase II, open-label trials, the response rate was at 6.3% (ClinicalTrials.gov Identifier: NCT00076024).

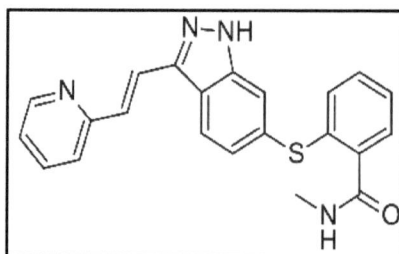

Fig. (9). Axitinib chemical structure.

Pazopanib

The tyrosine kinases vascular endothelial growth factors I, II, III, platelet-derived growth factors receptor- a and b, and c-kit tyrosine kinases, are inhibited by the small molecule drug candidate pazopanib (Fig. **10**) [179]. The drug is effective for hormone receptor-positive (HR+), HER2-negative (HER2-), FGFR1 amplified with resistant to endocrine therapy breast cancers. The therapeutic target is fibroblast growth factor receptor 1 (FGFR1). It also showed *in vitro* growth inhibition in Ras-Raf-ERK1/2 pathway on breast carcinoma and melanoma cell lines. The maximum tolerated dose observed at 800 mg/day was defined through phase II clinical trials [180] with adverse effects showing the symptoms of hypertension, nausea, vomiting, diarrhea, and fatigue with decoloration of hairs. The random phase II study on group of 76 participants with ErbB-2 (gene encoding EGFR member, HER2, tyrosine kinase receptor family) positive MBC administered pazopanib with lapatinib, and lapatinib as a stand-alone drug as the first line of therapeutic intervention. The results showed a decrease in the progression of tumor after 12 weeks which is an increased response rate in case of pazopanib and lapatinib as compared to the lapatinib standalone (36.2 and 22.2%, respectively) therapy [181]. The clinical studies on pazopanib with vinorelbine for metastatic breast cancer remained terminated. However, the pazopanib trials, in combination with capecitabine for metastatic breast cancer, exhibited around 25% clinical benefits (ClinicalTrials.gov Identifier: NCT014 98458).

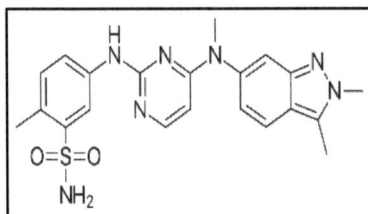

Fig. (10). Pazopanib chemical structure.

In another study on pazopanib for recurring MBC, the tumor was static for 5.3 months (1/21). The PFS and overall survival rates were at 22% in a year (ClinicalTrials.gov Identifier: NCT00509587). Moreover, other studies evaluating pazopanib with lapatinib for inflammatory breast cancers (ClinicalTrials.gov Identifier: NCT00558103), or pazopanib as a stand-alone drug for patients with MBC with pre-treated chemotherapeutic agents [ClinicalTrials.gov Identifier: NCT00509587] did not show significant results. Nonetheless, trials undergoing with pazopanib in combination with exemestane in postmenopausal breast cancer cases were also annulled probably due to high toxicity manifestations [ClinicalTrials.gov Identifier: NCT00615524]. However, in advanced breast cancer stages, pazopanib provided disease stability.

Following is the list of undertrial drugs and drug leads for different forms of breast cancers (Table **5**). The commercial products listed in the Table **5** have registered propriety names.

Drugs Approved to Treat Breast Cancers

The commercial name list includes the following chemical and biochemical drugs which acts as anti-angiogenic, hormonal, and recombinant-based therapeutic agents for first, second, and a further third line of treatment for naïve, metastatic and, refractory tumors. The drugs are used as monotherapy and also as part of combination therapies. However, drug combinations sometimes are not separately approved by USFDA but are widely used. The approved combinations are indicated in the listing below. These commercial drug names are registered (®) and protected. Following is the list of the anti-angiogenic and other drugs:

- Abemaciclib, Abraxane, Ado-Trastuzumab Emtansine, Afinitor (Everolimus), Anastrozole, Aredia (Pamidronate Disodium), Arimidex (Anastrozole), Aromasin (Exemestane), Atezolizumab, Trastuzumab
- Capecitabine, Cyclophosphamide (also in combination with Doxorubicin and Fluorouracil; also with Methotrexate and Fluorouracil)
- Docetaxel (also in combination with Doxorubicin and Cyclophosphamide),

Doxorubicin.HCl (also in combination with Cyclophosphamide; and also with Cyclophosphamide and Paclitaxel)

- Ellence (Epirubicin.HCl), Epirubicin.HCl, Eribulin Mesylate, Everolimus, Exemestane
- Fluorouracil (5-FU) (also in combination with Epirubicin Hydrochloride and Cyclophosphamide), Fareston (Toremifene), Faslodex (Fulvestrant), Femara (Letrozole), Fulvestrant
- Gemcitabine.HCl, Gemzar (Gemcitabine. HCl), Goserelin Acetate
- Halaven (Eribulin Mesylate), Herceptin Hylecta (Trastuzumab and Hyaluronidase-oysk), Herceptin (Trastuzumab)
- Ibrance (Palbociclib), Ixabepilone, Ixempra (Ixabepilone),
- Kadcyla (Ado-Trastuzumab Emtansine), Kisqali (Ribociclib)
- Lapatinib Ditosylate, Letrozole, Lynparza (Olaparib)
- Megestrol Acetate, Methotrexate
- Neratinib Maleate, Nerlynx (Neratinib Maleate)
  Olaparib
- Paclitaxel, Pamidronate Disodium, Palbociclib
- Perjeta (Pertuzumab), Pertuzumab
- Ribociclib
- Talazoparib Tosylate, Talzenna (Talazoparib Tosylate), Tamoxifen Citrate, Taxol (Paclitaxel)
- Taxotere (Docetaxel), Tecentriq (Atezolizumab), Thiotepa, Toremifene, Trastuzumab, Trastuzumab and Hyaluronidase-oysk, Trexall (Methotrexate), Tykerb (Lapatinib Ditosylate)
- Verzenio (Abemaciclib), Vinblastine Sulfate
- Xeloda (Capecitabine)
- Zoladex (Goserelin Acetate)

Some of the recently approved anti-angiogenic drugs are listed in Table **6**. More detailed information on generic and brand names, dose, drug strength, and drug form/route is available at https://www.empr.com/home/clinical-charts/fda-approved-breast-cancer-treatments/, which is very recent. The products listed in Table **6** have registered propriety names.

Table 5. The undertrial chemical/biochemical agents.

Drug	Trial	Condition	Treatment	Trail Number	Sponsor
Bevacizumab	Phase 2	Breast Cancer	Trastuzumab; Bevacizumab; Docetaxel	NCT00428922	B Ramaswamy
	Phase 2	Metastatic Breast Cancer	Low-dose Bevacizumab; Pemetrexed	NCT02829008	Chinese Academy of Medical Sciences
	Phase 2	Breast Cancer	Bevacizumab; Paclitaxel	NCT01722968	T Foukakis
	Phase 2	Breast Cancer	Bevacizumab; Docetaxel; Cyclophosphamide; Epirubicin.HCl; Fluorouracil	NCT00820547	Unicancer
	Phase 2	Breast Cancer	Everolimus; Liposomal Doxorubicin; Bevacizumab	NCT02456857	MD Anderson Cancer Center
	Early Phase 1	Metastatic Breast Cancer	Durvalumab; Bevacizumab	NCT02802098	Centro Nacional de Investig. Oncologicas, CARLOS III
	Phase 1 Phase 2	Breast Cancer	Carboplatin; Bevacizumab; Paclitaxel	NCT00691379	Hellenic Oncology Research Group
Cilengitide	Phase 1	Recurrent Breast Carcinoma	Cilengitide; Paclitaxel	NCT01276496	National Cancer Institute (NCI)
Aflibercept	Phase 1	Metastatic Breast Cancers	Capecitabine; Aflibercept; Capecitabine	NCT01843725	Jules B. Institute
Ramucirumab	Phase 3	Breast Cancer	Ramucirumab; Docetaxel	NCT00703326	Eli Lilly
Sorafenib	Phase ½	Metastatic Breast Cancer	Sorafenib; Letrozole	NCT00634634	State University of New Jersey, Rutgers
	Phase 2	Breast Cancer, Metastatic, Recurrent	Pemetrexed; Sorafenib	NCT02624700	Virginia Commonwealth University
	Phase 2	Breast Cancer	Paclitaxel; Sorafenib Tosylate	NCT00499525	Northwestern University
	Phase 1	Breast Cancer	Radiation; Sorafenib	NCT01724606	Memorial Sloan Kettering Cancer Institute
Sunitinib	Phase 1	Breast Cancer	Crizotinib + Sunitinib	NCT02074878	M Rimawi
	Phase 2	Breast Cancer	Doxorubicin/ Cyclophosphamide or/ plus + Sunitinib	NCT02790580	National University Hospital, Singapore
	Phase 2	Breast Cancer	Docetaxel; Sunitinib	NCT01803503	NU Hospital, Singapore

(Table 5) cont.....

Drug	Trial	Condition	Treatment	Trail Number	Sponsor
Vandetanib	Phase 2	Invasive Breast Cancer	Vandetanib	NCT01934335	R Weigel
	Phase 2	Neoplasms	Fulvestrant; Vandetanib	NCT02530411	Velindre NHS
	Phase 2	Metastatic Breast Cancer	Vandetanib; Selumetinib; plus others	NCT02299999	Unicancer
Pazopanib	Phase 2	Breast Cancer	Pazopanib; Lapatinib, P 86034	NCT00347919	GlaxoSmithKline
	Phase 1	Breast Cancer	Pazopanib; Paclitaxel; Carboplatin	NCT01407562	Rutgers, TSU, New Jersey
	Phase I	Malignant Breast Neoplasm	Alisertib; Pazopanib	NCT01639911	University Illinois at Chicago

Table 6. List of anti-angiogenesis drugs recently approved by US-FDA.

Serial	Drug	Condition/ Treatment	Approval Date	Pharma Company
1.	Alpelisib (PIQRAY) in combination with Fulvestrant	Postmenopausal women, and men with $HR^{(+)}$, $HER2^{(-)}$, PIK3CA-mutated, advanced/metastatic breast cancer	May 24, 2019	Novartis
2.	Ado-Trastuzumab emtansine (KADCYLA)	Adjuvant treatment for patients with $HER2^{(+)}$ early breast cancer with the residual invasive disease after neoadjuvant taxane and trastuzumab-based treatment.	May 3, 2019	Genentech
3.	Atezolizumab	PD-L1(+), unresectable, locally advanced/ metastatic, triple-negative breast cancer	March 8, 2019	Genentech
4.	Trastuzumab and Hyaluronidase-oysk (Herceptin Hylecta, injection)	HER2 overexpressing breast cancer	Feb. 28, 2019	Genentech
5.	Olaparib	$HER-2^{(-)}$, (human epidermal growth factor receptor), metastatic breast cancer	January 12, 2018	AstraZeneca
6.	Pertuzumab	$HER-2^{(+)}$, early breast cancer	Dec. 20, 2017	Genentech
7.	Ogivri (Biosimilar to Herceptin)	HER-2-overexpressing breast	Dec.1, 2017	Mylan
8.	Abemaciclib (Combination with Fulvestrant	$HR^{(+)}$, $HER-2^{(-)}$, advanced/ metastatic breast cancer	Sep. 28, 2017	Eli Lilly
9.	Neratinib	Early stage HER---overexpressed/amplified breast cancer	July 17, 2017	Puma Biotech

(Table 6) cont.....

Serial	Drug	Condition/ Treatment	Approval Date	Pharma Company
10.	Palbociclib	HR$^{(+)}$, HER-2$^{(-)}$, advanced/ metastatic breast cancer	March 31, 2017	Pfizer
11.	Ribociclib	HR$^{(+)}$, HER-2$^{(-)}$, advanced/ metastatic breast cancer in post-menopausal women	March 13, 2017	Novartis

*Sourced from https://www.fda.gov/Drugs/InformationOnDrugs/ApprovedDrugs/ucm279174.htm

However, a vast majority of anti-breast cancer drugs failed to improve overall survival rates in the early stages of metastatic breast cancers. The case of bevacizumab, approved in 2008 for treating metastatic breast cancers and the HER-2 negative breast cancers, wherein various clinical trials showed improved survival, although it was not as expected and contrary to expectations and claims, the approval was withdrawn by FDA in 2011. Furthermore, in this context, the corrective measures, such as predictive biomarkers, play an essential role in cancer diagnosis, and these factors are helping to improve the clinical efficacy of the API (active pharmaceutical ingredient) of interest. In one of the trials, the VEGF at a high concentration level generated encouraging treatment effects with bevacizumab while in numerous other trials, without the VEGF presence, no substantial outcome was observed. Moreover, some of the promising results from certain biomarkers, *i.e.*, tumor-neuropilin-1, and carbonic anhydrase IX, need to be further substantiated in this regard [182].

RELATIONSHIP BETWEEN INFLAMMATION, ANGIOGENESIS, AND COAGULATION IN PROSTATE CANCERS

The prostate cancer is one of highest frequency cancers [183], and can be noticed at 30-40 years of age by the gland exhibiting locus heterogeneity, or diagnosed late at age 60-70. Studies revealed that men having a family member with the first degree of prostate cancer are on high risk [184]. The rise of the disease takes place after prolonged exposure of the epithelium to genome-oxidative destructive actions followed by numerous involved sites inflammations [185]. The endothelial cells respond quickly to vasoactive agents, thrombin, or TNF-α. This response is enough for signaling the receptor-mediated cells. The influx of calcium ions and phosphorylation initiation results in activating enzymes for platelet ligature, leukocyte survival, and inflammation inflection. Thus, continuous exposure may develop the disease (precancerous wounds in epithelium) rather than healing. Recent work has shown that the cellular aging of epithelial cells of prostate gland help cytokines to express [186]. It further initiates connective tissues to release FGFs to provide the environment for cancer cells to grow and progress. Variation in degree in cell aging may create a difference in the occurrence of disease. However, oxidative DNA damage is the main ingredient of endothelium cell aging of the prostate. The dietary habits and lifestyle of the patient play an essential protective role in controlling the high incidence of prostate cancers [187]. This fact is supported by many pieces of evidence that indicate that diet is the determining factor of diminishing prostate cancer and the probability of survival [188]. The plant-based foods are considered as cancer-protective while animal-based meat products have been implicated, primarily, for the cancers which are although inconclusive and may differ case by case [189 - 192]. The anti-oxidants, selenium, vitamin E, and carotenoids help in reducing the effects of oxidative DNA damage. Several clinical trials are running on Selenium, Vitamin E (Selenium and Vitamin E Chemoprevention Trial; SELECT) in addition to the clinical studies on carotenoids and tomato products. In parallel to such prophylactic agents, new classes of drugs are required to control inflammation of prostate endothelial cells. Resveratrol, a polyphenol found in grapes, has anti-angiogenesis and anti-inflammatory activities. It stops cancer metastasis and helps in preventing DNA damage from oxidation. When it works with quercetin with anti-hormonal agent indole-3-carbinol (I3C), it is suggested to be the best combination approach for preventing cancer [193]. Upon withdrawal of rofecoxib for being deleterious in cardiac diseases, several non-steroidal anti-inflammatory drugs have been tested as possible alternative for prostate cancer.

ANGIOGENESIS, THROMBOSIS AND INFLAMMATION MEDIATORS' CROSSTALK

6.1. Angiogenesis and Inflammation Mediators' Crosstalk

At another side, with evidence, there exists crosstalk between angiogenesis, inflammation, and thrombosis, which ultimately connecting those to invasive diseases (Fig. **11**). It is of the utmost importance to state on targets considered during the past decades to illuminate how the targets of anti-angiogenic treatment might change as a purpose of tumor progression.

The angiogenic factors, VEGF, FGF-2, TGF-b, and COX-2 (cyclooxygenase-2) along with metalloproteinases are involved in prostate cancer while the most common factor is VEGF-A[164.] The isoform VEGF-A[164-165] forms large tumor masses when overexpressed by blood vessels, and various growth factors and cytokines help tumor epithelial cells and stromal cells to communicate during metastasis [194] which stimulates VEFG production with help from several other factors. Numerous other stimuli govern the VEGF expression wherein the hypoxia, along with nitric oxide (NO), up-regulates the VEGF gene by enhancing HIF-1 [195]. Positive feedback existing in these factors governed by the NO also affects permeability and blood vessel vasodilation. Another cross-interaction takes place under the regulation of both inducible Nitric Oxide Synthase (iNOS) and COX-2 under stress conditions, resulting in the stimulation of angiogenesis and perhaps cancer development [196].

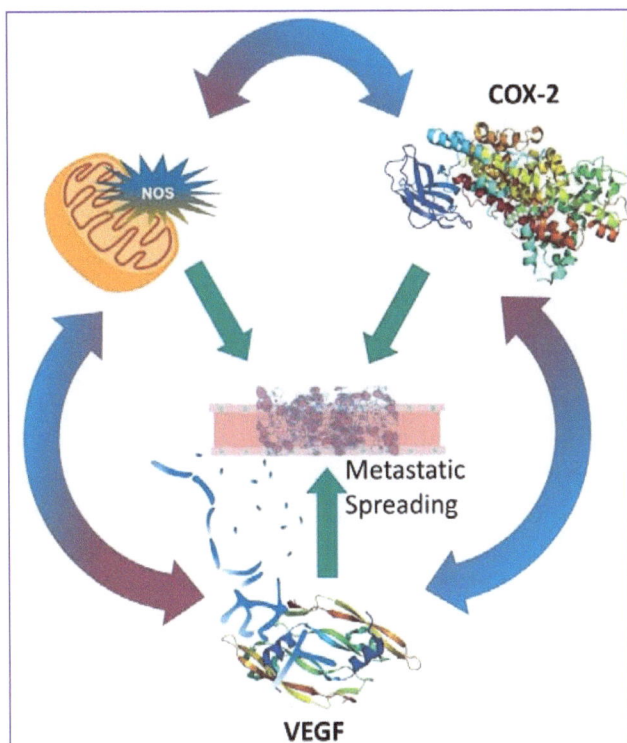

Fig. (11). Angiogenesis-inflammation crosstalk.

The COX-2 and LOX (lysyl oxidase) 5/12-LOX and 15-LOX-1 are involved in the biogenesis of eicosanoids and up-regulate the initiation as well as the progression of the prostate cancers. The 15-LOX-2 is involved in the tumor metastasis [197] whereby at first, the selective COX-2 inhibitor, *i.e.*, NS-398, controls the growth of PC-3 (prostate tumor-initiating cells, FAM65B high/MFI 2low/LEF 1, low angiogenesis increase) tumors by controlling the angiogenesis [198]. Second, the overexpression of 12-LOX in PC-3 cells helps in tumor cells adhesion as well as endothelial cells migration along with cancerous mass metastasis [198, 199] while also promoting the VEGF expressions [200]. Finally, the expression of 15-LOX-1 in PC-3 cells is stimulatory for tumor angiogenesis and growth [201]. The dual COX/LOX inhibitors have been designed to optimize therapeutic response [202]. However, further work was curtailed due to stimulating adverse cardiac effects of rofecoxib, but the findings of inflammation resolvers, an innovative mediating agent, autacoids, *i.e.*, lipoxins, and resolvins are still under considerations [203]. The results corroborated the over-expression of VEGF which is organ/site specific for prostrate cancer, and it is suspected that it could be a major player in organ tropism for metastatic spread of the cancer [204]. Unfortunately, every tumor keeps the equilibrium between proangiogenic and antiangiogenic factors. These factors are vibrant over time; hence, when drug and one of the factors interact, they may not provide steady momentum in the same direction as in any other tumor, or tumor condition. Thus, for all the cases, a general model cannot work, as each case is unique. The anti-angiogenic alone would not cause significant antitumor effects. Instead, it may facilitate the delivery of a chemotherapeutic agent and re-oxygenate the interstitium, which also increases the chemo-sensitivity [205]. Hence, angiogenesis is the only phenomenon common to all kind of tumors.

Angiogenic Capability of Tumors and Thromboembolic Crosstalk

The hemostatic proteins play essential roles in tumor neo-angiogenesis along with other hemostasis related functions. The tissue factor (TF) induces angiogenesis through clotting-dependent biomechanism in downstream processing of generation of thrombin and fibrin, followed by thrombin-induced platelets activation. The fibrin upregulates the TF and ECs (endothelial cells) with the secretion of a pro-angiogenic factor, IL-8, which leads to clotting and tumor growth [206] wherein angiogenesis related genes upregulation and VEGF, vascular endothelial growth factor receptors (VEGFR), TF, bFGF, and metalloproteinase-2 contribute significantly. The thrombin is known to contribute in a major way towards more malignant phenotype through induction of platelet/tumor aggregation, tumor adhesion to ECs, ECM, tumor cell proliferation and the metastases. The activity of thrombin in triggering release of growth factors [207], chemokines and extracellular proteins [208] which promote the proliferation and migration of tumor cells is another important factor in angiogenesis. The formation of fibrin, new tumor vessels with inputs from inflammatory and tumor cells facilitate in the progression of tumor. The cancer-related thrombosis is a unique phenomenon of the imbalances of coagulation and fibrinolysis along with the formation and deactivation of fibrins. The organ-specific endothelial ECs (endothelial cells) are also involved in regulating thrombosis, hemostasis, and angiogenesis. The adhesion molecules belonging to the integrin family mediate interactions in the ECs and its environment.

The hemostatic proteins, pro-coagulant, anti-fibrinolytic activities, along with the presence of inflammatory cytokines, activation of vascular cells, adhesion of tumor cells to healthy cells, including platelets, endothelial cells (ECs) and monocytes are the main characteristics steps in tumor growth [209]. Interestingly, on a more subtle progenesis, the tumor growth is influenced by neo-angiogenesis while the dissemination is put up by the coagulation, activation, and feedback of the coagulation cascade which enhances the thrombogenesis [210]. Some patients with malignancy represent an acquired thrombophilic condition with a high risk of venous thromboembolism (VTE) which is a fervent complication in patients with cancers encountered in about 5-10% of all cancer patients [211, 212]. The cancer-inflicted patients with thrombotic conditions have been found to have lower survival rates as compared to cancers without thrombosis and attributed to more aggressive tumor behavior as compared to the thrombotic condition [213]. Alarmingly, patients with VTE and cancerous conditions showed unusual complications from anticoagulants with ever increasing risks of recurrent VTE [214], which is a common cause of morbidity and mortality [215 - 217].

Several of the clinical situations resulting in the highest risk of VTE, such as those associated with major orthopedic or other surgeries or hospitalization for acute medical illnesses, have been transitory; and in consequence, the guidelines recommend for short-term VTE prophylaxis, has most often been achieved with parenteral anticoagulant [218]. These drugs may also be prescribed to keep blood clots from forming in AF (Atrial Fibrillation). These agents include heparin and low molecular weight heparins (LMWH), which carry a low but severe risk of thrombocytopenia [219]. By their very nature, the parenteral agents are not likely to be appropriately used by patients after hospital discharge compared with a simple *per os* (delivery through the mouth) regimens. Thus, an unmet medical need for safe and effective agents for administration *per os* exists. These observations justified the new concept of isolating, characterizing, and inhibiting the protease factor X in the activated state as a step forward in anti-angiogenesis treatments. In the middle of the blood coagulation process, the factor X associates as a complex to the already formed, Factor VIIa, a tissue factor complex to form the protease-activated factor X (FXa), which acts at the convergence zone of the coagulation pathways. Not all patients undergoing orthopedic surgery receive appropriate thrombo-prophylaxis because there are concerns about the bleeding risks [220]. In 2001, Fondaparinux was approved as a parenteral indirect FXa tissue factor inhibitor for short-term VTE prophylaxis because it inhibited FXa by interacting with antithrombin. Further research work on oral FXa inhibitors yielded the discovery and advancement of *per-os*, direct-acting FXa inhibitors that progressed to clinical trials.

The FXa L-shaped binding site has been reported to have the S1 and S4 pockets at the edge positions in the protease [221]. The S1 described being a deep, mostly hydrophobic pocket, bearing Asp189 and Tyr228 residues. The S4 was described to be a highly hydrophobic pocket bearing the aryl-binding Tyr99, Phe174, and

Trp215 amino acids [222]. Other features include His57, Asp102, and Ser195, which were found to play a catalytic role and the β-strand region that covers Trp215 (S4 region) (Figs. **12-14**). To discover new direct FXa inhibitors, based on small molecule structures, an initial strategy was to design compounds with functional groups that could interact strongly and invariably with the edging pockets (S1, S4) of the catalytic site, and thus stabilize the ligand-protease interactions, thereby preventing the enzyme from any catalytic action.

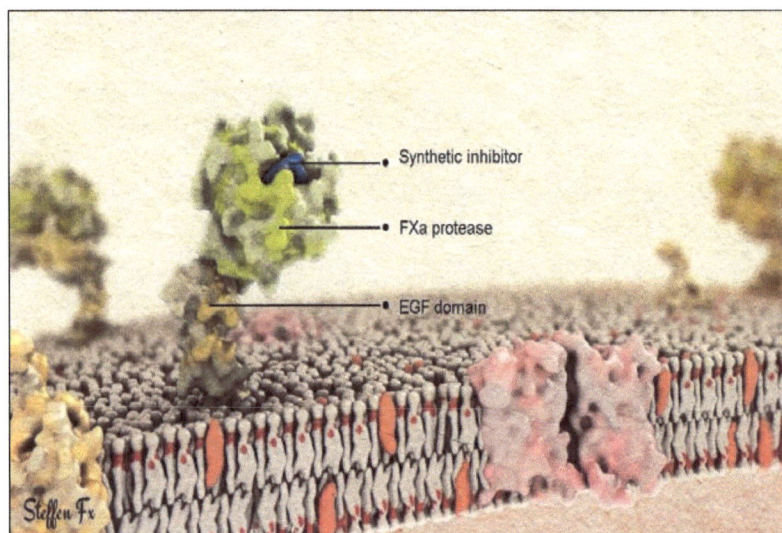

Fig. (12). The Factor Xa model in complexation with a synthetic inhibitor attached to the lipid bilayers of cells; *Reprinted with permission from Steffen VFX, and from Pinto DJP, Smallheer JM, Cheney DL, Knabb RM, Wexler RR. Factor Xa Inhibitors: Next-Generation Antithrombotic Agents. J Med Chem 2010;53: 6243-74. Copyright© 2014 American Chemical Society.*

CLINICAL TRIALS FOR ANTI-ANGIOGENIC PROSTATE CANCER DRUG DEVELOPMENT

Anti-angiogenic therapy as a potent minimal tumor burden model was shown through selective tumor growth inhibition by VEGFR antagonists prior to the production of high VEGF levels by prostate cancer in a murine model [223]. However, the anti-angiogenic drug development faced with the inverse relationship between prostate-specific antigen response and the clinical outcomes. However, cabazitaxel- a cytotoxic agent, abiraterone acetate – the androgen biosynthesis inhibitor, enzalutamide – the anti-androgen, and alpha-particle emitting ^{223}Ra (Radium-223) have shown treatment promise in randomized phase III clinical trials. Some of the VEGF inhibitors, *e.g.*, sunitinib, bevacizumab, and aflibercept as combination therapy with docetaxel, a standard first-line anti-cancer agent, for mCRPC (metastatic castration-resistant prostate cancer) were used. In clinical trials phase II, both the drugs, sunitinib, and bevacizumab did not show any significant activity in monotherapy, and docetaxel combination. The aflibercept and bevacizumab in combination with docetaxel and prednisone showed better results in extending survival in comparison with the docetaxel and prednisone, respectively, alone, in specifically-designed phase III clinical trials, CALGB 90401 and VENICE, although bevacizumab showed extended PFS with higher ORR rate [224 - 226].

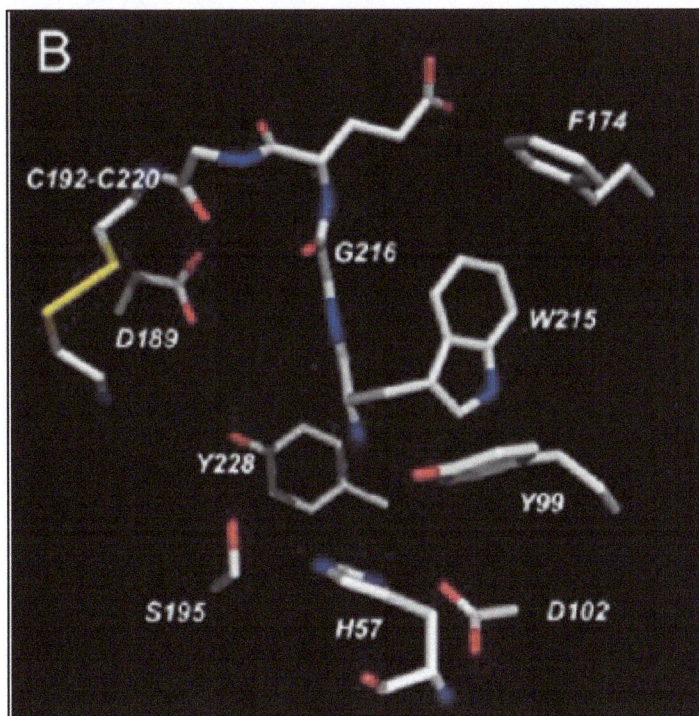

Fig. (13). A zoomed view of the amino acids surrounding the active site without inhibitor; *Reprinted with permission from Steffen VFX, and from Pinto DJP, Smallheer JM, Cheney DL, Knabb RM, Wexler RR. Factor Xa Inhibitors: Next-Generation Antithrombotic Agents. J Med Chem 2010;53: 6243-74. Copyright© 2014 American Chemical Society.*

Studies on both types, castration sensitive (CSPC) and castration-resistant prostate cancers (CRPC) drug are available. In an open-label, randomized, phase II clinical trial, vandetanib 300 mg/oral (P.O)/ Once daily (O.D) with bicalutamide 50 mg/ P.O/O.D, or bicalutamide 50 mg/ P.O/O.D with cross-over trial protocol to vandetanib monotherapy at tumor progression, as required at this condition, was conducted wherein the PSA response was at under 50% decline from the baseline chosen for the conclusion. For 39 patients, the PSA response was nearly equal (18 and 19% respectively) with PSA (Prostate Specific Antigen) progression times at 3.16 months for both with 95% confidence intervals wherein treatment was discontinued owing to adverse reactions. The vandetanib along with bicalutamide were linked with substantial toxicity but without any higher efficacy over the bicalutamide alone treatment [227]. The abiraterone acetate in CRPC has been recommended at 500 mg/ once daily, or in combination with methylprednisolone at 4 mg/ twice daily with GnRH (Gonadotropin-releasing hormone) analog or with bilateral orchiectomy. The abiraterone acetate at 5 mg/once daily for CSPC with GnRH analog or with bilateral orchiectomy is recommended. The trials of vandetanib in combination with prednisolone and docetaxel (NCT00498797), vandetanib with bicalutamide (NCT00757692 and NCT00659438), have been reported (https://clinicaltrials.gov/ct2/show/NCT00498797;/NCT00659438).

USE OF ANTIANGIOGENIC AGENTS IN PROSTATE CANCER

Studies have shown promising results involving VEGF inhibition in tumor models with higher concentrations of soluble growth factors [228]. Microvessel density [229, 230], prostate biopsies, Gleason scores, and prostate-specific antigen (PSA) levels [231, 232] are indicative of the prostate cancer. Various therapeutic agents that are employed in the remedy of prostate cancer are outlined below.

Thalidomide

Thalidomide, alpha-N-phthalimido-glutarimide, is a potent therapeutic agent with questionable anti-angiogenic properties. Nonetheless, its immunomodulatory properties and downregulation of integrins seemingly resulted in inhibition of endothelial cells migration and adhesion [233]. The agent has been used as a monotherapy, or as part of combination with chemotherapy in the CRPC. A phase II randomized trial reduced the PSA levels by 40% in 27% patients at 1200 mg/day dose while low-dose at 200 mg/day resulted in weak response, and four patients exhibited sustained response of 150 days and PSA reduction of 50% [234]. A chemotherapeutic enhancement with docetaxel in combination showed over 50% more reduction in PSA levels as compared with a prior study involving only docetaxel with better survival [235 - 237]. A thalidomide analog, lenalidomide, was also tested in phase I and II. The phase I showed manageable toxicity with stable disease and nearly 50% PSA reduction in untreated and pre-treated patients at 47% and 50% patients population. The phase II trial constituting lenalidomide, docetaxel, prednisolone, and bevacizumab as combination therapy for chemotherapy-naive patients with metastatic CRPC at the National Cancer Institute showed encouraging results [238, 239].

Bevacizumab

Bevacizumab, a humanized IgG1 mAb, targets the human VEGF-A. The bevacizumab monotherapy did not show significant bioactivity in prostate cancer. However, in another study evaluating bevacizumab in prostate cancer with standard docetaxel (75 mg/m^2) and prednisone (5 mg) every 21 and twice daily, respectively, compared to docetaxel, and prednisone at earlier doses with bevacizumab at 15 mg/kg/21 days, was found to detect increased overall survival of more than 25% in the bevacizumab arm for chemotherapy-naive metastatic CRPC men in CALGB 90401 trial. Bevacizumab with the sipuleucel-T vaccine has shown promising activity with increased overall survival rate in comparison to placebo in phase III trial for patients with metastatic CRPC [240 - 244].

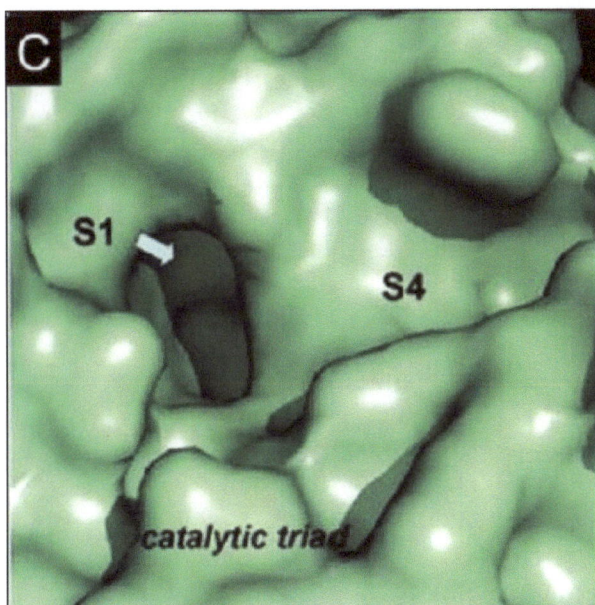

Fig. (14). The space-filling model showing the S1 site, the S4 site, and the catalytic triad; *Reprinted with permission from Steffen VFX, and from Pinto DJP, Smallheer JM, Cheney DL, Knabb RM, Wexler RR. Factor Xa Inhibitors: Next-Generation Antithrombotic Agents. J Med Chem 2010;53: 6243-74. Copyright© 2014 American Chemical Society.*

VEGF Trap

The VEGF Trap (Aflibercept), a human fusion protein, binds VEGF isoforms VEGF-A, VEGF-B, and (PlGF) [245]. The phase III trial in metastatic CRPC patients is designed with standard docetaxel, or prednisone or docetaxel and prednisone [246].

Tyrosine Kinase Inhibitors (TKI)

Several TKIs, including sorafenib and sunitinib, used in treating hormone therapy-resistant prostate cancers are owing to their multi-tyrosine kinase and VEGF inhibitions. These products also inhibit p38, c-kit, VEGFR-2, and PDGFR pathways and affect the tumor growth along with promoting the apoptosis through downstream events of c-Raf [159, 247, 248]. However, the sorafenib has only shown modest anti-prostate cancer activity with nearly insignificant PSA reductions [249 - 254] while sunitinib has shown some anti-prostate cancer activity but with few PSA reductions. Another drug candidate, cediranib with 30 mg dose-limiting toxicity and a finalized dose of 20 mg/day [255] showed better activity in docetaxel-resistant metastatic CRPC wherein 13 of 23 patients showed a decrease in soft tissue lesions, and 4 of them met partial response criteria [256].

USFDA APPROVED DRUGS FOR PROSTATE CANCER

Following is the alphabetically-listed, USFDA approved drugs and therapeutic agents for treating prostate cancers of either castration resistant/refractory or castration-sensitive, and both types. The commercial drug names are registered (®), and protected. The list includes generic and brand names as followings:

- Abiraterone Acetate, Apalutamide
- Bicalutamide
- Cabazitaxel, Casodex (Bicalutamide)
- Degarelix, Docetaxel
- Eligard (Leuprolide Acetate), Enzalutamide, Estradiol
- Firmagon (Degarelix), Flutamide
- Goserelin Acetate
- Jevtana (Cabazitaxel)
- Lupron (Leuprolide Acetate)
- Mitoxantrone.HCl
- Nilandron (Nilutamide), Nilutamide
- Provenge (Sipuleucel-T)
- Sipuleucel-T
- Taxotere (Docetaxel), Triptorelin
- Xofigo (^{223}Ra-Cl$_2$, Radium-223 Dichloride), Xtandi (Enzalutamide)
- Zoladex (Goserelin Acetate), Zytiga (Abiraterone Acetate)

A list of prostate cancer drugs including the anti-angiogenic, anti-androgenic are also available at https://www.empr.com/home/clinical-charts/fda-approv-d-prostate-cancer-treatments/ with details on drugs' generic and brand names, dose, strength, and mode of delivery.

CONCLUSIONS

The anti-angiogenesis based therapy for curing cancers is in clinical trial stages with low benefits to patients. However, in the case of breast cancer when anti-angiogenesis treatment combined with chemotherapeutic regimes, the progression-free survival has been achieved, though without any improvements in overall survival rates of the undertrial patients. Some of the developing drugs in different phases of clinical trials also affected the healthy and non-cancerous tissues which induced vascular changes in several other organs and tissues in the vicinity of existing cancers which led to generate adverse effects, including hypertension, hypothyroidism, gastrointestinal perforation, and cardiovascular problems [257 - 259]. Therefore, designing new generation of targeted angiogenic drugs is pertinent in light of the cancer etiology, and the work is continuously in progress.

CONSENT FOR PUBLICATION

Not applicable.

CONFLICT OF INTEREST

The author confirms that this chapter contents have no conflict of interest.

ACKNOWLEDGEMENTS

Authors thank their respective institutions for infrastructure support.

REFERENCES

[1]   Boyce BF, Yoneda T, Guise TA. Factors regulating the growth of metastatic cancer in bone. Endocr Relat Cancer 1999; 6(3): 333-47.
[http://dx.doi.org/10.1677/erc.0.0060333] [PMID: 10516850]

[2]   Burri PH, Hlushchuk R, Djonov V. Intussusceptive angiogenesis: its emergence, its characteristics, and its significance. Dev Dyn 2004; 231(3): 474-88.
[http://dx.doi.org/10.1002/dvdy.20184] [PMID: 15376313]

[3]   Nishida N, Yano H, Nishida T, Kamura T, Kojiro M. Angiogenesis in cancer. Vasc Health Risk Manag 2006; 2(3): 213-9.
[http://dx.doi.org/10.2147/vhrm.2006.2.3.213] [PMID: 17326328]

[4]   do Amaral RJFC, Cavanagh B, O'Brien FJ, Kearney CJ. Platelet-derived growth factor stabilises vascularisation in collagen-glycosaminoglycan scaffolds *in vitro*. J Tissue Eng Regen Med 2019; 13(2): 261-73.
[http://dx.doi.org/10.1002/term.2789] [PMID: 30554484]

[5]   Allard WJ, Matera J, Miller MC, *et al.* Tumor cells circulate in the peripheral blood of all major carcinomas but not in healthy subjects or patients with nonmalignant diseases. Clin Cancer Res 2004;

10(20): 6897-904.
[http://dx.doi.org/10.1158/1078-0432.CCR-04-0378] [PMID: 15501967]

[6] Senger DR, Galli SJ, Dvorak AM, Perruzzi CA, Harvey VS, Dvorak HF. Tumor cells secrete a vascular permeability factor that promotes accumulation of ascites fluid. Science 1983; 219(4587): 983-5.
[http://dx.doi.org/10.1126/science.6823562] [PMID: 6823562]

[7] Dvorak HF, Nagy JA, Feng D, Brown LF, Dvorak AM. Vascular Permeability Factor/Vascular Endothelial Growth Factor and the Significance of Microvascular Hyperpermeability in Angiogenesis. Current Topics Microbiol Immunol. Springer Berlin Heidelberg 1999; pp. 97-132.
[http://dx.doi.org/10.1007/978-3-642-59953-8_6]

[8] Soker S, Takashima S, Miao HQ, Neufeld G, Klagsbrun M. Neuropilin-1 is expressed by endothelial and tumor cells as an isoform-specific receptor for vascular endothelial growth factor. Cell 1998; 92(6): 735-45.
[http://dx.doi.org/10.1016/S0092-8674(00)81402-6] [PMID: 9529250]

[9] Tordjman R, Ortéga N, Coulombel L, Plouët J, Roméo PH, Lemarchandel V. Neuropilin-1 is expressed on bone marrow stromal cells: A novel interaction with hematopoietic cells? Blood 1999; 94(7): 2301-9. http://www.ncbi.nlm.nih.gov/pubmed/10498602
[PMID: 10498602]

[10] Carmeliet P, Mackman N, Moons L, *et al.* Role of tissue factor in embryonic blood vessel development. Nature 1996; 383(6595): 73-5.
[http://dx.doi.org/10.1038/383073a0] [PMID: 8779717]

[11] Nagy JA, Benjamin L, Zeng H, Dvorak AM, Dvorak HF. Vascular permeability, vascular hyperpermeability and angiogenesis. Angiogenesis 2008; 11(2): 109-19.
[http://dx.doi.org/10.1007/s10456-008-9099-z] [PMID: 18293091]

[12] Warren CM, Iruela-Arispe ML. Signaling circuitry in vascular morphogenesis. Curr Opin Hematol 2010; 17(3): 213-8.
[http://dx.doi.org/10.1097/moh.0b013e32833865d1] [PMID: 20216211]

[13] Arroyo AG, Iruela-Arispe ML. Extracellular matrix, inflammation, and the angiogenic response. Cardiovasc Res 2010; 86(2): 226-35.
[http://dx.doi.org/10.1093/cvr/cvq049] [PMID: 20154066]

[14] Nagy JA, Chang S-H, Shih S-C, Dvorak AM, Dvorak HF. Heterogeneity of the tumor vasculature. Semin Thromb Hemost 2010; 36(3): 321-31.
[http://dx.doi.org/10.1055/s-0030-1253454] [PMID: 20490982]

[15] Minchinton AI, Durand RE, Chaplin DJ. Intermittent blood flow in the KHT sarcoma--flow cytometry studies using Hoechst 33342. Br J Cancer 1990; 62(2): 195-200.
[http://dx.doi.org/10.1038/bjc.1990.259] [PMID: 2386734]

[16] Carmeliet P, Jain RK. Angiogenesis in cancer and other diseases. Nature 2000; 407(6801): 249-57.
[http://dx.doi.org/10.1038/35025220] [PMID: 11001068]

[17] Carmeliet P, Jain RK. Molecular mechanisms and clinical applications of angiogenesis. Nature 2011; 473(7347): 298-307.
[http://dx.doi.org/10.1038/nature10144] [PMID: 21593862]

[18] Ferrara N, Hillan KJ, Gerber H-P, Novotny W. Discovery and development of bevacizumab, an anti-VEGF antibody for treating cancer. Nat Rev Drug Discov 2004; 3(5): 391-400.
[http://dx.doi.org/10.1038/nrd1381] [PMID: 15136787]

[19] Fett JW, Strydom DJ, Lobb RR, *et al.* Isolation and characterization of angiogenin, an angiogenic protein from human carcinoma cells. Biochemistry 1985; 24(20): 5480-6.
[http://dx.doi.org/10.1021/bi00341a030] [PMID: 4074709]

[20] Kurachi K, Davie EW, Strydom DJ, Riordan JF, Vallee BL. A sequence of the cDNA and gene for

angiogenin, a human angiogenesis factor. Biochemistry 1985; 24(20): 5494-9.
[http://dx.doi.org/10.1021/bi00341a032] [PMID: 2866795]

[21]   Strydom DJ, Fett JW, Lobb RR, *et al.* Amino acid sequence of human tumor derived angiogenin. Biochemistry 1985; 24(20): 5486-94.
[http://dx.doi.org/10.1021/bi00341a031] [PMID: 2866794]

[22]   Tello-Montoliu A, Patel JV, Lip GYH. Angiogenin: a review of the pathophysiology and potential clinical applications. J Thromb Haemost 2006; 4(9): 1864-74.
[http://dx.doi.org/10.1111/j.1538-7836.2006.01995.x] [PMID: 16961595]

[23]   Zhang J, Zhang YP. Pseudogenization of the tumor-growth promoter angiogenin in a leaf-eating monkey. Gene 2003; 308: 95-101.
[http://dx.doi.org/10.1016/S0378-1119(03)00470-0] [PMID: 12711394]

[24]   Pilch H, Schlenger K, Steiner E, Brockerhoff P, Knapstein P, Vaupel P. Hypoxia-stimulated expression of angiogenic growth factors in cervical cancer cells and cervical cancer-derived fibroblasts. Int J Gynecol Cancer 2001; 11(2): 137-42.http://www.ncbi.nlm.nih.gov/pubmed/11328412
[http://dx.doi.org/10.1046/j.1525-1438.2001.011002137.x] [PMID: 11328412]

[25]   Hartmann A, Kunz M, Köstlin S, Gillitzer R, Toksoy A, Bröcker EB, *et al.* Hypoxia-induced up-regulation of angiogenin in human malignant melanoma. Cancer Res 1999; 7(2): 1578-83.
[PMID: 10197632]

[26]   Spong CY, Ghidini A, Sherer DM, Pezzullo JC, Ossandon M, Eglinton GS. Angiogenin: A marker for preterm delivery in mid-trimester amniotic. Fluid Am J Obstet Gynecol 1997; 176(2): 415-8.
[PMID: 9065191]

[27]   Skog J, Würdinger T, van Rijn S, Meijer DH, Gainche L, Curry WT, *et al.* Glioblastoma microvesicles transport RNA and proteins that promote tumor growth and provide diagnostic biomarkers. Nat Cell Biol 2008;10(12): 1470-6.
[PMID: 19011622]

[28]   Hooper LV, Stappenbeck TS, Hong CV, Gordon JI. Angiogenins: a new class of microbicidal proteins involved in innate immunity. Nat Immunol 2003; 4(3): 269-73.
[http://dx.doi.org/10.1038/ni888] [PMID: 12548285]

[29]   Bräuer L, Paulsen FP. Tear Film and Ocular Surface Surfactants. J Epith Biol Pharmacol 2008.
https://benthamopen.com/contents/ pdf/ JEBP/JEBP-1-62.pdf
[http://dx.doi.org/10.2174/1875044300801010062]

[30]   Sack RA, Conradi L, Krumholz D, Beaton A, Sathe S, Morris C. Membrane Array Characterization of 80 Chemokines, Cytokines, and Growth Factors in Open- and Closed-Eye Tears: Angiogenin and other defense system constituents. Investig Opthalmology Vis Sci 2005; 46(4): 1228.
[PMID: 15790883]

[31]   Fang J, Huang S, Liu H, Crepin M, Xu T, Liu J. Role of the FGF-2/FGFR signaling pathway in cancer and its signification in breast cancer. Chin Sci Bull 2003; 48(15): 1539-47.
[http://dx.doi.org/10.1007/BF03183956]

[32]   Landt S, Mordelt K, Schwidde I, *et al.* Prognostic significance of the angiogenic factors angiogenin, endoglin and endostatin in cervical cancer. Anticancer Res 2011; 31(8): 2651-5.
[PMID: 21778318]

[33]   Yoshioka N, Wang L, Kishimoto K, Tsuji T, Hu GF. A therapeutic target for prostate cancer based on angiogenin-stimulated angiogenesis and cancer cell proliferation. Proc Natl Acad Sci USA 2006; 103(39): 14519-24.
[http://dx.doi.org/10.1073/pnas.0606708103] [PMID: 16971483]

[34]   Koutroubakis ie, Xidakis C, Karmiris K, Sfiridaki A, Kandidaki E, Kouroumalis EA. Serum angiogenin in inflammatory bowel disease. Dig Dis Sci 49(11–12): 1758-62.
[http://dx.doi.org/10.1007/s10620-004-9565-4] [PMID: 15628698]

[35] Neubauer-Geryk J, Kozera GM, Wolnik B, Szczyrba S, Nyka WM, Bieniaszewski L. Angiogenin in middle-aged type 1 diabetes patients. Microvasc Res 2012; 84(3): 387-9.
[http://dx.doi.org/10.1016/j.mvr.2012.08.005] [PMID: 22940420]

[36] Siebert J, Reiwer-Gostomska M, Mysliwska J, Marek N, Raczynska K, Glasner L. Glycemic control influences serum angiogenin concentrations in patients with type 2 diabetes. Diabetes Care 2010; 33(8): 1829-30.
[http://dx.doi.org/10.2337/dc10-0130] [PMID: 20484129]

[37] Suzumori N, Zhao XX, Suzumori K. Elevated angiogenin levels in the peritoneal fluid of women with endometriosis correlate with the extent of the disorder. Fertil Steril 2004; 82(1): 93-6.
[http://dx.doi.org/10.1016/j.fertnstert.2003.11.043] [PMID: 15236995]

[38] Lambrechts D, Storkebaum E, Morimoto M, Del-Favero J, Desmet F, Marklund SL, *et al.* VEGF is a modifier of amyotrophic lateral sclerosis in mice and humans and protects motoneurons against ischemic death. Nat Genet 2003; 34(4): 383-94.
[http://dx.doi.org/10.1038/ng1211] [PMID: 12847526]

[39] Gho YS, Chae CB. Anti-Angiogenic activity of the peptides complementary to the receptor-binding site of angiogenin. J Biol Chem 1997; 272(39): 24294-9.
[PMID: 9305884]

[40] Ibaragi S, Yoshioka N, Li S, Hu MG, Hirukawa S, Sadow PM, *et al.* Neamine Inhibits Prostate Cancer Growth by Suppressing Angiogenin-Mediated rRNA Transcription. Clin Cancer Res 2009; 15(6): 1981-8..
[PMID: 19276260] [http://dx.doi.org/10.1158/ 1078-0432.CCR-08-2593]

[41] Kao RYT, Jenkins JL, Olson KA, Key ME, Fett JW, Shapiro R. A small-molecule inhibitor of the ribonucleolytic activity of human angiogenin that possesses antitumor activity. Proc Natl Acad Sci 2002; 99(15): 10066-71.
[PMID: 12118120] [http://dx.doi.org/10.1073/pnas.152342999]

[42] Herzog B, Pellet-Many C, Britton G, Hartzoulakis B, Zachary IC. VEGF binding to NRP1 is essential for VEGF stimulation of endothelial cell migration, complex formation between NRP1 and VEGFR2, and signaling *via* FAK Tyr407 phosphorylation. Mol Biol Cell 2011; 22(15): 2766-76.
[http://dx.doi.org/10.1091/mbc.e09-12-1061] [PMID: 21653826]

[43] Duffy AM, Bouchier-Hayes DJ, Harmey JH. Vascular Endothelial Growth Factor (VEGF) and Its Role in Non-Endothelial Cells: Autocrine Signalling by VEGF. Springer, US: VEGF and Cancer 2004; pp. 133-44.

[44] Roskoski R Jr. Vascular endothelial growth factor (VEGF) signaling in tumor progression. Crit Rev Oncol Hematol 2007; 62(3): 179-213.
[http://dx.doi.org/10.1016/j.critrevonc.2007.01.006] [PMID: 17324579]

[45] Ferrara N, Gerber H-P, LeCouter J. The biology of VEGF and its receptors. Nat Med 2003; 9(6): 669-76.
[http://dx.doi.org/10.1038/nm0603-669] [PMID: 12778165]

[46] Shibuya M. Vascular Endothelial Growth Factor (VEGF) and Its Receptor (VEGFR) Signaling in Angiogenesis: A Crucial Target for Anti- and Pro-Angiogenic Therapies. Genes Cancer 2011; 2(12): 1097-105.
[http://dx.doi.org/10.1177/1947601911423031] [PMID: 22866201]

[47] Longatto Filho A, Lopes JM, Schmitt FC. Angiogenesis and breast cancer. J Oncol 2010; 2010: 1-7.
[http://dx.doi.org/10.1155/2010/576384] [PMID: 20953378]

[48] Sa-Nguanraksa D, O-Charoenrat P. The role of vascular endothelial growth factor a polymorphisms in breast cancer. Int J Mol Sci 2012; 13(11): 14845-64.
[http://dx.doi.org/10.3390/ijms131114845] [PMID: 23203097]

[49] Srabovic N, Mujagic Z, Mujanovic-Mustedanagic J, *et al.* Vascular endothelial growth factor receptor-

1 expression in breast cancer and its correlation to vascular endothelial growth factor a. Int J Breast Cancer 2013; 2013746749.
[http://dx.doi.org/10.1155/2013/746749] [PMID: 24416596]

[50]   Guo S, Colbert LS, Fuller M, Zhang Y, Gonzalez-Perez RR. Vascular endothelial growth factor receptor-2 in breast cancer. Biochim Biophys Acta 2010; 1806(1): 108-21.
[http://dx.doi.org/10.1016/j.bbcan.2010.04.004] [PMID: 20462514]

[51]   Lushnikova AA, Nasunova IB, Parokonnaya AA, Lyubchenko LN, Kampova-Polevaya EB. VEGFR-2 expression in tumor tissue of breast cancer patients. Dokl Biol Sci 2010; 434(1): 363-7.
[http://dx.doi.org/10.1134/S0012496610050194] [PMID: 20963665]

[52]   Claesson-Welsh L, Welsh M. VEGFA and tumour angiogenesis. J Intern Med 2013; 273(2): 114-27.
[http://dx.doi.org/10.1111/joim.12019] [PMID: 23216836]

[53]   Linardou H, Kalogeras KT, Kronenwett R, *et al.* The prognostic and predictive value of mRNA expression of vascular endothelial growth factor family members in breast cancer: a study in primary tumors of high-risk early breast cancer patients participating in a randomized Hellenic Cooperative Oncology Group trial. Breast Cancer Res 2012; 14(6): R145.
[http://dx.doi.org/10.1186/bcr3354] [PMID: 23146280]

[54]   Todorović-Raković N, Milovanović J. Interleukin-8 in breast cancer progression. J Interferon Cytokine Res 2013; 33(10): 563-70.
[http://dx.doi.org/10.1089/jir.2013.0023] [PMID: 23697558]

[55]   Ornitz DM, Itoh N. Fibroblast growth factors. Genome Biol 2001; 2(3): S3005.
[http://dx.doi.org/10.1186/gb-2001-2-3-reviews3005] [PMID: 11276432]

[56]   Blaber M, DiSalvo J, Thomas KA. X-ray crystal structure of human acidic fibroblast growth factor. Biochemistry 1996; 35(7): 2086-94.
[http://dx.doi.org/10.1021/bi9521755] [PMID: 8652550]

[57]   Partanen J, Mäkelä TP, Eerola E, *et al.* FGFR-4, a novel acidic fibroblast growth factor receptor with a distinct expression pattern. EMBO J 1991; 10(6): 1347-54.
[http://dx.doi.org/10.1002/j.1460-2075.1991.tb07654.x] [PMID: 1709094]

[58]   Yiangou C, Gomm JJ, Coope RC, *et al.* Fibroblast growth factor 2 in breast cancer: occurrence and prognostic significance. Br J Cancer 1997; 75(1): 28-33.
[http://dx.doi.org/10.1038/bjc.1997.5] [PMID: 9000594]

[59]   Powers CJ, McLeskey SW, Wellstein A. Fibroblast growth factors, their receptors and signaling. Endocr Relat Cancer 2000; 7(3): 165-97.
[http://dx.doi.org/10.1677/erc.0.0070165] [PMID: 11021964]

[60]   Jain VK, Turner NC. Challenges and opportunities in the targeting of fibroblast growth factor receptors in breast cancer. Breast Cancer Res 2012; 14(3): 208.
[http://dx.doi.org/10.1186/bcr3139] [PMID: 22731805]

[61]   Brady N, Chuntova P, Bade LK, Schwertfeger KL. The FGF/FGFR axis as a therapeutic target in breast cancer. Expert Rev Endocrinol Metab 2013; 8(4): 391-402.
[http://dx.doi.org/10.1586/17446651.2013.811910] [PMID: 25400686]

[62]   Vlodavsky I, Korner G, Ishai-Michaeli R, Bashkin P, Bar-Shavit R, Fuks Z. Extracellular matrix-resident growth factors and enzymes: possible involvement in tumor metastasis and angiogenesis. Cancer Metastasis Rev 1990; 9(3): 203-26.
[http://dx.doi.org/10.1007/BF00046361] [PMID: 1705486]

[63]   Granato AM, Nanni O, Falcini F, *et al.* Basic fibroblast growth factor and vascular endothelial growth factor serum levels in breast cancer patients and healthy women: useful as diagnostic tools? Breast Cancer Res 2004; 6(1): R38-45.
[http://dx.doi.org/10.1186/bcr745] [PMID: 14680499]

[64]   Woessner JF. The Family of Matrix Metalloproteinases. Ann N Y Acad Sci 1994; 732: 11-21.

[http://dx.doi.org/10.1111/j.1749-6632.1994.tb24720.x]

[65]   Nagase H, Woessner JF Jr. Matrix metalloproteinases. J Biol Chem 1999; 274(31): 21491-4.
[http://dx.doi.org/10.1074/jbc.274.31.21491] [PMID: 10419448]

[66]   McCawley LJ, Matrisian LM. Matrix metalloproteinases: multifunctional contributors to tumor progression. Mol Med Today 2000; 6(4): 149-56.
[http://dx.doi.org/10.1016/S1357-4310(00)01686-5] [PMID: 10740253]

[67]   Murray GI. Matrix metalloproteinases: a multifunctional group of molecules. J Pathol 2001; 195(2): 135-7.
[http://dx.doi.org/10.1002/1096-9896(200109)195:2<135::AID-PATH939>3.0.CO;2-G]   [PMID: 11592090]

[68]   Bartsch JE, Staren ED, Appert HE. Matrix metalloproteinase expression in breast cancer. J Surg Res 2003; 110(2): 383-92.
[http://dx.doi.org/10.1016/S0022-4804(03)00007-6] [PMID: 12788669]

[69]   Kousidou OC, Mitropoulou TN, Roussidis AE, Kletsas D, Theocharis AD, Karamanos NK. Genistein suppresses the invasive potential of human breast cancer cells through transcriptional regulation of metalloproteinases and their tissue inhibitors. Int J Oncol 2005; 26(4): 1101-9.
[http://dx.doi.org/10.3892/ijo.26.4.1101] [PMID: 15754008]

[70]   van Hinsbergh VWM, Engelse MA, Quax PHA. Pericellular proteases in angiogenesis and vasculogenesis. Arterioscler Thromb Vasc Biol 2006; 26(4): 716-28.
[http://dx.doi.org/10.1161/01.ATV.0000209518.58252.17] [PMID: 16469948]

[71]   Verma RP, Hansch C. Matrix metalloproteinases (MMPs): chemical-biological functions and (Q)SARs. Bioorg Med Chem 2007; 15(6): 2223-68.
[http://dx.doi.org/10.1016/j.bmc.2007.01.011] [PMID: 17275314]

[72]   Heppner KJ, Matrisian LM, Jensen RA, Rodgers WH. Expression of most matrix metalloproteinase family members in breast cancer represents a tumor-induced host response.Am J Pathol 1996; 149(1): 273–82 .
[PMID: 8686751]

[73]   Rundhaug JE. Matrix metalloproteinases, angiogenesis, and cancer: Commentary re A. C. Lockhart et al., Reduction of wound angiogenesis in patients treated with BMS-275291, a broad spectrum matrix metalloproteinase inhibitor. Clin. Cancer Res., 9: 00-00, 2003; 9(2): 551–4.
[PMID: 12576417]

[74]   Benson CS, Babu SD, Radhakrishna S, Selvamurugan N, Ravi Sankar B. Expression of matrix metalloproteinases in human breast cancer tissues. Dis Markers 2013; 34(6): 395-405.
[http://dx.doi.org/10.1155/2013/420914] [PMID: 23568046]

[75]   Singer CF, Kronsteiner N, Marton E, *et al.* MMP-2 and MMP-9 expression in breast cancer-derived human fibroblasts is differentially regulated by stromal-epithelial interactions. Breast Cancer Res Treat 2002; 72(1): 69-77.
[http://dx.doi.org/10.1023/A:1014918512569] [PMID: 12000221]

[76]   Patel BP, Shah SV, Shukla SN, Shah PM, Patel PS. Clinical significance of MMP-2 and MMP-9 in patients with oral cancer. Head Neck 2007; 29(6): 564-72.
[http://dx.doi.org/10.1002/hed.20561] [PMID: 17252594]

[77]   Haas TL, Milkiewicz M, Davis SJ, *et al.* Matrix metalloproteinase activity is required for activity-induced angiogenesis in rat skeletal muscle. Am J Physiol Heart Circ Physiol 2000; 279(4): H1540-7.
[http://dx.doi.org/10.1152/ajpheart.2000.279.4.H1540] [PMID: 11009439]

[78]   Thurston G. Role of Angiopoietins and Tie receptor tyrosine kinases in angiogenesis and lymphangiogenesis. Cell Tissue Res 2003; 314(1): 61-8.
[http://dx.doi.org/10.1007/s00441-003-0749-6] [PMID: 12915980]

[79]   Fagiani E, Christofori G. Angiopoietins in angiogenesis. Cancer Lett 2013; 328(1): 18-26.
[http://dx.doi.org/10.1016/j.canlet.2012.08.018] [PMID: 22922303]

[80]   Brooks P, Clark R, Cheresh D. Requirement of vascular integrin alpha v beta 3 for angiogenesis. Science 1994; 264(5158): 569-71.
[http://dx.doi.org/10.1126/science.7512751]

[81]   Tonnesen MG, Feng X, Clark RAF. Angiogenesis in wound healing. J Investig Dermatol Symp Proc 2000; 5(1): 40-6.
[http://dx.doi.org/10.1046/j.1087-0024.2000.00014.x] [PMID: 11147674]

[82]   Coradini D, Biffi A, Costa A, Pellizzaro C, Pirronello E, Di Fronzo G. Effect of sodium butyrate on human breast cancer cell lines. Cell Prolif 1997; 30(3-4): 149-59.
[http://dx.doi.org/10.1111/j.1365-2184.1997.tb00931.x] [PMID: 9375027]

[83]   Tiwari RK, Wong GY, Mukhopadhyay B, *et al.* Interferon-alpha and gamma mediated gene responses in a human breast carcinoma cell line. Breast Cancer Res Treat 1991; 18(1): 33-41.
[http://dx.doi.org/10.1007/BF01975441] [PMID: 1713085]

[84]   Rehn M, Veikkola T, Kukk-Valdre E, *et al.* Interaction of endostatin with integrins implicated in angiogenesis. Proc Natl Acad Sci USA 2001; 98(3): 1024-9.
[http://dx.doi.org/10.1073/pnas.98.3.1024] [PMID: 11158588]

[85]   Scappaticci FA, Smith R, Pathak A, *et al.* Combination angiostatin and endostatin gene transfer induces synergistic antiangiogenic activity *in vitro* and antitumor efficacy in leukemia and solid tumors in mice. Mol Ther 2001; 3(2): 186-96.
[http://dx.doi.org/10.1006/mthe.2000.0243] [PMID: 11237675]

[86]   Yin G, Liu W, An P, *et al.* Endostatin gene transfer inhibits joint angiogenesis and pannus formation in inflammatory arthritis. Mol Ther 2002; 5(5 Pt 1): 547-54.
[http://dx.doi.org/10.1006/mthe.2002.0590] [PMID: 11991745]

[87]   Indraccolo S, Gola E, Rosato A, *et al.* Differential effects of angiostatin, endostatin and interferon-α(1) gene transfer on *in vivo* growth of human breast cancer cells. Gene Ther 2002; 9(13): 867-78.
[http://dx.doi.org/10.1038/sj.gt.3301703] [PMID: 12080381]

[88]   O'Reilly MS, Holmgren L, Shing Y, *et al.* Angiostatin: a novel angiogenesis inhibitor that mediates the suppression of metastases by a Lewis lung carcinoma. Cell 1994; 79(2): 315-28.
[http://dx.doi.org/10.1016/0092-8674(94)90200-3] [PMID: 7525077]

[89]   O'Reilly MS, Holmgren L, Chen C, Folkman J. Angiostatin induces and sustains dormancy of human primary tumors in mice. Nat Med 1996; 2(6): 689-92.
[http://dx.doi.org/10.1038/nm0696-689] [PMID: 8640562]

[90]   Wahl ML, Moser TL, Pizzo SV. Angiostatin and anti-angiogenic therapy in human disease. Recent Prog Horm Res 2004; 59(1): 73-104.
[http://dx.doi.org/10.1210/rp.59.1.73] [PMID: 14749498]

[91]   Harris AL, Generali D. Biological Therapies for Metastatic Breast Cancer: Antiangiogenesis [Internet]. Breast Cancer and Molecular Medicine>. 671-704. Available from:
[http://dx.doi.org/10.1007/978-3-540-28266-2_33]

[92]   Wajih N, Sane DC. Angiostatin selectively inhibits signaling by hepatocyte growth factor in endothelial and smooth muscle cells. Blood 2003; 101(5): 1857-63.
[http://dx.doi.org/10.1182/blood-2002-02-0582] [PMID: 12406896]

[93]   Lawler J, Detmar M. Tumor progression: the effects of thrombospondin-1 and -2. Int J Biochem Cell Biol 2004; 36(6): 1038-45.
[http://dx.doi.org/10.1016/j.biocel.2004.01.008] [PMID: 15094119]

[94]   Armstrong LC, Björkblom B, Hankenson KD, Siadak AW, Stiles CE, Bornstein P. Thrombospondin 2 inhibits microvascular endothelial cell proliferation by a caspase-independent mechanism. Mol Biol

Cell 2002; 13(6): 1893-905.
[http://dx.doi.org/10.1091/mbc.e01-09-0066] [PMID: 12058057]

[95] Lawler PR, Lawler J. Molecular basis for the regulation of angiogenesis by thrombospondin-1 and -2. Cold Spring Harb Perspect Med 2012; 2(5): a006627-7.
[http://dx.doi.org/10.1101/cshperspect.a006627] [PMID: 22553494]

[96] Roberts DD, Isenberg JS, Ridnour LA, Wink DA. Nitric oxide and its gatekeeper thrombospondin-1 in tumor angiogenesis. Clin Cancer Res 2007; 13(3): 795-8.
[http://dx.doi.org/10.1158/1078-0432.CCR-06-1758] [PMID: 17289869]

[97] Goldoni S, Seidler DG, Heath J, et al. An antimetastatic role for decorin in breast cancer. Am J Pathol 2008; 173(3): 844-55.
[http://dx.doi.org/10.2353/ajpath.2008.080275] [PMID: 18688028]

[98] Iozzo RV, Sanderson RD. Proteoglycans in cancer biology, tumour microenvironment and angiogenesis. J Cell Mol Med 2011; 15(5): 1013-31.
[http://dx.doi.org/10.1111/j.1582-4934.2010.01236.x] [PMID: 21155971]

[99] Iozzo RV, Murdoch AD. Proteoglycans of the extracellular environment: clues from the gene and protein side offer novel perspectives in molecular diversity and function. FASEB J 1996; 10(5): 598-614.
[http://dx.doi.org/10.1096/fasebj.10.5.8621059] [PMID: 8621059]

[100] Schaefer L, Iozzo RV. Biological functions of the small leucine-rich proteoglycans: from genetics to signal transduction. J Biol Chem 2008; 283(31): 21305-9.
[http://dx.doi.org/10.1074/jbc.R800020200] [PMID: 18463092]

[101] Iozzo RV, Bolender RP, Wight TN. Proteoglycan changes in the intercellular matrix of human colon carcinoma: An integrated biochemical and stereologic analysis. Lab Invest 1982; 47(2): 124–38.
[PMID: 7109538]

[102] Adany R, Iozzo RV. Altered methylation of versican proteoglycan gene in human colon carcinoma. Biochem Biophys Res Commun 1990; 171(3): 1402-13.
[http://dx.doi.org/10.1016/0006-291X(90)90841-A] [PMID: 2222452]

[103] Moscatello DK, Santra M, Mann DM, McQuillan DJ, Wong AJ, Iozzo RV. Decorin suppresses tumor cell growth by activating the epidermal growth factor receptor. J Clin Invest 1998; 101(2): 406-12.
[http://dx.doi.org/10.1172/JCI846] [PMID: 9435313]

[104] Csordás G, Santra M, Reed CC, et al. Sustained down-regulation of the epidermal growth factor receptor by decorin. A mechanism for controlling tumor growth in vivo. J Biol Chem 2000; 275(42): 32879-87.
[http://dx.doi.org/10.1074/jbc.M005609200] [PMID: 10913155]

[105] Santra M, Reed CC, Iozzo RV. Decorin binds to a narrow region of the epidermal growth factor (EGF) receptor, partially overlapping but distinct from the EGF-binding epitope. J Biol Chem 2002; 277(38): 35671-81.
[http://dx.doi.org/10.1074/jbc.M205317200] [PMID: 12105206]

[106] Santra M, Eichstetter I, Iozzo RV. An anti-oncogenic role for decorin. Down-regulation of ErbB2 leads to growth suppression and cytodifferentiation of mammary carcinoma cells. J Biol Chem 2000; 275(45): 35153-61.
[http://dx.doi.org/10.1074/jbc.M006821200] [PMID: 10942781]

[107] Santra M, Skorski T, Calabretta B, Lattime EC, Iozzo RV. De novo decorin gene expression suppresses the malignant phenotype in human colon cancer cells. Proc Natl Acad Sci USA 1995; 92(15): 7016-20.
[http://dx.doi.org/10.1073/pnas.92.15.7016] [PMID: 7624361]

[108] De Luca A, Santra M, Baldi A, Giordano A, Iozzo RV. Decorin-induced growth suppression is associated with up-regulation of p21, an inhibitor of cyclin-dependent kinases. J Biol Chem 1996;

271(31): 18961-5.
[http://dx.doi.org/10.1074/jbc.271.31.18961] [PMID: 8702560]

[109] Santra M, Mann DM, Mercer EW, Skorski T, Calabretta B, Iozzo RV. Ectopic expression of decorin protein core causes a generalized growth suppression in neoplastic cells of various histogenetic origin and requires endogenous p21, an inhibitor of cyclin-dependent kinases. J Clin Invest 1997; 100(1): 149-57.
[http://dx.doi.org/10.1172/JCI119507] [PMID: 9202067]

[110] Patel S, Santra M, McQuillan DJ, Iozzo RV, Thomas AP. Decorin activates the epidermal growth factor receptor and elevates cytosolic Ca2+ in A431 carcinoma cells. J Biol Chem 1998; 273(6): 3121-4.
[http://dx.doi.org/10.1074/jbc.273.6.3121] [PMID: 9452417]

[111] Goldoni S, Humphries A, Nyström A, *et al.* Decorin is a novel antagonistic ligand of the Met receptor. J Cell Biol 2009; 185(4): 743-54.
[http://dx.doi.org/10.1083/jcb.200901129] [PMID: 19433454]

[112] Buraschi S, Pal N, Tyler-Rubinstein N, Owens RT, Neill T, Iozzo RV. Decorin antagonizes Met receptor activity and down-regulates β-catenin and Myc levels. J Biol Chem 2010; 285(53): 42075-85.
[http://dx.doi.org/10.1074/jbc.M110.172841] [PMID: 20974860]

[113] Zhu J-X, Goldoni S, Bix G, *et al.* Decorin evokes protracted internalization and degradation of the epidermal growth factor receptor *via* caveolar endocytosis. J Biol Chem 2005; 280(37): 32468-79.
[http://dx.doi.org/10.1074/jbc.M503833200] [PMID: 15994311]

[114] Kermorgant S, Parker PJ. c-Met signalling: spatio-temporal decisions. Cell Cycle 2005; 4(3): 352-5.
[http://dx.doi.org/10.4161/cc.4.3.1519] [PMID: 15701970]

[115] Liu Z-X, Yu CF, Nickel C, Thomas S, Cantley LG. Hepatocyte growth factor induces ERK-dependent paxillin phosphorylation and regulates paxillin-focal adhesion kinase association. J Biol Chem 2002; 277(12): 10452-8.
[http://dx.doi.org/10.1074/jbc.M107551200] [PMID: 11784715]

[116] Lupo G, Caporarello N, Olivieri M, *et al.* Anti-angiogenic Therapy in Cancer: Downsides and New Pivots for Precision Medicine. Front Pharmacol [Internet] 2017; 7:519.
[http://dx.doi.org/10.3389/fphar.2016.00519.]

[117] Miller KD. Recent translational research: antiangiogenic therapy for breast cancer - where do we stand? Breast Cancer Res 2004; 6(3): 128-32.
[http://dx.doi.org/10.1186/bcr782] [PMID: 15084233]

[118] Samant RS, Shevde LA. Recent advances in anti-angiogenic therapy of cancer. Oncotarget 2011; 2(3): 122-34.
[http://dx.doi.org/10.18632/oncotarget.234] [PMID: 21399234]

[119] Kim KJ, Li B, Winer J, *et al.* Inhibition of vascular endothelial growth factor-induced angiogenesis suppresses tumour growth *in vivo.* Nature 1993; 362(6423): 841-4.
[http://dx.doi.org/10.1038/362841a0] [PMID: 7683111]

[120] Rüegg C, Hasmim M, Lejeune FJ, Alghisi GC. Antiangiogenic peptides and proteins: from experimental tools to clinical drugs. Biochim Biophys Acta 2006; 1765(2): 155-77.
[http://dx.doi.org/10.1016/j.bbcan.2005.09.003] [PMID: 16263219]

[121] Hsu JY, Wakelee HA. Monoclonal antibodies targeting vascular endothelial growth factor: current status and future challenges in cancer therapy. BioDrugs 2009; 23(5): 289-304.
[http://dx.doi.org/10.2165/11317600-000000000-00000] [PMID: 19754219]

[122] Gordon MS, Margolin K, Talpaz M, Sledge GW, Holmgren E, Benjamin R, et al. Phase I Safety and Pharmacokinetic Study of Recombinant Human Anti-Vascular Endothelial Growth Factor in Patients With Advanced Cancer. J Clin Oncol 2001; 19(3): 843-50.
[http://dx.doi.org/10.1200/jco.2001.19.3.843]

[123]   Cobleigh MA, Langmuir VK, Sledge GW, *et al.* A phase I/II dose-escalation trial of bevacizumab in previously treated metastatic breast cancer. Semin Oncol 2003; 30(5) (Suppl. 16): 117-24.
[http://dx.doi.org/10.1053/j.seminoncol.2003.08.013] [PMID: 14613032]

[124]   Bukowski RM, Kabbinavar FF, Figlin RA, *et al.* Randomized phase II study of erlotinib combined with bevacizumab compared with bevacizumab alone in metastatic renal cell cancer. J Clin Oncol 2007; 25(29): 4536-41.
[http://dx.doi.org/10.1200/JCO.2007.11.5154] [PMID: 17876014]

[125]   Herbst RS, O'Neill VJ, Fehrenbacher L, *et al.* Phase II study of efficacy and safety of bevacizumab in combination with chemotherapy or erlotinib compared with chemotherapy alone for treatment of recurrent or refractory non small-cell lung cancer. J Clin Oncol 2007; 25(30): 4743-50.
[http://dx.doi.org/10.1200/JCO.2007.12.3026] [PMID: 17909199]

[126]   de Groot JF, Yung WKA. Bevacizumab and irinotecan in the treatment of recurrent malignant gliomas. Cancer J 2008; 14(5): 279-85.
[http://dx.doi.org/10.1097/PPO.0b013e3181867bd6] [PMID: 18836331]

[127]   Dickler MN, Rugo HS, Eberle CA, *et al.* A phase II trial of erlotinib in combination with bevacizumab in patients with metastatic breast cancer. Clin Cancer Res 2008; 14(23): 7878-83.
[http://dx.doi.org/10.1158/1078-0432.CCR-08-0141] [PMID: 19047117]

[128]   Li WW, Hutnik M, Gehr G. Antiangiogenesis in haematological malignancies. Br J Haematol 2008; 143(5): 622-31.
[http://dx.doi.org/10.1111/j.1365-2141.2008.07372.x] [PMID: 19036013]

[129]   Manegold C. Bevacizumab for the treatment of advanced non-small-cell lung cancer. Expert Rev Anticancer Ther 2008; 8(5): 689-99.
[http://dx.doi.org/10.1586/14737140.8.5.689] [PMID: 18471042]

[130]   Sachdev JC, Jahanzeb M. Evolution of bevacizumab-based therapy in the management of breast cancer. Clin Breast Cancer 2008; 8(5): 402-10.
[http://dx.doi.org/10.3816/CBC.2008.n.048] [PMID: 18952553]

[131]   Torrisi R, Bagnardi V, Cardillo A, *et al.* Preoperative bevacizumab combined with letrozole and chemotherapy in locally advanced ER- and/or PgR-positive breast cancer: clinical and biological activity. Br J Cancer 2008; 99(10): 1564-71.
[http://dx.doi.org/10.1038/sj.bjc.6604741] [PMID: 18941458]

[132]   Arkenau H-T, Brunetto AT, Barriuso J, *et al.* Clinical benefit of new targeted agents in phase I trials in patients with advanced colorectal cancer. Oncology 2009; 76(3): 151-6.
[http://dx.doi.org/10.1159/000195884] [PMID: 19169046]

[133]   Thomas MB, Morris JS, Chadha R, *et al.* Phase II trial of the combination of bevacizumab and erlotinib in patients who have advanced hepatocellular carcinoma. J Clin Oncol 2009; 27(6): 843-50.
[http://dx.doi.org/10.1200/JCO.2008.18.3301] [PMID: 19139433]

[134]   Yang JC, Haworth L, Sherry RM, *et al.* A randomized trial of bevacizumab, an anti-vascular endothelial growth factor antibody, for metastatic renal cancer. N Engl J Med 2003; 349(5): 427-34.
[http://dx.doi.org/10.1056/NEJMoa021491] [PMID: 12890841]

[135]   Greenberg S, Rugo HS. Triple-negative breast cancer: role of antiangiogenic agents. Cancer J 2010; 16(1): 33-8.
[http://dx.doi.org/10.1097/PPO.0b013e3181d38514] [PMID: 20164688]

[136]   Hurwitz H, Fehrenbacher L, Novotny W, *et al.* Bevacizumab plus irinotecan, fluorouracil, and leucovorin for metastatic colorectal cancer. N Engl J Med 2004; 350(23): 2335-42.
[http://dx.doi.org/10.1056/NEJMoa032691] [PMID: 15175435]

[137]   Johnson DH, Fehrenbacher L, Novotny WF, *et al.* Randomized phase II trial comparing bevacizumab plus carboplatin and paclitaxel with carboplatin and paclitaxel alone in previously untreated locally advanced or metastatic non-small-cell lung cancer. J Clin Oncol 2004; 22(11): 2184-91.

[http://dx.doi.org/10.1200/JCO.2004.11.022] [PMID: 15169807]

[138] Blagosklonny MV. How Avastin potentiates chemotherapeutic drugs: action and reaction in antiangiogenic therapy. Cancer Biol Ther 2005; 4(12): 1307-10.
[http://dx.doi.org/10.4161/cbt.4.12.2315] [PMID: 16322683]

[139] de Gramont A, Van Cutsem E. Investigating the potential of bevacizumab in other indications: metastatic renal cell, non-small cell lung, pancreatic and breast cancer. Oncology 2005; 69(3) (Suppl. 3): 46-56.
[http://dx.doi.org/10.1159/000088483] [PMID: 16301835]

[140] Herbst RS, Johnson DH, Mininberg E, *et al.* Phase I/II trial evaluating the anti-vascular endothelial growth factor monoclonal antibody bevacizumab in combination with the HER-1/epidermal growth factor receptor tyrosine kinase inhibitor erlotinib for patients with recurrent non-small-cell lung cancer. J Clin Oncol 2005; 23(11): 2544-55.
[http://dx.doi.org/10.1200/JCO.2005.02.477] [PMID: 15753462]

[141] Miller KD, Chap LI, Holmes FA, *et al.* Randomized phase III trial of capecitabine compared with bevacizumab plus capecitabine in patients with previously treated metastatic breast cancer. J Clin Oncol 2005; 23(4): 792-9.
[http://dx.doi.org/10.1200/JCO.2005.05.098] [PMID: 15681523]

[142] Hochster HS. Bevacizumab in combination with chemotherapy: first-line treatment of patients with metastatic colorectal cancer. Semin Oncol 2006; 33(5) (Suppl. 10): S8-S14.
[http://dx.doi.org/10.1053/j.seminoncol.2006.08.005] [PMID: 17145525]

[143] Dyar S, Moreno-Aspitia A. Efficacy of Bevacizumab-Capecitabine in Combination for the First-Line Treatment of Metastatic Breast Cancer. Breast Cancer Basic Clin Res 2011; 5 BCBCR.S 7379.
[http://dx.doi.org/10.4137/BCBCR.S7379]

[144] Miller K, Wang M, Gralow J, *et al.* Paclitaxel plus bevacizumab versus paclitaxel alone for metastatic breast cancer. N Engl J Med 2007; 357(26): 2666-76.
[http://dx.doi.org/10.1056/NEJMoa072113] [PMID: 18160686]

[145] Miles DW, Chan A, Dirix LY, *et al.* Phase III study of bevacizumab plus docetaxel compared with placebo plus docetaxel for the first-line treatment of human epidermal growth factor receptor 2-negative metastatic breast cancer. J Clin Oncol 2010; 28(20): 3239-47.
[http://dx.doi.org/10.1200/JCO.2008.21.6457] [PMID: 20498403]

[146] Gianni L, Romieu GH, Lichinitser M, *et al.* AVEREL: a randomized phase III Trial evaluating bevacizumab in combination with docetaxel and trastuzumab as first-line therapy for HER2-positive locally recurrent/metastatic breast cancer. J Clin Oncol 2013; 31(14): 1719-25.
[http://dx.doi.org/10.1200/JCO.2012.44.7912] [PMID: 23569311]

[147] Bäuerle T, Komljenovic D, Merz M, Berger MR, Goodman SL, Semmler W. Cilengitide inhibits progression of experimental breast cancer bone metastases as imaged noninvasively using VCT, MRI and DCE-MRI in a longitudinal *in vivo* study. Int J Cancer 2011; 128(10): 2453-62.
[http://dx.doi.org/10.1002/ijc.25563] [PMID: 20648558]

[148] Lautenschlaeger T, Perry J, Peereboom D, *et al. In vitro* study of combined cilengitide and radiation treatment in breast cancer cell lines. Radiat Oncol 2013; 8(1): 246.
[http://dx.doi.org/10.1186/1748-717X-8-246] [PMID: 24153102]

[149] Burke PA, DeNardo SJ, Miers LA, Kukis DL, DeNardo GL. Combined modality radioimmunotherapy. Promise and peril. Cancer 2002; 94(4) (Suppl.): 1320-31.
[http://dx.doi.org/10.1002/cncr.10303] [PMID: 11877763]

[150] Stupp R, Hegi ME, Gorlia T, *et al.* Cilengitide combined with standard treatment for patients with newly diagnosed glioblastoma with methylated MGMT promoter (CENTRIC EORTC 26071-22072 study): a multicentre, randomised, open-label, phase 3 trial. Lancet Oncol 2014; 15(10): 1100-8.
[http://dx.doi.org/10.1016/S1470-2045(14)70379-1] [PMID: 25163906]

[151] Manegold C, Vansteenkiste J, Cardenal F, *et al.* Randomized phase II study of three doses of the integrin inhibitor cilengitide versus docetaxel as second-line treatment for patients with advanced non-small-cell lung cancer. Invest New Drugs 2013; 31(1): 175-82.
[http://dx.doi.org/10.1007/s10637-012-9842-6] [PMID: 22752690]

[152] Bradley DA, Daignault S, Ryan CJ, *et al.* Cilengitide (EMD 121974, NSC 707544) in asymptomatic metastatic castration resistant prostate cancer patients: a randomized phase II trial by the prostate cancer clinical trials consortium. Invest New Drugs 2011; 29(6): 1432-40.
[http://dx.doi.org/10.1007/s10637-010-9420-8] [PMID: 20336348]

[153] Eskens FAL, Dumez H, Hoekstra R, *et al.* Phase I and pharmacokinetic study of continuous twice weekly intravenous administration of Cilengitide (EMD 121974), a novel inhibitor of the integrins alphavbeta3 and alphavbeta5 in patients with advanced solid tumours. Eur J Cancer 2003; 39(7): 917-26.
[http://dx.doi.org/10.1016/S0959-8049(03)00057-1] [PMID: 12706360]

[154] Mas-Moruno C, Rechenmacher F, Kessler H. Cilengitide: the first anti-angiogenic small molecule drug candidate design, synthesis and clinical evaluation. Anticancer Agents Med Chem 2010; 10(10): 753-68.
[http://dx.doi.org/10.2174/187152010794728639] [PMID: 21269250]

[155] Stupp R, Hegi ME, Gorlia T, Erridge SC, Perry J, Hong Y-K, et al. Cilengitide combined with standard treatment for patients with newly diagnosed glioblastoma with methylated MGMT promoter (CENTRIC EORTC 26071-22072 study): A multicentre, randomized, open-label, phase 3 trial. Lancet Oncol. 2014; 15(10): 1100–8.

[156] Wu FT, Paez-Ribes M, Xu P, Man S, Bogdanovic E, Thurston G, *et al.* Aflibercept and Ang1 supplementation improve neoadjuvant or adjuvant chemotherapy in a preclinical model of resectable breast cancer. Sci Rep 2016; 6: 36694
[http://dx.doi.org/10.1038/srep36694]

[157] Lu D, Jimenez X, Zhang H, Bohlen P, Witte L, Zhu Z. Selection of high affinity human neutralizing antibodies to VEGFR2 from a large antibody phage display library for antiangiogenesis therapy. Int J Cancer 2002; 97(3): 393-9.
[http://dx.doi.org/10.1002/ijc.1634] [PMID: 11774295]

[158] Adnane L, Trail PA, Taylor I, Wilhelm SM. Sorafenib (BAY 43-9006, Nexavar), a dual-action inhibitor that targets RAF/MEK/ERK pathway in tumor cells and tyrosine kinases VEGFR/PDGFR in tumor vasculature. Methods Enzymol 2006; 407: 597-612.
[http://dx.doi.org/10.1016/S0076-6879(05)07047-3] [PMID: 16757355]

[159] Wilhelm SM, Carter C, Tang L, *et al.* BAY 43-9006 exhibits broad spectrum oral antitumor activity and targets the RAF/MEK/ERK pathway and receptor tyrosine kinases involved in tumor progression and angiogenesis. Cancer Res 2004; 64(19): 7099-109.
[http://dx.doi.org/10.1158/0008-5472.CAN-04-1443] [PMID: 15466206]

[160] Moreno-Aspitia A, Morton RF, Hillman DW, *et al.* Phase II trial of sorafenib in patients with metastatic breast cancer previously exposed to anthracyclines or taxanes: North Central Cancer Treatment Group and Mayo Clinic Trial N0336. J Clin Oncol 2009; 27(1): 11-5.
[http://dx.doi.org/10.1200/JCO.2007.15.5242] [PMID: 19047293]

[161] Baselga J, Zamagni C, Gómez P, Bermejo B, Nagai SE, Melichar B. RESILIENCE: Phase III Randomized, Double-Blind Trial Comparing Sorafenib With Capecitabine Versus Placebo With Capecitabine in Locally Advanced or Metastatic HER2-Negative Breast Cancer. Clin Breast Cancer 2017; 17(8): 585-94.
[http://dx.doi.org/10.1016/j.clbc.2017.05.006]

[162] Aogi K, Masuda N, Ohno S, *et al.* First-line bevacizumab in combination with weekly paclitaxel for metastatic breast cancer: efficacy and safety results from a large, open-label, single-arm Japanese

study. Breast Cancer Res Treat 2011; 129(3): 829-38.
[http://dx.doi.org/10.1007/s10549-011-1685-x] [PMID: 21805309]

[163] Pierga J-Y, Petit T, Delozier T, *et al.* Neoadjuvant bevacizumab, trastuzumab, and chemotherapy for primary inflammatory HER2-positive breast cancer (BEVERLY-2): an open-label, single-arm phase 2 study. Lancet Oncol 2012; 13(4): 375-84.
[http://dx.doi.org/10.1016/S1470-2045(12)70049-9] [PMID: 22377126]

[164] Mavratzas A, Baek S, Gerber B, *et al.* Sorafenib in combination with docetaxel as first-line therapy for HER2-negative metastatic breast cancer: Final results of the randomized, double-blind, placebo-controlled phase II MADONNA study. Breast 2019; 45: 22-8.
[http://dx.doi.org/10.1016/j.breast.2019.02.002] [PMID: 30822621]

[165] Bronte G, Andreis D, Bravaccini S, *et al.* Sorafenib for the treatment of breast cancer. Expert Opin Pharmacother 2017; 18(6): 621-30.
[http://dx.doi.org/10.1080/14656566.2017.1309024] [PMID: 28335647]

[166] Zafrakas M, Papasozomenou P, Emmanouilides C. Sorafenib in breast cancer treatment: A systematic review and overview of clinical trials. World J Clin Oncol 2016; 7(4): 331-6.
[http://dx.doi.org/10.5306/wjco.v7.i4.331] [PMID: 27579253]

[167] Loibl S, Rokitta D, Conrad B, *et al.* Sorafenib in the Treatment of Early Breast Cancer: Results of the Neoadjuvant Phase II Study - SOFIA. Breast Care (Basel) 2014; 9(3): 169-74.
[http://dx.doi.org/10.1159/000363430] [PMID: 25177258]

[168] Bronte G, Andreis D, Bravaccini S, Maltoni R, Cecconetto L, Schirone A, *et al.* Sorafenib for the treatment of breast cancer. Drug Evaluation 2017; pp. 621-30.

[169] Demetri GD, van Oosterom AT, Garrett CR, *et al.* Efficacy and safety of sunitinib in patients with advanced gastrointestinal stromal tumour after failure of imatinib: a randomised controlled trial. Lancet 2006; 368(9544): 1329-38.
[http://dx.doi.org/10.1016/S0140-6736(06)69446-4] [PMID: 17046465]

[170] Sun B, Zhao X, Ding L, Meng X, Song S, Wu S. Sunitinib as salvage treatment including potent anti-tumor activity in carcinomatous ulcers for patients with multidrug-resistant metastatic breast cancer. Oncotarget 2016; 7(36): 57894-902.
[http://dx.doi.org/10.18632/oncotarget.11082] [PMID: 27506945]

[171] Elgebaly A, Menshawy A, El Ashal G, *et al.* Sunitinib alone or in combination with chemotherapy for the treatment of advanced breast cancer: A systematic review and meta-analysis. Breast Dis 2016; 36(2-3): 91-101.
[http://dx.doi.org/10.3233/BD-160218] [PMID: 27612040]

[172] Wragg JW, Heath VL, Bicknell R. Sunitinib treatment enhances metastasis of innately drug-resistant breast tumors. Cancer Res 2017; 77(4): 1008-20.
[http://dx.doi.org/10.1158/0008-5472.CAN-16-1982] [PMID: 28011623]

[173] Tamura T, Minami H, Yamada Y, *et al.* A phase I dose-escalation study of ZD6474 in Japanese patients with solid, malignant tumors. J Thorac Oncol 2006; 1(9): 1002-9.
[http://dx.doi.org/10.1097/01243894-200611000-00014] [PMID: 17409986]

[174] Miller KD, Trigo JM, Wheeler C, *et al.* A multicenter phase II trial of ZD6474, a vascular endothelial growth factor receptor-2 and epidermal growth factor receptor tyrosine kinase inhibitor, in patients with previously treated metastatic breast cancer. Clin Cancer Res 2005; 11(9): 3369-76.
[http://dx.doi.org/10.1158/1078-0432.CCR-04-1923] [PMID: 15867237]

[175] Hatem R, Labiod D, Château-Joubert S, de Plater L, El Botty R, Vacher S, *et al.* Vandetanib as a potential new treatment for estrogen receptor-negative breast cancers. Int J Cancer 2016; 15;138(10): 2510-1.
[http://dx.doi.org/10.1002/ijc.29974]

[176] Boér K, Láng I, Llombart-Cussac A, *et al.* Vandetanib with docetaxel as second-line treatment for

advanced breast cancer: a double-blind, placebo-controlled, randomized Phase II study. Invest New Drugs 2012; 30(2): 681-7.
[http://dx.doi.org/10.1007/s10637-010-9538-8] [PMID: 20830502]

[177] Gee JMW, Goddard L, Mottram HJ, Burmi RS, Pumford SL, Dutkowski CM, *et al.* Increased Ret signaling and impact of vandetanib in acquired tamoxifen-resistant breast cancer. Cancer Res 2014; 74(19): 738.

[178] Trimboli P, Castellana M, Virili C, Giorgino F, Giovanella L. Efficacy of Vandetanib in Treating Locally Advanced or Metastatic Medullary Thyroid Carcinoma According to RECIST Criteria: A Systematic Review and Meta-Analysis. Front Endocrinol (Lausanne) 2018; 3; 9: 224.
[http://dx.doi.org/10.3389/fendo.2018.00224]

[179] Friedlander M, Brooks PC, Shaffer RW, Kincaid CM, Varner JA, Cheresh DA. Definition of Two Angiogenic Pathways by Distinct alpha(v) Integrins Science (80-) [Internet] 1995; 270(5241): 1500-2. Available from:
[http://dx.doi.org/10.1126/science.270.5241.1500]

[180] Brooks PC, Strömblad S, Klemke R, Visscher D, Sarkar FH, Cheresh DA. Antiintegrin alpha v beta 3 blocks human breast cancer growth and angiogenesis in human skin. J Clin Invest 1995; 96(4): 1815-22.
[http://dx.doi.org/10.1172/JCI118227] [PMID: 7560073]

[181] Cristofanilli M, Johnston SRD, Manikhas A, *et al.* A randomized phase II study of lapatinib + pazopanib versus lapatinib in patients with HER2+ inflammatory breast cancer. Breast Cancer Res Treat 2013; 137(2): 471-82.
[http://dx.doi.org/10.1007/s10549-012-2369-x] [PMID: 23239151]

[182] Aalders KC, Tryfonidis K, Senkus E, Cardoso F. Anti-angiogenic treatment in breast cancer: Facts, successes, failures and future perspectives. Cancer Treat Rev 2017; 53: 98-110.
[http://dx.doi.org/10.1016/j.ctrv.2016.12.009] [PMID: 28088074]

[183] Siegel RL, Miller KD, Jemal A. Cancer statistics, 2015. CA Cancer J Clin 2015; 65(1): 5-29.
[http://dx.doi.org/10.3322/caac.21254] [PMID: 25559415]

[184] Bratt O, Damber JE, Emanuelsson M, Grönberg H. Hereditary prostate cancer: clinical characteristics and survival. J Urol 2002; 167(6): 2423-6.
[http://dx.doi.org/10.1016/S0022-5347(05)64997-X] [PMID: 11992050]

[185] Khandrika L, Kumar B, Koul S, Maroni P, Koul HK. Oxidative stress in prostate cancer. Cancer Lett 2009; 282(2): 125-36.
[http://dx.doi.org/10.1016/j.canlet.2008.12.011] [PMID: 19185987]

[186] McLaren ID, Jerde TJ, Bushman W. Role of interleukins, IGF and stem cells in BPH. Differentiation 2011; 82(4-5): 237-43.
[http://dx.doi.org/10.1016/j.diff.2011.06.001] [PMID: 21864972]

[187] Wilson KM, Giovannucci EL, Mucci LA. Lifestyle and dietary factors in the prevention of lethal prostate cancer. Asian J Androl 2012; 14(3): 365-74.
[http://dx.doi.org/10.1038/aja.2011.142] [PMID: 22504869]

[188] Mandair D, Rossi RE, Pericleous M, Whyand T, Caplin ME. Prostate cancer and the influence of dietary factors and supplements: a systematic review. Nutr Metab (Lond) 2014; 11(1): 30.
[http://dx.doi.org/10.1186/1743-7075-11-30] [PMID: 24976856]

[189] Cohen JH, Kristal AR, Stanford JL. Fruit and vegetable intakes and prostate cancer risk. J Natl Cancer Inst 2000; 92(1): 61-8.
[http://dx.doi.org/10.1093/jnci/92.1.61] [PMID: 10620635]

[190] Jain MG, Hislop GT, Howe GR, Ghadirian P. Plant foods, antioxidants, and prostate cancer risk: findings from case-control studies in Canada. Nutr Cancer 1999; 34(2): 173-84.
[http://dx.doi.org/10.1207/S15327914NC3402_8] [PMID: 10578485]

[191] Michaud DS, Augustsson K, Rimm EB, Stampfer MJ, Willet WC, Giovannucci E. A prospective study on intake of animal products and risk of prostate cancer. Cancer Causes Control 2001; 12(6): 557-67. [http://dx.doi.org/10.1023/A:1011256201044] [PMID: 11519764]

[192] Veierød MB, Laake P, Thelle DS. Dietary fat intake and risk of prostate cancer: a prospective study of 25,708 Norwegian men. Int J Cancer 1997; 73(5): 634-8. [http://dx.doi.org/10.1002/(SICI)1097-0215(19971127)73:5<634::AID-IJC4>3.0.CO;2-Y] [PMID: 9398038]

[193] Rostoka E, Baumane L, Isajevs S, Line A, Silina K, Dzintare M, *et al.* Effects of Indole-3-Carbinol and Flavonoids Administered Separately and in Combination on Nitric Oxide Production and iNOS Expression in Rats. Chin Med 2010; 01(01): 5-17. [http://dx.doi.org/10.4236/cm.2010.11002]

[194] Elenbaas B, Weinberg RA. Heterotypic signaling between epithelial tumor cells and fibroblasts in carcinoma formation. Exp Cell Res 2001; 264(1): 169-84. [http://dx.doi.org/10.1006/excr.2000.5133] [PMID: 11237532]

[195] Kimura H, Esumi H. Reciprocal regulation between nitric oxide and vascular endothelial growth factor in angiogenesis. Acta Biochim Pol 2003; 50(1): 49-59.http://www.ncbi.nlm.nih.gov/pubmed/12673346 [PMID: 12673346]

[196] Alexanian A, Miller B, Chesnik M, Mirza S, Sorokin A. Post-translational regulation of COX2 activity by FYN in prostate cancer cells. Oncotarget 2014; 5(12): 4232-43. [http://dx.doi.org/10.18632/oncotarget.1983] [PMID: 24970799]

[197] Shappell SB, Boeglin WE, Olson SJ, Kasper S, Brash AR. 15-lipoxygenase-2 (15-LOX-2) is expressed in benign prostatic epithelium and reduced in prostate adenocarcinoma. Am J Pathol 1999; 155(1): 235-45. [http://dx.doi.org/10.1016/S0002-9440(10)65117-6] [PMID: 10393855]

[198] Xinhua L, Kirschenbaum A, Yao S, Lee R, Holland JF, Levine AC. Inhibition of cyclooxygenase-2 suppresses angiogenesis and the growth of prostate cancer *in vivo* J Urol 2000; 164(3 Part 1): 820-5. [http://dx.doi.org/10.1016/s0022-5347(05) 67321-1]

[199] Tang DG, Honn KV. 12-Lipoxygenase, 12(S)-HETE, and Cancer Metastasis Ann N Y Acad Sci 1994; 744(1 Cellular Gene): 199-215. [http://dx.doi.org/10.1111/j.1749-6632.1994.tb52738.x]

[200] Nie D, Hillman GG, Geddes T, Tang K, Pierson C, Grignon DJ, *et al.* Platelet-Type 12-Lipoxygenase Regulates Angiogenesis in Human Prostate Carcinoma. Springer, US: Advances in Experimental Medicine and Biology 1999; pp. 623-30. Internet [http://dx.doi.org/10.1007/978-1-4615-4793-8_90]

[201] Kelavkar UP, Nixon JB, Cohen C, Dillehay D, Eling TE, Badr KF. Overexpression of 15-lipoxygenase-1 in PC-3 human prostate cancer cells increases tumorigenesis. Carcinogenesis 2001; 22(11): 1765-73. [http://dx.doi.org/10.1093/carcin/22.11.1765] [PMID: 11698337]

[202] Charlier C, Michaux C. Dual inhibition of cyclooxygenase-2 (COX-2) and 5-lipoxygenase (5-LOX) as a new strategy to provide safer non-steroidal anti-inflammatory drugs. Eur J Med Chem 2003; 38(7-8): 645-59. [http://dx.doi.org/10.1016/S0223-5234(03)00115-6] [PMID: 12932896]

[203] Kohli P, Levy BD. Resolvins and protectins: mediating solutions to inflammation. Br J Pharmacol 2009; 158(4): 960-71. [http://dx.doi.org/10.1111/j.1476-5381.2009.00290.x] [PMID: 19594757]

[204] Krupski T, Harding MA, Herce ME, Gulding KM, Stoler MH, Theodorescu D. The role of vascular endothelial growth factor in the tissue specific *in vivo* growth of prostate cancer cells. Growth Factors

2001; 18(4): 287-302.
[http://dx.doi.org/10.3109/08977190109029117] [PMID: 11519827]

[205] Hernández-Agudo E, Mondejar T, Soto-Montenegro ML, *et al.* Monitoring vascular normalization induced by antiangiogenic treatment with (18)F-fluoromisonidazole-PET. Mol Oncol 2016; 10(5): 704-18.
[http://dx.doi.org/10.1016/j.molonc.2015.12.011] [PMID: 26778791]

[206] Rickles FR. Mechanisms of cancer-induced thrombosis in cancer. Pathophysiol Haemost Thromb 2006; 35(1-2): 103-10.
[http://dx.doi.org/10.1159/000093551] [PMID: 16855354]

[207] Daniel TO, Gibbs VC, Milfay DF, Garovoy MR, Williams LT. Thrombin stimulates c-sis gene expression in microvascular endothelial cells. J Biol Chem 1986; 261(21): 9579-82.http://www.ncbi.nlm.nih.gov/pubmed/2426251
[PMID: 2426251]

[208] Papadimitriou E, Manolopoulos VG, Hayman GT, *et al.* Thrombin modulates vectorial secretion of extracellular matrix proteins in cultured endothelial cells. Am J Physiol 1997; 272(4 Pt 1): C1112-22.
[http://dx.doi.org/10.1152/ajpcell.1997.272.4.C1112] [PMID: 9142835]

[209] Rickles FR, Falanga A. Molecular basis for the relationship between thrombosis and cancer. Thromb Res 2001; 102(6): V215-24.
[http://dx.doi.org/10.1016/S0049-3848(01)00285-7] [PMID: 11516455]

[210] Rickles FR, Patierno S, Fernandez PM. Tissue factor, thrombin, and cancer. Chest 2003; 124(3) (Suppl.): 58S-68S.
[http://dx.doi.org/10.1378/chest.124.3_suppl.58S] [PMID: 12970125]

[211] Kröger K, Weiland D, Ose C, *et al.* Risk factors for venous thromboembolic events in cancer patients. Ann Oncol 2006; 17(2): 297-303.
[http://dx.doi.org/10.1093/annonc/mdj068] [PMID: 16282243]

[212] Silverstein MD, Heit JA, Mohr DN, Petterson TM, O'Fallon WM, Melton LJ III. Trends in the incidence of deep vein thrombosis and pulmonary embolism: a 25-year population-based study. Arch Intern Med 1998; 158(6): 585-93.
[http://dx.doi.org/10.1001/archinte.158.6.585] [PMID: 9521222]

[213] Sørensen HT, Mellemkjaer L, Olsen JH, Baron JA. Prognosis of cancers associated with venous thromboembolism. N Engl J Med 2000; 343(25): 1846-50.
[http://dx.doi.org/10.1056/NEJM200012213432504] [PMID: 11117976]

[214] Prandoni P, Lensing AW, Bagatella P, Simioni P, Girolami A. Low rate of warfarin-related major bleeding in patients with recurrent venous thromboembolism. Thromb Haemost 1999; 82(1): 158-9.
[http://dx.doi.org/10.1055/s-0037-1614653] [PMID: 10456478]

[215] Lyman GH, Culakova E, Poniewierski MS, Kuderer NM. Morbidity, mortality and costs associated with venous thromboembolism in hospitalized patients with cancer. Thromb Res 2018; 164 (Suppl. 1): S112-8.
[http://dx.doi.org/10.1016/j.thromres.2018.01.028] [PMID: 29703467]

[216] Budhiparama NC, Abdel MP, Ifran NN, Parratte S. Venous Thromboembolism (VTE) Prophylaxis for Hip and Knee Arthroplasty: Changing Trends. Curr Rev Musculoskelet Med 2014; 7(2): 108-16.
[http://dx.doi.org/10.1007/s12178-014-9207-1] [PMID: 24706152]

[217] Kappelle LJ. Preventing deep vein thrombosis after stroke: strategies and recommendations. Curr Treat Options Neurol 2011; 13(6): 629-35.
[http://dx.doi.org/10.1007/s11940-011-0147-4] [PMID: 21909622]

[218] Fareed J, Adiguzel C, Thethi I. Differentiation of parenteral anticoagulants in the prevention and treatment of venous thromboembolism. Thromb J 2011; 9(1): 5.
[http://dx.doi.org/10.1186/1477-9560-9-5] [PMID: 21443789]

[219] Junqueira DR, Zorzela LM, Perini E. Unfractionated heparin versus low molecular weight heparins for avoiding heparin-induced thrombocytopenia in postoperative patients. Cochrane Database Syst Rev 2017; 4CD007557
[http://dx.doi.org/10.1002/14651858.CD007557.pub3] [PMID: 28431186]

[220] Solayar GN, Shannon FJ. Thromboprophylaxis and orthopaedic surgery: options and current guidelines. Malays J Med Sci 2014; 21(3): 71-7.
[PMID: 25246838]

[221] Sidhu PS. QSAR Study of Thiophene-Anthranilamides Based Factor Xa Direct Inhibitors. Postdoc J 2014.
[http://dx.doi.org/10.14304/SURYA.JPR.V2N3.4]

[222] Rai R, Sprengeler PA, Elrod KC, Young WB. Perspectives on factor Xa inhibition. Curr Med Chem 2001; 8(2): 101-19.
[http://dx.doi.org/10.2174/0929867013373822] [PMID: 11172669]

[223] Isayeva T, Chanda D, Kallman L, Eltoum ie, Ponnazhagan S. Effects of sustained antiangiogenic therapy in multistage prostate cancer in TRAMP model. Cancer Res 2007; 67(12): 5789-97.
[http://dx.doi.org/10.1158/0008-5472.CAN-06-3637] [PMID: 17575146]

[224] Zurita AJ, George DJ, Shore ND, *et al.* Sunitinib in combination with docetaxel and prednisone in chemotherapy-naive patients with metastatic, castration-resistant prostate cancer: a phase 1/2 clinical trial. Ann Oncol 2012; 23(3): 688-94.
[http://dx.doi.org/10.1093/annonc/mdr349] [PMID: 21821830]

[225] Kelly WK, Halabi S, Carducci M, *et al.* Randomized, double-blind, placebo-controlled phase III trial comparing docetaxel and prednisone with or without bevacizumab in men with metastatic castration-resistant prostate cancer: CALGB 90401. J Clin Oncol 2012; 30(13): 1534-40.
[http://dx.doi.org/10.1200/JCO.2011.39.4767] [PMID: 22454414]

[226] Tannock IF, Fizazi K, Ivanov S, *et al.* VENICE investigators. Aflibercept versus placebo in combination with docetaxel and prednisone for treatment of men with metastatic castration-resistant prostate cancer (VENICE): a phase 3, double-blind randomised trial. Lancet Oncol 2013; 14(8): 760-8.
[http://dx.doi.org/10.1016/S1470-2045(13)70184-0] [PMID: 23742877]

[227] Azad AA, Beardsley EK, Hotte SJ, *et al.* A randomized phase II efficacy and safety study of vandetanib (ZD6474) in combination with bicalutamide versus bicalutamide alone in patients with chemotherapy naïve castration-resistant prostate cancer. Invest New Drugs 2014; 32(4): 746-52.
[http://dx.doi.org/10.1007/s10637-014-0091-8] [PMID: 24671507]

[228] Shariat SF, Anwuri VA, Lamb DJ, Shah NV, Wheeler TM, Slawin KM. Association of preoperative plasma levels of vascular endothelial growth factor and soluble vascular cell adhesion molecule-1 with lymph node status and biochemical progression after radical prostatectomy. J Clin Oncol 2004; 22(9): 1655-63.
[http://dx.doi.org/10.1200/JCO.2004.09.142] [PMID: 15117988]

[229] Borre M, Offersen BV, Nerstrøm B, Overgaard J. Microvessel density predicts survival in prostate cancer patients subjected to watchful waiting. Br J Cancer 1998; 78(7): 940-4.
[http://dx.doi.org/10.1038/bjc.1998.605] [PMID: 9764587]

[230] Borre M, Bentzen SM, Nerstrøm B, Overgaard J. Tumor cell proliferation and survival in patients with prostate cancer followed expectantly. J Urol 1998; 159(5): 1609-14.
[http://dx.doi.org/10.1097/00005392-199805000-00054] [PMID: 9554364]

[231] Bostwick DG, Wheeler TM, Blute M, *et al.* Optimized microvessel density analysis improves prediction of cancer stage from prostate needle biopsies. Urology 1996; 48(1): 47-57.
[http://dx.doi.org/10.1016/S0090-4295(96)00149-5] [PMID: 8693651]

[232] Mucci LA, Powolny A, Giovannucci E, *et al.* Prospective study of prostate tumor angiogenesis and cancer-specific mortality in the health professionals follow-up study. J Clin Oncol 2009; 27(33): 5627-

33.
[http://dx.doi.org/10.1200/JCO.2008.20.8876] [PMID: 19858401]

[233] Dredge K, Marriott JB, Macdonald CD, *et al.* Novel thalidomide analogues display anti-angiogenic activity independently of immunomodulatory effects. Br J Cancer 2002; 87(10): 1166-72.
[http://dx.doi.org/10.1038/sj.bjc.6600607] [PMID: 12402158]

[234] Figg WD, Dahut W, Duray P, *et al.* A randomized phase II trial of thalidomide, an angiogenesis inhibitor, in patients with androgen-independent prostate cancer. Clin Cancer Res 2001; 7(7): 1888-93.
[PMID: 11448901]

[235] Figg WD, Arlen P, Gulley J, *et al.* A randomized phase II trial of docetaxel (taxotere) plus thalidomide in androgen-independent prostate cancer. Semin Oncol 2001; 28(4) (Suppl. 15): 62-6.
[http://dx.doi.org/10.1016/S0093-7754(01)90157-5] [PMID: 11685731]

[236] Dahut WL, Gulley JL, Arlen PM, *et al.* Randomized phase II trial of docetaxel plus thalidomide in androgen-independent prostate cancer. J Clin Oncol 2004; 22(13): 2532-9.
[http://dx.doi.org/10.1200/JCO.2004.05.074] [PMID: 15226321]

[237] Figg WD, Retter A, Steinberg SM, Dahut WL. In reply. J Clin Oncol 2005; 23(9): 2113-4.
[http://dx.doi.org/10.1200/JCO.2005.05.296] [PMID: 15774812]

[238] Petrylak DP, Resto-Garces K, Tibyan M, Mohile SG. A phase I open-label study using lenalidomide and docetaxel in castration-resistant prostate cancer. J Clin Oncol 2009; 27(Suppl.15) Abs 5156.

[239] Phase A. 2 Trial of Bevacizumab, Lenalidomide, Docetaxel, and Prednisone (ART-P) for Treatment of Metastatic Castrate-Resistant Prostate Cancer. October. 2009.

[240] Docetaxel and Prednisone With or Without Bevacizumab in Treating Patients with Prostate Cancer That Did Not Respond to Hormone Therapy October 2009,. http://clinicaltrials.gov/ct2/show/NCT00110214?term=prostate+avastin+ docetaxel&rank=3www.aua2009.org/program /lbsciforum.asp

[241] Kelly WK, Halabi S, Carducci M, *et al.* Randomized, double-blind, placebo-controlled phase III trial comparing docetaxel and prednisone with or without bevacizumab in men with metastatic castration-resistant prostate cancer: CALGB 90401. J Clin Oncol 2012; 30(13): 1534-40.
[http://dx.doi.org/10.1200/JCO.2011.39.4767] [PMID: 22454414]

[242] Patel JN, Jiang C, Hertz DL, *et al.* Bevacizumab and the risk of arterial and venous thromboembolism in patients with metastatic, castration-resistant prostate cancer treated on Cancer and Leukemia Group B (CALGB) 90401 (Alliance). Cancer 2015; 121(7): 1025-31.
[http://dx.doi.org/10.1002/cncr.29169] [PMID: 25417775]

[243] Hertz DL, Owzar K, Halabi S, Kelly WK, Zembutsu H, Jiang C, *et al.* A Genome-Wide Association Study (GWAS) of Docetaxel-Induced Peripheral Neuropathy in CALGB 90401 (Alliance). 2013 ASCO Annual Meeting J Clin Oncol. 31 (suppl; abstr 11053).

[244] Hertz DL, Jiang C, Owzar K, Halabi S, Kelly WK, Mulkey F, *et al.* A Genome-Wide Association Study (GWAS) of Docetaxel-Induced Neutropenia in CALGB 90401/60404 (Alliance). 2014 ASCO Annual Meeting J Clin Oncol. 32 5s (suppl; abstr 9612)

[245] Chu QS-C. Aflibercept (AVE0005): an alternative strategy for inhibiting tumour angiogenesis by vascular endothelial growth factors. Expert Opin Biol Ther 2009; 9(2): 263-71.
[http://dx.doi.org/10.1517/14712590802666397] [PMID: 19236257]

[246] Aflibercept in Combination with Docetaxel in Metastatic Androgen Independent Prostate Cancer (VENICE) 10/2009;. www.clinicaltrials.gov/ct2/show/NCT00519285? term= Aflibercept+prostate&rank=1

[247] Wilhelm S, Chien D-S. BAY 43-9006: preclinical data. Curr Pharm Des 2002; 8(25): 2255-7.
[http://dx.doi.org/10.2174/1381612023393026] [PMID: 12369853]

[248] Dahut WL, Scripture C, Posadas E, *et al.* A phase II clinical trial of sorafenib in androgen-independent prostate cancer. Clin Cancer Res 2008; 14(1): 209-14.
[http://dx.doi.org/10.1158/1078-0432.CCR-07-1355] [PMID: 18172272]

[249] Aragon-Ching JB, Jain L, Gulley JL, *et al.* Final analysis of a phase II trial using sorafenib for metastatic castration-resistant prostate cancer. BJU Int 2009; 103(12): 1636-40.
[http://dx.doi.org/10.1111/j.1464-410X.2008.08327.x] [PMID: 19154507]

[250] Chi KN, Ellard SL, Hotte SJ, *et al.* A phase II study of sorafenib in patients with chemo-naive castration-resistant prostate cancer. Ann Oncol 2008; 19(4): 746-51.
[http://dx.doi.org/10.1093/annonc/mdm554] [PMID: 18056648]

[251] Colloca G, Checcaglini F, Venturino A. About sorafenib in castration-resistant prostate cancer. Ann Oncol 2008; 19(10): 1812-3.
[http://dx.doi.org/10.1093/annonc/mdn546] [PMID: 18689865]

[252] Chi KN. Seymour l. Reply to the letter - About sorafenib in castration-resistant prostate cancer by G. Colloca, F. Checcaglini, and A. Venturino. Ann Oncol 2008; 19(10): 1813-4.
[http://dx.doi.org/10.1093/annonc/mdn549]

[253] Steinbild S, Mross K, Frost A, *et al.* A clinical phase II study with sorafenib in patients with progressive hormone-refractory prostate cancer: a study of the CESAR Central European Society for Anticancer Drug Research-EWIV. Br J Cancer 2007; 97(11): 1480-5.
[http://dx.doi.org/10.1038/sj.bjc.6604064] [PMID: 18040273]

[254] Safarinejad MR. Safety and efficacy of sorafenib in patients with castrate resistant prostate cancer: a Phase II study. Urol Oncol 2010; 28(1): 21-7.
[http://dx.doi.org/10.1016/j.urolonc.2008.06.003] [PMID: 18789732]

[255] Ryan CJ, Stadler WM, Roth B, *et al.* Phase I dose escalation and pharmacokinetic study of AZD2171, an inhibitor of the vascular endothelial growth factor receptor tyrosine kinase, in patients with hormone refractory prostate cancer (HRPC). Invest New Drugs 2007; 25(5): 445-51.
[http://dx.doi.org/10.1007/s10637-007-9050-y] [PMID: 17458505]

[256] Karakunnel JJ, Gulley JL, Arlen PM, *et al.* Phase II trial of cediranib (AZD2171) in docetaxel-resistant, castrate-resistant prostate cancer (CRPC). J Clin Oncol 2008; 26(Sup 15) abs 5136.

[257] Yang Y, Zhang Y, Cao Z, *et al.* Anti-VEGF- and anti-VEGF receptor-induced vascular alteration in mouse healthy tissues. Proc Natl Acad Sci USA 2013; 110(29): 12018-23.
[http://dx.doi.org/10.1073/pnas.1301331110] [PMID: 23818623]

[258] Perren TJ, Swart AM, Pfisterer J, *et al.* ICON7 Investigators. A phase 3 trial of bevacizumab in ovarian cancer. N Engl J Med 2011; 365(26): 2484-96.
[http://dx.doi.org/10.1056/NEJMoa1103799] [PMID: 22204725]

[259] Tol J, Koopman M, Cats A, *et al.* Chemotherapy, bevacizumab, and cetuximab in metastatic colorectal cancer. N Engl J Med 2009; 360(6): 563-72.
[http://dx.doi.org/10.1056/NEJMoa0808268] [PMID: 19196673]

CHAPTER 3

Microbe-based Antiangiogenesis Therapies for Cancer Management

Samman Munir[1], **Usman Ali Ashfaq**[1], **Asad Ali Shah**[1], **Muhammad Shahid**[1], **Muhammad Sajid Hamid Akash**[2] and **Mohsin Khurshid**[3,*]

[1] *Department of Bioinformatics & Biotechnology, Government College University Faisalabad, Pakistan*

[2] *Department of Pharmaceutical Chemistry, Government College University Faisalabad, Pakistan*

[3] *Department of Microbiology, Government College University Faisalabad, Pakistan*

Abstract: The recent scientific advancements have aroused the attention towards the role of microbes in the therapeutic management of various maladies that have transformed the pharmaceutical research. Although certain bacteria are widely known to cause cancer, recent research has shown exciting outcomes signifying the role of bacteria as an effective therapeutic agent for cancer. Different bacterial strains have been scrutinized for their inherent potentials to colonize the tumors environment and subsequent oncolytic properties in animal models. Moreover, their inherent anti-cancer properties can be boosted through genetic engineering, which allows the bacterial species to transfer the therapeutic molecules into tumor cells. During the previous few years, the studies have focused on the use of genetically modified bacteria for cancer therapy with an emphasis on blocking tumor angiogenesis. Although the studies regarding the microbial-based anti-angiogenesis therapy for cancer management are quite a few, it seems to be an innovative and attractive approach, particularly for solid tumors which usually possess increased vascularization. This chapter aimed to provide recent information relating to the candidates for anti-angiogenesis therapy, including angiostatin, tumstatin, endostatin, interleukin-12, metargidin peptide with a focus on recent developments in the newly identified field of microbe-based angiogenesis suppression. The advanced approaches for the use of modified bacteria as anti-cancer therapeutics have been discussed, particularly the DNA vaccination, bactofection, alternative gene therapy, and RNA interference with an emphasis on their anti-angiogenesis potential.

* **Corresponding author Mohsin Khurshid:** Department of Microbiology, Government College University Faisalabad, Pakistan; E-mail: mohsin.mic@gmail.com

Atta-ur-Rahman & M. Iqbal Choudhary (Eds.)

Keywords: Angiogenesis, Gene therapy, RNA Interference, Tumor vaccines, Vascularization.

INTRODUCTION

Regardless of the development in cancer diagnosis and therapy, cancer has been retained as a leading health issue and considered as the primary cause of death throughout the world. Approximately, 0.6 million deaths were estimated within the US, in the year 2016, from a total of 16,00000 reported cases of cancer [1]. Likewise, almost 3,000,000 deaths were projected within China, in the year 2015, from a total of 4,000,000 reported cases of cancer [2]. Different treatment therapies are available for cancer, although the selection of therapy involves various factors, for example, the tumor type, time of detection along with the capability of the patient to endure the prescribed therapy [3]. Currently, surgical treatments are combined with radiotherapy and chemotherapy to prevent the growth of undetectable tumors after the completion of surgical resection [4]. However, these traditional techniques for the treatment of cancer possess poor bioavailability, specificity, and dosage sensitivity. Moreover, such techniques do not completely distinguish the normal cells and cancer cells [5].

One borderland, in the battle against cancer cells, is the regulation of the angiogenesis, *i.e* ., the development of new vasculature. Targeting the angiogenesis can serve as an effective technique for the prevention as well as the formation of new vasculature and is also an important modality to normalize the tumor-associated vessels. Therefore, it can inhibit the formation of tumor cells and can act as a potential therapeutic theory for cancer treatment [6, 7].

The first contemporary attempt for using bacteria as a therapeutic purpose was made almost forty centuries ago. It is now clear that bacteria can dominantly replicate within solid tumors [8]. The first evidence of this fact originated in the 19th century and these outcomes remained mysterious till the 20th century when an oncolytic bacteria, responsible for the host cell lysing, was first investigated by different research groups [9, 10]. Therefore, the apparent drawbacks of conventional therapies can be overcome through the potential applications of facultative and obligate anaerobic strains of bacteria. Furthermore, using the bacterial system as therapeutic options can be improved through genetic engineering, which renders them a very promising tool for the targeted transfer of genes and their products. The precise advantages of utilizing bacteria as anticancer therapy involve the intrinsic oncolytic capability of several species or strains, directly targeting the tumor tissues along with the simplicity of eradication and regulation.

Regardless of recent advancements, few recent investigations regarding bacterial therapy have particularly focused on antiangiogenic therapy. In this chapter, we explain the nature of the tumor vasculature and how these antiangiogenic drugs can be used in view of their advantages. We also summarize the latest studies of cancer therapy employing bacterial strains with a specific focus on their prospects as tumor angiogenesis inhibitors. Further, the critical areas, along with the future targets of bacteria-based therapies have also been discussed.

TUMOR ANGIOGENESIS

In 1971, a hypothesis was proposed by Folkman that the process of angiogenesis is necessary for the growth as well as the development of the solid tumors above 1-2mm3 size [11]. Afterward, they exhibited certain incomplete proof to signify that the solid tumors are dependent on the neo-vascularization for constant growth [12]. Thereafter, the antiangiogenic approach, which can evolve as an innovative therapeutic technique, became a spotlight for the research groups [13]. Simultaneously, the complicated process of angiogenesis has now been progressively studied, owing to a lot of efforts that have been made into this area of investigation. The angiogenesis process is based on the dynamic homeostasis, strictly controlled by various anti and pro-angiogenic factors. If this homeostasis is disturbed then the 'angiogenic switch' that is connected with the phenotype will be activated and the process of angiogenesis will initiate [14].

Through several investigations, the tumor angiogenesis has extensively been studied and various kinds of regulators have been described [15, 16]. These regulating factors are released from the stromal cells, endothelial cells (ECs), blood cells, extracellular matrix, and tumor cells [17, 18]. These angiogenesis factors can co-exist or else, switch with another during the proliferation and growth of tumors [19, 20]. Several widely known proangiogenic factors include the VEGF (vascular endothelium growth factor), bFGF (basic-fibroblast growth factor), epidermal growth factor, transforming growth factor-alpha and beta, angiopoietin-1 and-2, and platelet-derived growth factor. Certain, frequently examined antiangiogenic factors include tumstatin, angiostatin, interleukin-12, endostatin, interferon-alpha, interferon-beta, interferon-gamma, and thrombospondin-1. Different biological events activate the angiogenic switch including the metabolic stress like hypoxia, hypoglycemia and low pH. Moreover, genetic mutations such as loss of the tumor-suppressing genes or triggering of oncogenes which regulate the synthesis of angiogenesis factors, inflammatory or immune response *i.e* . inflammatory or immune cells which have penetrated into tissue and mechanical stress like pressure produced by various proliferating cells are all vital stimuli of the angiogenic signaling pathway and possess the tendency to cause the tumor development [21]. Among these, hypoxia is classified as the major factor which direct tumor angiogenesis, producing increased VEGF expression along with the other stimulators of angiogenesis from the hypoxic cells [22]. Concomitantly, the extracellular matrix (ECM) remodeling enzymes, specifically matrix metalloproteinases, regulate several changes within the tumor microenvironment (TME) through the degradation of ECM [23]. Upon the hypoxia-induced upregulation of VEGF, the angiogenesis is started with further activation of the HIF (hypoxia inaudible factor) signaling that activates the ECs of pre-existing blood vessels to develop and migrate within hypoxic tissues [24]. Consequently, the ECs are differentiated in various cell types, involving the tip, tube, and stalk cells [25]. During further vascular formation, the progenitor cells of endothelial are responsible for the development of the inner layer in the new vasculature, with pericytes, for example specified muscle cells that stabilize the tubes of vessels by providing the structural support along with the formation of outer layer over the ECs [26]. Afterward, the ECs attach to one another for the formation of continuous endothelium, which is indicated by the complex tight junctions along with the formation of loops that permit the blood circulation within adhesion molecules, accompanied by the production of the basement membrane [27]. Lastly, the vessel becomes mature as well as capable of transferring the oxygen along with the nutrition to fulfill the needs of hypoxic tissues [28].

TUMOR MICROENVIRONMENT

A solid tumor is homogenous in rare instances, rather, it possesses a different microenvironment, which can strongly affect the therapeutic procedures. Probably the well-studied component of the tumor microenvironment (TME) is the occurrence of hypoxia or low oxygen level [29]. An aggressive tumor mostly does not have an adequate supply of blood, partially due to the fast growth of tumor cells in comparison to endothelial cells (ECs), which forms the lining of blood vessels and partly due to the disorganized supply of newly formed blood vessels [30]. This leads to nutrient deprivation and acidity, along with the hypoxic regions within TME. The tumors usually have a microenvironment with the oxygen level of below 2.5 mmHg. the concentration where cells are threefold resistant to the radiations in comparison to the aerated cells. The regions of tumor hypoxia have lesser sensitivity for ionizing radiations since their effects depend upon oxygen; they also have less sensitivity for chemotherapeutic drugs because the agent concentration in these areas could be suboptimal [29]. The regions of tumor hypoxia have a poor supply of blood vessels and their treatment with traditional anticancer drugs is not easy. The hypoxia also results in more malignant phenotype, for example, apoptosis, metastasis, angiogenesis, and genetic stability [31]. Therefore, hypoxia is believed to be a major obstacle in treatment. In different studies, the anaerobic and the facultative anaerobic bacteria have been used for the administration of anticancer drugs owing to their selective mode of growth in necrotic or hypoxic areas of the tumors. The bacteria can actively move out of the blood vessels and penetrate the necrotic area of solid tumors.

VASCULAR NORMALIZATION

The body maintains the balance between pro-angiogenic and anti-angiogenic regulators within normal tissues. The excess formation of angiogenic regulators, such as VEGF or decreased production of the angiogenic inhibitors, for example, thrombospondin-1, can lead to the formation of various kinds of infectious diseases, inflammations, and malignancies [32]. The maintenance of the angiogenic regulators can result in the reduction of interstitial fluid pressure (IFP) along with improved tumor oxygenation, hence ultimately improving the drug distribution within the targeted tissues [33]. Usually, a normal vasculature carries less intricate, less dilated, and less leaky blood vessels that have a properly structured and firm basement membrane. Studying the molecular pattern of these alternate methods of vessel growth could be extremely useful to improve the effectiveness of antiangiogenic therapy [34]. Significant success has been made in the past two decades. The VEGF pathway has been directed to stimulate the vessel normalization within tumors, cutting the unessential immature blood vessels, enhanced perfusion, decreased blood vessel diameter, and tortuosity [35]. The latest research has exhibited that blocking the placental-growth factor that is a member of the VEGF family, normalized the vessels of the tumor within models of hepatocellular carcinoma up to a certain extent by the decrease in vessel tortuosity along with the formation of hypoperfusion in the string vessels [36]. The results validated that this kind of blockage can sequentially enhance the effectiveness of VEGF directed therapy [37].

The other factors, for example, angiopoietin family, nitric oxide, integrins family, can also be suppressed and eventually participate in regulating the vessel normalization [38 - 40]. Moreover, numerous other agents responsible for vascular normalization involving numerous proteolytic enzymes exhibit their potential effects *via* indirect antiangiogenic action. For instance, the trastuzumab has the capability to mimic the anti-angiogenesis and hence, considerably reduce the diameter, volume as well as the tumor cells permeability along with the generation of more networks [41]. Therefore, the angiogenic pathways can be targeted with antiangiogenic drugs that will enhance the vessel normalization, rendering them more capable for the transport of drugs as well as oxygen.

BASIS OF ANTI-ANGIOGENESIS THERAPY

Currently, the antiangiogenic therapies for cancer have mainly adopted the two principles *i.e* . gene blockage and gene augmentation. The first one inhibits the overexpression of the proangiogenic genes within ECs and several other tumor cells, while the second one introduces the exogenous genes for anti-angiogenesis in the target cells ensuring the termination of tumor angiogenesis as a result of their expression. Hence, the particular genes can be divided into corresponding categories: pro-angiogenic genes used for gene blockage; and the antiangiogenic genes employed for gene therapy.

Current Antiangiogenic Agents

The antiangiogenic drugs currently being employed either as anticancer therapeutic agents or entering clinical trials are produced with the objective of preventing the access of tumor cells to the nutrients through the eradication of vessels in various tumor types along with the inhibition of new vasculature formation [42, 43]. Owing to the central role of vessels in the whole process, one evident benefit of the antiangiogenic treatment could be that a few steps can be compromised, specifically within primary tumors, for example by destroying the immature blood vessels to suppress or prevent the intravasation, and in the distant areas, for example, hindrance of angiogenic switch during vascular metastasis. The approved Antiangiogenic drugs for the treatment of different cancers are shown in Table 1.

Table 1. Approved Antiangiogenic drugs for Cancer therapy

Clinical Condition	Drugs	References
Lungs Cancer	Sunitinib, Bevacizumab, Endostatin, Erlotinib, Nintedanib, Gefitinib, Cediranib, and Axitinib.	[199, 200]
Ovarian Cancer	Bevacizumab, Sorafenib and Pazopanib	[201, 202]
Colorectal Cancer	Aflibercept, Bevacizumab, Endostatin, Regorafenib, Vatalanib, Brivanib, Cetuximab and Cediranib	[203 - 205]
Breast Cancer	Axitnib and Bevacizumab	[200]
Hepatocellular Carcinoma	Sorafenib, Sunitinib, Erlotinib and Brivanib	[206, 207]
Glioblastoma Cancer	Cediranib and Bevacizumab	[205]
Renal Cancer	Pazopanib, Sunitinib, Axitinib, Bevacizumab, Temsirolimus and Sorafenib	[208, 209]
Prostate Cancer	Sunitinib, Aflibercept and Bevacizumab	[210]
Thyroid Cancer	Pazopanib, Sorafenib, Axitnib, and Vandetanib	[200, 211]
Pancreatic Cancer	Erlotinib, Sunitinib, and Axitnib	[200, 212]
Malignant Melanoma Cancer	Endostatin and Dasatinib	[213, 214]
Gastric Cancer	Cetuximab	[215]

Moreover, the vascular pruning as the potent antiangiogenic strategy can successfully enhance the effectiveness of chemotherapeutic agents in various ways, such as, by partially normalizing the vessels associated with tumor through the differentiation among tumor cells and tumor linked vessels along with their enhanced bioavailability, improved drug delivery and selective targeting of tumor sites [44, 45].

The VEGF activity is usually inhibited by the humanized monoclonal antibody called bevacizumab or Avastin [46]. In comparison to the placebo, the bevacizumab more efficiently delayed the progression period within patients of kidney cancer [47]. Because of its enhanced effectiveness, as validated by the phase II clinical tests, a concomitant therapy involving irinotecan along with bevacizumab is strongly advised and has been authorized for the management of recurrent glioblastoma [48]. Another investigation has exhibited that combining chemotherapy with VEGF inhibitors successfully extended the life of patients affected with colorectal carcinoma, metastatic breast carcinoma, and lung carcinoma [49]. Nevertheless, the clinical studies have exposed that bevacizumab as a single agent is less efficient as compared to concomitant therapy and also involved in arterial and venous thrombosis, hypertension, and bleeding [50]. Furthermore, Avastin does not work immediately to block the process of angiogenesis but instead treats the condition of disease by normalizing the tumor vessels [45]. The signaling pathway of VEGF can be blocked by inhibiting the PDGF as well as VEGF with the usage of a small agent, such as TKI (tyrosine kinase inhibitor). So far, four distinct inhibitors for various applications have been authorized by the FDA: pazopanib and sunitinib for renal cell cancer and gastrointestinal tumor, vandetanib for thyroid cancer and sorafenib for hepatocellular cancer [34]. Numerous other drugs are also under clinical studies.

Regardless of the major developments in a clinical study of the antiangiogenic suppressors, a suitable dosing pattern along with the time period of VEGFR for the management of cancer cells is still to be demonstrated in clinical studies. Earlier investigations have revealed that inhibitors of angiogenesis, like TKI, are usually not capable of getting access to tumor-associated vasculature hence, these inhibitors sometimes show an inadequate biodistribution along with the pharmacokinetic profile besides having serious side effects [51, 52]. Moreover, these inhibitors have developed resistance along with the improved invasiveness during therapy, which has restricted effects on OS and validated biomarkers are not available to monitor the response against the treatment. The mechanism of action of various angiogenesis inhibitors is shown in Fig. (1).

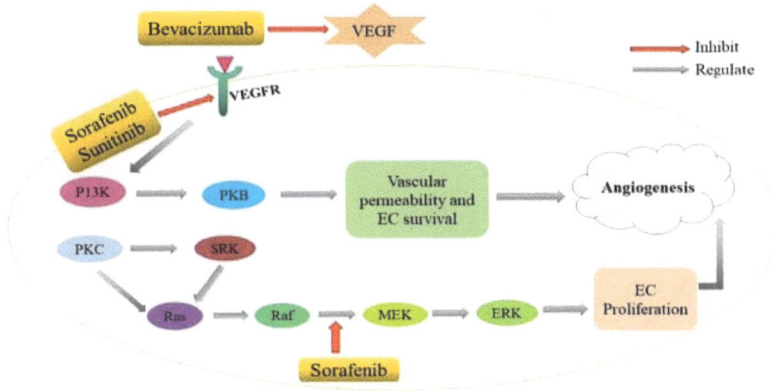

Fig. (1). The mechanism of action of various angiogenesis inhibitors. The bevacizumab binds with the VEGF, which results in its inability to activate the VEGF receptors. The sorafenib and sunitinib inhibit the VEGF receptors. The sorafenib can also act on the downstream pathway.

GENE THERAPY USING ANGIOGENESIS INHIBITORS

Gene therapy is an experimental approach that is used to prevent the diseases through the transfer of exogenous DNA into an individual cell that can alter or improve the defective gene, otherwise cause cell death. Overall, there are four different techniques that are used in gene therapy, comprising gene augmentation, gene replacement, gene blockage, and gene modification [53]. As of July 2015, more than 2200 clinical trials have been performed and authorized throughout the world [54, 55]. Among them, more than 60% are involved in gene therapy of cancer, which signifies that gene therapy is not restricted to genetic diseases only, but can also be exploited for acquired diseases for example cancer and has become a potential approach for the its' treatment. In recent years, several gene therapy techniques for cancer have been introduced, for example, suicide gene therapy, pro-apoptotic (PAP) gene therapy, anti-angiogenesis gene therapy, siRNA gene therapy, oncolytic virus gene therapy, and immune-modulatory gene therapy [56, 57]. The tumorigenesis is a complicated process that involves several signaling pathways along with different procedures, and many times a certain gene might induce numerous biological reactions and activate different signaling pathways, sometimes no specific barrier exists between these above-mentioned therapies. Such as, the p53 gene can not only provoke apoptotic activities within cells of the tumor, but has also exhibited anti-angiogenic activity in several reports [58 - 60]. Hence, gene therapy using the tumor protein p53 can be considered as a PAP and anti-angiogenic therapy. In general, either the gene therapy can be employed effectively or not, is dependent upon two conditions: first, the identification of suitable gene to alleviate the symptoms of the disease; secondly, the delivery of this gene in the right place for the expression of the gene product to manage the disorder without producing any side effects. Since gene therapy seems an effective therapeutic intervention at a molecular level, there are still many technical difficulties that need to be overcome, for example, the potential to design an appropriate delivery system for gene therapy. Fig. (**2**) describes the anti-angiogenesis potential of gene therapy in the endothelial cells (ECs).

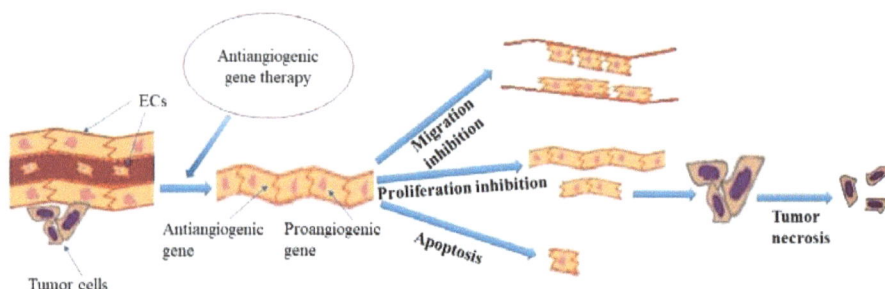

Fig. (2). Gene therapy as an anti-angiogenesis therapy in the endothelial cells (ECs). The figure describes that gene therapy can target the angiogenesis in the ECs as the growth of tumor cells is supported by the surrounding ECs by the provision of nutrients, oxygen, and growth factors. The gene-therapy based approach can inhibit the proliferation and migration of ECs and increase the EC apoptosis leading to the blood vessel destruction that initiates the tumor necrosis.

With the advancement of biotechnology and the improved knowledge of the angiogenic processes, several anti-angiogenic as well as pro-angiogenic genes have now been distinguished and employed in various studies exploring the gene therapy for cancer [61, 62]. Overall, more than 300 inhibitors of angiogenesis have been found and more than 30 candidate drugs have been widely investigated for gene therapy [63]. Since many studies have already discussed several antiangiogenic agents [63 - 65], only the more frequently examined molecules will be discussed in this chapter.

Angiostatin

Angiostatin has been documented as a powerful endogenous inhibitor of angiogenesis and its antitumor activity has also been extensively validated [66]. The major barrier restricting its future application in the clinical experiments is its limited therapeutic effectiveness along with the shortest half-life [67]. To overcome this deficiency, studies are now paying attention to clarify the effective delivery system as well as the different viral and non-viral techniques for the delivery of the angiostatin gene. Currently, the angiostatin protein has been expressed within adenovirus, vaccinia virus, HSV, and Adeno associated virus vectors or plasmids using the cationic liposomes [68 - 70]. Simultaneously, angiostatin is usually transferred along with the other genes to enhance the antitumor effectiveness, such as Fas gene, HIF-1α, IL-12, soluble VEGFR-2 sFIK-1, p53, and angiostatin-endostatin gene fusion so as to work in a synergistic manner [68, 69, 71]. The earlier investigations have shown that angiostatin mimic proteins seem more effective in comparison to angiostatin with respect to metastasis inhibition as well as tumor suppression, possibly as a result of synergistic activity of the Kringle domain of the plasminogen [72, 73].

Tumstatin

Tumstatin: a fragment that is cleaved from the alpha-3 chain of collagen type-IV is another endogenous inhibitor of angiogenesis that seems to be an appealing candidate for the gene therapy of cancer. The anti-angiogenic capability of tumstatin is ten-times greater in comparison to the endostatin [74, 75]. Tumstatin put on its antiangiogenic activity by binding with α3β1 and αVβ3 integrins through the inhibition of tubulogenesis and cell proliferation in ECs and induction of apoptosis in ECs. An earlier study has detected that tumstatin promotes the EC apoptosis *via* the FAS-receptor pathway [76, 77]. The antitumor, as well as antiangiogenic activity of tumstatin, has been extensively exhibited through gene therapy carried out in different xenograft models, for example, S180 tumor, renal cell carcinoma, hepatocellular carcinoma, and lung carcinoma [75, 78]. In recent years, attempts are being made to design and test the delivery system of tumstatin-gene therapy. As an example, the lentivirus expression system comprising of TNF-alpha tumstatin in the mesenchymal stem cells has been employed as an innovative delivery method in prostate cancer cell lines. The findings have revealed substantial antitumor effects in cell lines of prostate cancer, denoting that this approach can exhibit a promising solution towards prostate cancer [79]. In another investigation, naked (plasmid) DNA transferred through gene electro-transfer comprising of tumstatin cDNA has been implemented for the exploration of the antitumor activity of tumstatin in B16F1 melanoma tumor-bearing mice. A significant decrease in the growth of the tumor along with improved survival of mice was detected, revealing that this approach appears exquisite in regards to tumor suppression as well as gene delivery [80]. Moreover, pET-15b vector designed for expressing the fusion protein VTF (synthetic), which consist of tumstatin and vasostatin, using a (Gly-Ser-Gly)2 linker exhibited the suppression in the growth of B16 melanoma tumor, along with the powerful inhibition of the development of tumor vasculature *in vivo*, in comparison to the one inhibitor, while the chimeric proteins of various angiogenesis inhibitors directing various pathways demonstrated enhanced therapeutic effects [81]. Furthermore, for T42, which has been derived from the two adenovirus vectors along with the genes of T42 and quadruple T42 peptide to assess their anticancer activity in breast cancer cells *in-vivo* as well as *in-vitro*, the findings proposed that this method can be a possible substitute for the management of the breast cancer [82].

Endostatin

Endostatin, a 20 Kilodalton C-terminal fragment cleaved from the alpha1 chain of collagen type XVIII, is considered among the most widely investigated endogenous inhibitors of angiogenesis [83, 84]. Endostar (YH-16) is a protein agent of the rh-endostatin that was adopted by the China Food and Drug Administration to manage the non-small lung cancer cell in 2005, signifying the prospective use of endostatin for the treatment of cancer [85]. A gene-based approach of endostatin has also grasped the attention and significant improvement has been observed in the pre-clinical and the clinical trials during the past few years. Earlier studies have mainly focused on two approaches that include either the combinational use of endostatin with other genes or chemotherapeutic agent or the selection of a suitable delivery method for the expression of endostatin protein. For instance, the therapeutic activity of fusing the endostatin therapy with the radiotherapy, using 32P colloid on the cells of HCC (hepatocellular carcinoma), was examined and found that the fusion of these therapeutic agents exhibited an enhanced therapeutic activity on HCC in comparison to either one of the therapies alone [86]. Moreover, combination therapy of endostatin with an antiangiogenic gene, sFIK1, and angiostatin, was investigated and an enhanced therapeutic effect was observed compared to a single-drug administration, owing to the capability of these genes directing various signaling pathways of the endothelium growth factor [68]. In another investigation, it was detected that fusing the endostatin and the soluble TRAIL gene delivery showed an increased tumor-suppressing activity through PAP and antiangiogenic processes [87]. In regards to delivery methods, an earlier investigation has established that UTMD (ultrasound targeted microbubble destruction) mediated gene delivery might improve the transfection efficacy of the endostatin, demonstrating that this delivery method displays the capability as a suitable gene therapy directing the retinal neovascularization [88]. Furthermore, some other prior studies regarding the effectiveness of gene transfer and combination therapy, using endostatin, have validated advancement in cancer management up to a particular level [89, 90].

Interleukin-12 (IL-12)

IL-12, initially identified as the inflammatory cytokine having immune-regulatory functions, has been proposed to employ the antiangiogenic effect during various investigations [91, 92]. Owing to its potential to induce immunity along with the inhibition of tumor angiogenesis, IL-12 has also been recognized among the most useful antitumor cytokine as well as antiangiogenic agents [93]. Even though the previous investigations have revealed its antitumor potential in both *in-vivo* as well as *in-vitro* studies, the antitumor activity of the IL-12 distinctly varies among the strains of the mouse, however, the mechanisms that result in these altered responses are still unclear [94]. Nevertheless, a previous investigation exhibited that elevated expression of the IL-12 receptor on the C3H/HeJ mice spleen cells leads to a significantly greater response for IL-12 in comparison to the other strains of the mouse that show a possible mechanism for the altered antitumor response to IL-12 among various individuals [94]. The side effects involving toxicity has also been reported in numerous clinical trials during the systemic use of rH (recombinant Human) IL-12 that advocate the use of gene therapy because of its potential to attain higher concentrations within the local TME with less systemic side effects [95, 96]. Although several previous clinical studies regarding gene therapy using IL-12 have reported the potential of IL-12 for the management of tumors, a comprehensive report has used the intra-tumoral electroporation mediated plasmid IL-12 delivery among 24 people affected with the malignant melanoma. The investigation has reported an enhanced survival rate and efficacy of pIL-12 electroporation technique with fewer side effects in this clinical trial [97]. A different study from the same group revealed the effectiveness of intra-tumoral electroporation of pIL-12 during a phase II trial involving melanoma cases and found that electroporation monotherapy was effective and no critical systemic or local toxicity was detected during the treatment [98]. Simultaneously, several gene therapies involving the IL-12 have used diverse delivery methods to highlight the therapeutic strategies using the local expression of IL-12 and have reported higher tumor specificity with minimal systematic toxicity. These studies have mainly involved the T-cells, plasmids, bacteria, such as *Lactococcus lactis,* and viruses, mainly helper-dependent adenovirus (HDAd) and HSV-1 [99 - 101]. Many other studies have concentrated on the use of IL-12 along with the antitumor genes, suicide gene therapy, oncolytic viruses, and chemotherapy for its efficacy and safety in pre-clinical trials [102, 103].

NK4

NK4 was initially obtained as a product of proteolytic digestion of the HGF (hepatocyte growth factor). NK4 is considered as an excellent antitumor drug owing to the bifunctional properties of the HGF antagonist as well as antiangiogenesis [104]. Reports have revealed that NK4 has the capability to exert its powerful antiangiogenic effects through the indirect inhibition of VEGF expression in tumor cells, along with the direct effect on ECs [105]. The remarkable antitumor effects along with the antiangiogenic capability of NK4 has been validated in different cancer, for example, pancreatic cancer, lung cancer, gall bladder cancer, biliary gastric carcinomas, and colon cancers. This antiangiogenic drug seems therapeutically good enough as the human carcinomas are more complicated and require management with numerous targets [106 - 108]. The later reports have revealed the prospects of the use of NK4 along with the traditional chemotherapeutic drugs and several other inhibitor molecules directing various signaling pathways. It was found that the antitumor effect by fusion of the plasmid of NK4 with the cisplatin for the treatment of squamous cell cancer was enhanced in comparison to NK4 therapy alone [109]. One more finding has validated that 5-FU (fluorouracil) increased the NK4 mediated apoptosis in cells of colon cancer through downregulation of the intracellular signaling pathway of HGF/c-Met [110]. The investigations have revealed a more suitable and effective method for the transfer of NK4 and found that MSC-mediated NK4 therapy can significantly suppress the gastric cancer growth in xenograft models and the MSCs serve as a better agent for NK4 therapy in comparison to lentiviral vectors [111]. Moreover, the initial clinical study in humans was carried out to analyze the protective as well as the probable clinical advantages of an adenovirus vector expressing the NK4 [112].

Metargidin peptide

Antiangiogenesis Metargidin Peptide (AMEP), the recombinant domain of human metargidin is another innovative anti-cancer drug, which employs its activity by combining to αVβ3 and α5β1 through its binding sequence of RGD (Arginylglycylaspartic acid) integrin [113, 114]. The antiangiogenic, in addition to the antitumor activities of AMEP, was initially proposed *in vitro* by using the recombinant protein [114]. Afterward, it was established *in vivo* with the use of a plasmid AMEP gene therapy, which showed greater antitumor efficacy of AMEP in comparison to tyrosine kinase and TSP1, as a considerable decrease in the tumor metastasis was observed. This shows that AMEP can not only suppress tumor cell proliferation but can also inhibit tumor metastasis [115]. Consequently, the phase 1 clinical assessment trial was carried out to explore the acceptability as well as the safety of plasmid AMEP mediated by the intra-tumoral gene electrotransfer within the epidermal metastatic melanoma. The findings revealed a good safety in addition to the efficiency of gene electrotransfer using AMEP plasmid into the metastatic melanoma [116]. Moreover, an investigation reported that antitumor effects of the plasmid AMEP gene electrotransfer within cells of murine melanoma were associated with the integrins levels in the melanoma cells rather than the AMEP expression level, although the antiangiogenic activity was partly dependent on the integrin concentrations and was mainly associated with the quantity of AMEP plasmid [117]. Moreover, a previous study has found that the quantity of integrin in the cells of melanoma can also function as a biological marker for the efficiency of antitumor treatments targeting the integrins and the efficacy of antiangiogenic activity of the plasmid AMEP can be estimated through the AMEP expression levels during the therapeutic management of melanoma [118]. This also proposed that the intra-tumoral transfer of plasmid AMEP had been more effective, in comparison to the intra-muscular approach. On the basis of these aforesaid studies, it can be anticipated that forthcoming studies exploring the electro-transfer of plasmid AMEP will be better targeted towards a specific cancer type in which the integrins overexpression is found.

Endoglin

Endoglin is a TGF-β co-receptor that is responsible for activating the complicated signaling pathway involving the adhesion, migration as well as the proliferation of ECs, specifically in tumor vessels. Due to the fact that the endoglin expression is significantly enhanced within ECs of the tumor vasculature, it is a prospective prognostic marker [119, 120]. Therefore, endoglin has been considered to act as a promising target in cancer therapy. Various anti-endoglin antibody products, involving the radiolabeled antibodies, antibodies conjugated immunotoxins along with the monoclonal antibodies that exhibited great antitumor as well as antiangiogenic responses have also been reported [121, 122]. For gene therapy, the silencing of endoglin through RNAi seems to be an alternate and promising technique. The therapeutic efficacy of the siRNA (small interfering RNA) molecules towards the endoglin were examined *in-vivo* as well as *in-vitro*, and findings signify that molecules of siRNA, which target the endoglin have shown great antitumor as well as antiangiogenic effectiveness on the ECs *in-vitro* and *in-vivo* on the tumor cells [123]. Furthermore, for the purpose of selectively silencing the endoglin in the tumor vessels, a tissue-specific approach was used by designing a plasmid with an hTERT promoter that was endothelin-1(ET) dependent and responsible for the migration of ECs [124, 125]. The findings of the investigation signify that this particular plasmid can attain high safety as well as specificity levels with the same effect similar to a plasmid that possesses the constitutive promoter. In an earlier investigation, it was validated that melanoma and ET cells have expressed higher endoglin levels, and after the silencing of endoglin with the gene electro-transfer, the viability of these particular cells was reduced, whereas the tumor cells having low endoglin expression, just an uncertain decrease in viability of cells was found after the electro-transfer. The findings suggest an innovative approach for the treatment of melanoma with a targeted approach using gene therapy [126].

INHERENT RESISTANCE AGAINST ANTIANGIOGENIC THERAPY

The resistance against cancer is the main hindrance in the angiogenesis therapies for various cancer types that need to be handled carefully. The rise of resistance among the tumor cells against the antiangiogenic drugs could be either intrinsic or acquired. In comparison to the acquired resistance mechanism, the phenomenon of the intrinsic resistance towards antiangiogenic drugs is complex events that pose a greater impact on the TME [35, 127].

Compared to the few cases of intrinsic resistance towards antiangiogenic treatments, the tumors usually attain resistance against the therapies by upregulating the signals involved in tumor growth, progression, and metastasis [51]. Vessel co-option is one of the leading mechanisms associated with the progression of cancer that involves the existing vasculature for growth and nutrients. This mechanism is also important in the intrinsic resistance to anti-angiogenic drugs [128]. Although these processes were found to contribute towards the intrinsic resistance, the impact of this mechanism has not been completely validated in the clinical studies [127, 129]. Therefore, it is necessary to figure out why most patients have stopped responding or become unresponsive completely against the antiangiogenic agents and how these shortcomings can be resolved.

BACTERIA AS TUMORICIDAL AGENTS

The utilization of living, non-infectious, genetically modified or attenuated bacteria has started to arise as promising antitumor drugs, for providing immediate tumoricidal effects and for transferring the tumoricidal agents. M55, a non-infectious *Clostridium* strain, has exhibited that it can colonize the anaerobic areas of the tumor through the intravenous drug administration, however, it did not give considerable tumor regression [130]. Lately, several anaerobic species of bacteria, such as lactobacilli, pathogenic clostridia, and bifidobacteria, have been investigated for their potential to accumulate in the tumor microenvironment (TME) during animal trials of the tumor. *Clostridium novyi* exhibited considerable antitumor activities, although the results of clinical studies were not satisfactory. *C. novyi*-NT; an attenuated strain was used after the deletion of a gene that codes for a toxin, demonstrated excellent effects, but also produced toxicity. Moreover, the spores of *C. novyi*-NT were administered along with the traditional chemotherapeutic drugs, such as mitomycin C, docetaxel, dolastatin-10, and vinorelbine. This technique leads to considerable antitumor effects but was associated with significant deaths in animal studies [131]. *C. novyi* has been examined in combination with radioimmunotherapy, radiotherapy, and more chemotherapy in the experimental animal models of the different tumors [132]. The findings have validated the prospects of combined treatment methodologies as the "future of cancer therapies". *C. novyi*-NT has been utilized to improve the liposome-encapsulated drug delivery in tumors owing to its explicit membrane disrupting capability [133].

The VNP20009 is a strain derived from *Salmonella typhimurium* that has been used for the targeted drug delivery for therapeutic management of cancer. VNP20009 has been explored effectively in Phase one clinical study within cancer patients. Moreover, new bacterial strains being studied for anticancer therapy include *Listeria monocytogenes*, *Salmonella choleraesuis*, *Escherichia coli,* and *Vibrio cholerae* [134]. The bacteria mediated inhibition of tumor cells is shown in Fig. (**3**).

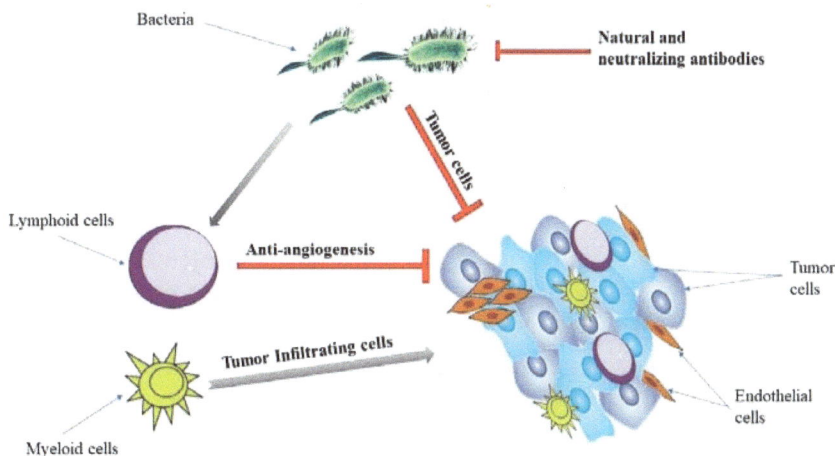

Fig. (3). Bacteria mediated inhibition of tumor cells. Following the accumulation of bacteria inside the tumor microenvironment, the death of tumor cells can occur due to an increased number of infiltrating cells, or increased production of anti-angiogenic cytokines. The neutralizing antibodies or the natural antibodies can, however, block the ability of tumor-targeting bacteria.

BACTERIA MEDIATED ANTI-ANGIOGENESIS GENE THERAPY

The growth and metastasis of the tumor tissue depend upon the new blood vessel formation (angiogenesis). Therefore, blocking tumor angiogenesis could be a practical approach for the treatment of solid tumors. A therapy was used with a low dose of rh-endostatin and *Salmonella* (auxotrophic, attenuated) in the murine melanoma model, which leads to a reduction in the growth of tumors [135]. The treatment is claimed to be effective and safer as well as economically suitable, as it reduces the possible adverse effects and lessens the therapeutic cost. Furthermore, a non-pathogenic *Bifidobacterium adolescentis* strain has been employed as the vector to express the endostatin (anti-angiogenic agent) in tumors [136]. The findings exhibited that *Bifidobacterium adolescentis* based therapy significantly inhibited the tumor angiogenesis and the growth of the tumor tissue. The *Bifidobacterium longum* effectively transported the endostatin in the murine model of liver cancer and resulted in an anti-cancer activity [137, 138]. Moreover, the oral administration of the anti-angiogenic (bacteria-based) vaccines targeted against the VEGFR-2 (vascular endothelium growth factor receptor-2) has been proven effectual in the animal (mouse) models of lung tumors, malignant melanoma, and colorectal cancer [139].

The combination therapy of anti-angiogenic along with bacteriolytic using the tumor-targeting bacteria has also exhibited promising results. The bacteria have the capability to infect the weakly perfused areas of the tumor that cannot be accessed through systemically administered antimicrobial agents, exploiting their distinctive metabolic properties. They also induce the inhibition of angiogenesis to kill the residual tumor cells and thus, substantially contribute towards the clearance of the tumor cells [140]. Additionally, the antitumor activity can be improved by co-administering the endostatin and tumor necrosis factor (TNF) related apoptosis-inducing ligand (TRAIL) [141].

BACTERIA BASED DELIVERY SYSTEMS FOR TUMOR ENDOTHELIAL VACCINES

There are a number of potential tumor EC vaccines, the efficacy of which has been validated in different animal models. These vaccines were delivered through different vectors/techniques, involving the direct introduction of naked DNA or peptides, gold particles in gene gun, tumor-based vectors, attenuated bacterial vectors, and intradermal electroporation. The specific delivery system for the antiangiogenic based vaccine therapy needs to be carefully selected and this depends upon the nature of vaccines *i.e* . proteins or peptides vaccines DNA or RNA. In case of gene therapy-based vaccine methods, the rDNA can be introduced alone, through various viral or non-viral vectors, or through the prokaryotic/eukaryotic cells. Though the delivery system designed for vaccines targets particular tumor ECs, there are still some exceptions, especially for viruses which can infect normal tissue along with tumor EC [142 - 144].

Bacteria been reported as the most commonly employed delivery method for plasmid-based DNA vaccines [145, 146]. Numerous animal trials have validated that oral administration of the bacterial vectors using the attenuated strains of *Salmonella* and *Listeria* possess the capability to treat as well as prevent cancer by inhibiting the angiogenesis [147, 148]. Though safety issues are a big factor while considering these bacteria-based methods for delivery, however, it will be of utmost importance that one strain of *Salmonella enterica* has been authorized by FDA for the usage of the vaccine [146, 149]. Furthermore, numerous bacterial vaccines that had significant antitumor, as well as antiangiogenic effect, exhibited little or no immunological response during animal studies [150, 151]. Besides proteins, rDNA, peptides, and mRNA have been explored as the potential technique to improve cellular immunity [152]. Even though the majority of studies did not compare various delivery systems with each other, it is obvious that the method of administration, as well as carrier system, are important for the effectiveness of the vaccine in animal studies and the clinical trials [153]. The mode of delivery is as critical as the particular angiogenic drug, to achieve a positive response in humans against the tumor. The Bacterial mediated delivery of anti-angiogenic vaccines and their targets are explained in Table **2**.

Table 2. Bacterial mediated delivery of vaccines and their targets with anti-angiogenic effect

Bacterial Vector	Vaccine Type	Target	Route	References
Salmonella typhimurium	DNA vaccine	VEGFR2	Oral	[139]
Bifidobacterium adolescentis	Alternative gene therapy	Endostatin	Intravenous	[136]
Listeria monocytogenes	DNA vaccine	VEGFR2	Oral	[148]
Escherichia coli	tkRNAi	B-catenin	Intravenous	[165]
Salmonella choleraessuis	Bactofection	Endostatin	Intravenous	[154]
Salmonella typhimurium	Alternative gene therapy	LIGHT	Intravenous	[191]
Salmonella typhimurium	Bactofection	IL-12	Oral	[216]
Salmonella enterica	Bactofection	Thrombospondin-1	Intraperitoneal	[157]
Bifidobacterium longum	Alternative gene therapy	Endostatin	Oral	[138]
Salmonella typhimurium	tkRNAi	STAT3	Intravenous	[163]

TECHNIQUES FOR THE USE OF MODIFIED BACTERIA AS ANTICANCER THERAPEUTICS

Using the genetically engineered bacteria for the effective inhibition of tumors, the bacterial gene-targeted enzyme prodrug treatment has exhibited promising results. Here, we will discuss the most promising techniques for employing the engineered bacteria as an anticancer therapy, for example, DNA vaccination, trans-kingdom RNAi, autofiction, and gene alternative therapy, with an emphasis on their anti-angiogenesis potential.

Bactofection

The bacteria used as a biological vector for the transfer of a therapeutic gene into the target cells of patients is termed as bactofection. There are several reports that have utilized this technique for transferring the genes containing antiangiogenic agents into the cells of the tumor *in-vivo*. An investigation was carried out using *S. choleraesuis* strain carrying the endostatin expression plasmid. The endostatin expression was directed particularly within bacterial colonized tumor tissues and considerable suppression in the growth of the tumor with reduced microvessel density (MVD) and decreased expression of the VEGF was observed [154]. The bactofection, using the *Salmonella* (auxotrophic) as a vector, has been successfully used for the treatment of clinical models of the tumor with the use of expression plasmids bearing numerous cytokine genes, for example, IL-18, IL-12, IL-4, GM-CSF and other genes having a function in angiogenesis, for example, Fit-3 ligand [155, 156]. Moreover, a dual antiangiogenic and tumorigenic activity of *S. choleraesuis,* holding the expression plasmid consisting of thrombospondin (TSP)-1 gene controlled by the eukaryotic promoter, have been reported within the murine melanoma model [157]. Nevertheless, based on different studies exploiting bactofection for the management of cancer, it appears that this technique is more appropriate for targeting the other tissues and cells, for example of lungs and colonic mucosa [158, 159]. A possible drawback of using bactofection for the treatment of cancer is possibly that effector molecule is presumably expressed particularly in cells that are infected by the bacteria, as a result, a large amount of the tumor cells remains untreated. Nonetheless, if the transgene product is excreted outside of the targeted cell then it can have a significant therapeutic impact on the non-infected cells of the tumor.

RNA Interference

Another encouraging technique for the bacteria mediated cancer therapy is the fusion of two different approaches: RNAi along with bacteriotherapy. The bacteria have been modified to generate and transfer the siRNA for the effective introduction of RNAi within the host cells [160]. This idea was based on the observations that the invasive strain of *E. coli* can produce RNAi within the cultures of the mammalian cell [161, 162]. During the initial experiments, it was found that the invasive *E. coli* was responsible for producing the beta-catenin shRNA (small hairpin RNA), which can stimulate RNAi within the intestinal epithelial cells as well as colonic tumors xeno-transplanted within nude mice. The technique is called trans-kingdom RNAi because this report presented the first proof of delivering the effector molecules of RNAi between the mammals as well as bacteria *in-vivo*. In another study, the attenuated strain of *S. Typhimurium* was effectively used as a suitable vector for the delivery of MDR1-siRNA within the tumor cells *in-vivo* [161]. The combined therapy of siRNA along with oncolytic virus exploiting the systematic administration of *S. Typhimurium,* which expresses the siRNA targeting STAT3 transcription factor of the tumor, has also been assessed [163]. These reports revealed greater efficacy for combined treatment in comparison to the therapy with non-RNAi producing bacteria. Apart from the production and transfer of the shRNA, the bacteria can be utilized for transferring the eukaryotic shRNA expression plasmids into the cells of the mammalian tumor [162]. The oral use of *S. Typhimurium* containing expression plasmid of shRNA for the anti-apoptotic protein, BCL-2, causes a remarkable delay in the growth of the tumor along with extended survival within the murine melanoma model [164]. So far, the trans-kingdom RNAi has not been employed for targeting the angiogenesis directly, even though some targets described above have been known to strengthen the process of angiogenesis owing to their effect upon the expression level of several pro-angiogenic growth factors [165, 166]. The antitumor activities of destroying these targets can, partially, be associated with the inhibition of angiogenesis. Conversely, certain investigations using the non-bacterial therapy of siRNA interfering with the HIF1a, VEGF along with other molecules of angiogenesis signifies that the suppression of EC proliferation along with the formation of new vasculature is a strong target for the cancer therapy based on RNAi and for several other diseases [167 - 169]. Though the trans-kingdom RNAi explicitly provides an innovative pathway to investigate, further research will be needed to expose its imminent applications.

DNA Vaccination

It is well known that the tumor-specific antigens encoded by bactofection plasmids can result in the production of cellular as well as a humoral response within the host thus, providing protection against the tumors [170]. The technique, called DNA vaccination, has been effectively executed as antiangiogenic treatment. The oral administration of antiangiogenic related bacterial vaccines, targeted against the VEGFR2, has proved effective within models of lung cancer, malignant melanoma, colorectal cancer and non-malignant conditions, such as atherosclerosis and stromal keratitis [171 - 173]. Moreover, the *Salmonella* mediated DNA vaccination for a murine model of VEGFR2 has been effectively fused with the traditional gene therapy to treat malignant melanoma [174]. Furthermore, the oral vaccine strain containing plasmid, which encodes a chemokine IP10/CXCL10 leads to a considerable synergetic antitumor effect. Similarly, the inhibition of angiogenesis has been detected with the oral DNA vaccine, which was carried by the bacteria, *Salmonella typhimurium,* encoding Fos-mediated antigen 1 was found to be effective against the growth and metastasis of cancer [175]. The bacterial vaccines targeted against the survivin (apoptosis inhibitor) along with the endoglin (a co-receptor for the transforming-growth factor (TGF)-beta-1) have also proved effective for suppressing the tumor angiogenesis [176, 177]. Several studies for DNA vaccination directed for anticancer therapy have used *Salmonella* strains (attenuated), whereas other bacterial species, such as *Pseudomonas aeruginosa,* have also been explored widely [178].

Further investigations with a deeper understanding of the immune mechanisms are essential because similar strains of the vector are now utilized for the DNA vaccination as well as bactofection based methodologies. In bacterial gene transfer and bactofection techniques, immune activation (IA) is seen as the non-desired adverse effect, while in the case of DNA vaccination, the immunogenic characteristics of carrier bacteria are considered as a vital factor, which significantly contributes towards the therapeutic outcomes.

A major advantage of the DNA vaccination for the treatment of cancer is the capability for oral use of the bacterial therapeutic strains, which has proven to be effective in the animal models, therefore, the majority of the present investigations are focused to develop the clinically significant bacteria-based oral vaccines. Nevertheless, a considerable lack of knowledge is still present and the mode of action of the oral use of DNA vaccines has not been completely understood.

Alternative Gene Therapy (AGT)

One more method of exploiting the bacteria as gene therapy is referred to as the AGT technique, also called bacterial protein transfer [179]. This approach depends on the delivery of therapeutic proteins expressed by the bacteria into the host through genetically engineered bacteria. In contrast to DNA vaccination or bactofection based approaches, the existence of the bacteria within the targeted tissue might be required during the bacterial protein transfer. The persistent bacteria generate the therapeutic polypeptide locally, thereby magnificently offering a local drug delivery without increasing its systematic levels. Similar to bactofection, the AGT is also mainly employed for the management of various tumors and primarily exploits the tumor tissue and various cancer colonizing strains, such as Salmonella, Clostridia, and Bifidobacteria, have been used [9, 10]. The bifidobacteria, as well as clostridia strains, have been effectively employed as the enzyme pro-drug treatment [180]. As clostridia are considered obligate anaerobe, their potential for spore formation along with the simplicity of transformation have adapted to AGT against tumors [181, 182]. Moreover, their capability of colonizing the tumors in cells can be increased by deleting the genes, which are involved in the basal oxygen consumption, for example, SOD (superoxide dismutase) encoding gene [183]. The key benefit of using bifidobacterial strain is their non-pathogenic nature. In an investigation, *Bifidobacterium adolescentis* have been employed as a biological vector to express the endostatin in the tumor cells [136]. It was exhibited that powerful anti-angiogenesis can lead to effective inhibition of the local growth of tumor cells. Other studies have found that *Bifidobacterium longum* has been exhibited to efficaciously transfer the endostatin into a murine model of the liver tumor, which resulted in the induction of antitumor effect [137, 138]. Moreover, antitumor activity was improved through the concurrent use of the same strain, which expresses the TRAIL (Tumor necrosis factor-related apoptosis-inducing ligand) [141].

An essential element of various studies exploring AGT *in-vivo* is the potential to particularly regulate the bacterial expression associated with therapeutic protein. The precise spatial, along with the temporal control, is essential to enhance the therapeutic activity and reduce the possible side effects. A primary tool in this section is the utilization of various inducible promoters when a particular exogenously delivered compound is present, such as arabinose and IPTG (isopropyl thiogalactoside). The exogenous control of the expression of the therapeutic gene can be further enhanced with the utilization of bacteria bearing the suicide genes. A major investigation has validated the capability of regulating the *in-vivo* therapeutic genes expression through plasmids [184]. In this study, intravenously used *S. Typhimurium* bearing a plasmid consisting of GFP (green fluorescent protein) gene controlled by arabinose promoter (pBAD) was capable of selectively colonizing the tumors, however, only GFP was expressed after administering the L-arabinose. The bacteria mediated delivery of the therapeutic proteins within tumor cells with the use of the L-arabinose expression system have also been described for EcN (*E. coli* Nissle) 1917, the strain of probiotic bacteria which can colonize the humans [185]. The findings of this investigation considerably improve the usage of this bacterial strain and provide a good representation of the therapeutic capability of AGT. Nevertheless, in spite of the tremendous safety report of EcN 1917, it still seems quite difficult to genetically modify this strain owing to the occurrence of various plasmids. Moreover, a vast majority of studies regarding EcN 1917 have described its potential in the gastrointestinal tract disorders. Consequently, more investigations are required to reveal their perspective as antitumor therapeutic.

Another model being studied for improving the regulation of gene expression using hypoxia-inducible promoters within *Salmonella* colonized tumors [186, 187]. Moreover, a sub-group of promoters that are specifically triggered within tumors has been detected, indicating that more methods of regulation exist apart from the use of only hypoxia-based systems [188]. This is definitely attracting in view of current studies regarding the potential of bacteria, which target tumor for colonizing the necrotic as well as perfused areas of tumors [189]. All these findings further improve the possibility of exploiting bacteria as antitumor therapeutic, by offering a broad range of promoters which have the capability to target tumor as well as regulate the expression of the gene. Furthermore, bacteria have gained an edge on viruses when exploited as cancer therapeutic because the treatment can be promptly terminated with the use of antimicrobial agents. The bacterial strains, however, do not integrate within the genome of the host, considerably decreasing the possibility of therapy-induced tumorigenesis as well as mutagenesis. The in-situ formation of cytokines through bacteria signifies a safe as well as a cost-friendly alternative primarily for systematic administration [190].

In a study, the attenuated *S. Typhimurium* was modified to enhance their oncolytic effect by integrating a gene that encodes the LIGHT, a cytokine of TNF-family, which is known for promoting the tumor removal [191]. The LIGHT also performs several functions related to the immunological defense involving the stimulation of T as well as B cells along with the migration of natural killer (NK) cells. Most importantly, LIGHT can exhibit antiangiogenic activity by activating the receptors chemokine CXCL10, along with the CXCL9, for the activation of pathways responsible for the inhibition of angiogenesis. During a subsequent study, it was validated that interleukin-12 producing the *Salmonella* can inhibit the tumor [192]. Apart from its widely known activity against immune response, IL-18 can also inhibit the angiogenesis through the direct suppression of the fibroblast growth factor (FGF)-2, which induces the EC proliferation, thereby inhibiting several pathways responsible for tumor angiogenesis. Altogether, these investigations have provided proof that intravenously directed, non-malignant genetically engineered bacteria could be effectively used as a tool for the development of the antiangiogenic drugs within tumors. Moreover, it was shown that the engineered *S. Typhimurium,* which produces the chemokine CCL21 possesses anticancer properties with no evidence of toxicity [193]. Remarkably, a prominent antitumor activity of the *S. Typhimurium* strains producing IL-2 has been exhibited in the mouse melanoma model [194]. Furthermore, this activity was clearly associated with reduced tumor angiogenesis. Despite the great achievement in the non-clinical trials, the use of bacterial strains for the treatment of human tumors has not been exactly successful, even though this technique was highly endorsed in the majority of investigations [195, 196]. In view of all the above-stated results, it is proposed that the angiogenesis can be a significant target for new investigations, in course of bacteria based antitumor therapy, specifically if used along with oncolytic bacterial strains.

CONCLUSION AND FUTURE PROSPECTS

Regardless of the developments which have been achieved in recent years, traditional therapies of cancer exhibit two primary limitations: systemic toxicity due to the low sensitivity and specificity along with the difficulty of removing the residual cancer cells. The different biological properties of cancer are the main target for the treatment, however, hypoxia is one of the leading mechanisms to target, owing to its importance for the outcomes of cancer therapy. The hypoxic areas of the tumor can function as the niche for facultative along with the anaerobic bacteria. Such bacteria can particularly populate the hypoxic areas within the cancer cells and the surrounding areas and can result in the destruction of cancer cells [197]. On the other hand, bacteriolytic treatment alone is mostly deficient to completely destroy the cancer cells [198].

It is clear that cancer is one of the highly complicated diseases with significantly diverse biological events even in the same type of cancer, leading to substantial differences within their responses against the therapies. The interaction between the individual host and cancer types and the individual immune response makes the cancer therapy more difficult. Therefore, it is idealistic to expect that a single "miracle drug" will treat all cancer types or even a single cancer type. Successful cancer treatment in the coming years will possibly include a broad range of combinatorial methods, including both the novel ones as well as conventional treatments, for example, bacteriolytic therapy, immunotherapy, and therapies which are based on the specified molecular targets. From all the combinational possibilities, which can be assumed, the combination of angiogenesis inhibitors and bacteria-based oncolytic treatment hold a special position. The bacteria can eradicate a tumor cell from its root and the antiangiogenic drugs can affect the periphery of the tumor by turning off its supply of blood that can ultimately decrease the chances of survival for the cancer cells. Furthermore, it is generally believed that the chance of resistance against this combinatorial therapy is low compared to other treatment methodologies.

CONSENT FOR PUBLICATION

Not applicable.

CONFLICT OF INTEREST

The authors confirm that the contents of this chapter have no conflict of interest.

ACKNOWLEDGEMENTS

Declare none.

REFERENCES

[1]   Siegel RL, Miller KD, Jemal A. Cancer Statistics, 2017. CA Cancer J Clin 2017; 67(1): 7-30.
        [http://dx.doi.org/10.3322/caac.21387] [PMID: 28055103]

[2]   Chen W, Zheng R, Baade PD, *et al.* Cancer statistics in China, 2015. CA Cancer J Clin 2016; 66(2): 115-32.
        [http://dx.doi.org/10.3322/caac.21338] [PMID: 26808342]

[3]   Wolinsky JB, Colson YL, Grinstaff MW. Local drug delivery strategies for cancer treatment: gels, nanoparticles, polymeric films, rods, and wafers. J Control Release 2012; 159(1): 14-26.
        [http://dx.doi.org/10.1016/j.jconrel.2011.11.031] [PMID: 22154931]

[4]   Bellon JR, Come SE, Gelman RS, *et al.* Sequencing of chemotherapy and radiation therapy in early-stage breast cancer: updated results of a prospective randomized trial. J Clin Oncol 2005; 23(9): 1934-40.
        [http://dx.doi.org/10.1200/JCO.2005.04.032] [PMID: 15774786]

[5]   Ghadjar P, Vock J, Vetterli D, *et al.* Acute and late toxicity in prostate cancer patients treated by dose escalated intensity modulated radiation therapy and organ tracking. Radiat Oncol 2008; 3: 35.

[http://dx.doi.org/10.1186/1748-717X-3-35] [PMID: 18937833]

[6] Carmeliet P, Jain RK. Principles and mechanisms of vessel normalization for cancer and other angiogenic diseases. Nat Rev Drug Discov 2011; 10(6): 417-27.
[http://dx.doi.org/10.1038/nrd3455] [PMID: 21629292]

[7] Abdalla AME, Xiao L, Ullah MW, Yu M, Ouyang C, Yang G. Current Challenges of Cancer Anti-angiogenic Therapy and the Promise of Nanotherapeutics. Theranostics 2018; 8(2): 533-48.
[http://dx.doi.org/10.7150/thno.21674] [PMID: 29290825]

[8] Moese JR, Moese G. Oncolysis by Clostridia. I. Activity of Clostridium Butyricum (M-55) and Other Nonpathogenic Clostridia against the Ehrlich Carcinoma. Cancer Res 1964; 24: 212-6.
[PMID: 14115686]

[9] Zheng LM, Luo X, Feng M, *et al.* Tumor amplified protein expression therapy: Salmonella as a tumor-selective protein delivery vector. Oncol Res 2000; 12(3): 127-35.
[http://dx.doi.org/10.3727/096504001108747602] [PMID: 11216671]

[10] Theys J, Landuyt AW, Nuyts S, Van Mellaert L, Lambin P, Anné J. Clostridium as a tumor-specific delivery system of therapeutic proteins. Cancer Detect Prev 2001; 25(6): 548-57.
[PMID: 12132875]

[11] Folkman J. Tumor angiogenesis: therapeutic implications. N Engl J Med 1971; 285(21): 1182-6.
[http://dx.doi.org/10.1056/NEJM197111182852108] [PMID: 4938153]

[12] Folkman J. Anti-angiogenesis: new concept for therapy of solid tumors. Ann Surg 1972; 175(3): 409-16.
[http://dx.doi.org/10.1097/00000658-197203000-00014] [PMID: 5077799]

[13] Dimova I, Popivanov G, Djonov V. Angiogenesis in cancer - general pathways and their therapeutic implications. J BUON 2014; 19(1): 15-21.
[PMID: 24659637]

[14] Ribatti D, Nico B, Crivellato E, Roccaro AM, Vacca A. The history of the angiogenic switch concept. Leukemia 2007; 21(1): 44-52.
[http://dx.doi.org/10.1038/sj.leu.2404402] [PMID: 16990761]

[15] Moschetta M, Mishima Y, Sahin I, *et al.* Role of endothelial progenitor cells in cancer progression. Biochim Biophys Acta 2014; 1846(1): 26-39.
[PMID: 24709008]

[16] de la Puente P, Muz B, Azab F, Azab AK. Cell trafficking of endothelial progenitor cells in tumor progression. Clin Cancer Res 2013; 19(13): 3360-8.
[http://dx.doi.org/10.1158/1078-0432.CCR-13-0462] [PMID: 23665736]

[17] Ferrara N, Adamis AP. Ten years of anti-vascular endothelial growth factor therapy. Nat Rev Drug Discov 2016; 15(6): 385-403.
[http://dx.doi.org/10.1038/nrd.2015.17] [PMID: 26775688]

[18] Eelen G, de Zeeuw P, Simons M, Carmeliet P. Endothelial cell metabolism in normal and diseased vasculature. Circ Res 2015; 116(7): 1231-44.
[http://dx.doi.org/10.1161/CIRCRESAHA.116.302855] [PMID: 25814684]

[19] Bridgeman VL, Vermeulen PB, Foo S, *et al.* Vessel co-option is common in human lung metastases and mediates resistance to anti-angiogenic therapy in preclinical lung metastasis models. J Pathol 2017; 241(3): 362-74.
[http://dx.doi.org/10.1002/path.4845] [PMID: 27859259]

[20] Frentzas S, Simoneau E, Bridgeman VL, *et al.* Vessel co-option mediates resistance to anti-angiogenic therapy in liver metastases. Nat Med 2016; 22(11): 1294-302.
[http://dx.doi.org/10.1038/nm.4197] [PMID: 27748747]

[21] Kerbel RS. Tumor angiogenesis: past, present and the near future. Carcinogenesis 2000; 21(3): 505-

15.
[http://dx.doi.org/10.1093/carcin/21.3.505] [PMID: 10688871]

[22]   Dor Y, Porat R, Keshet E. Vascular endothelial growth factor and vascular adjustments to perturbations in oxygen homeostasis. Am J Physiol Cell Physiol 2001; 280(6): C1367-74.
[http://dx.doi.org/10.1152/ajpcell.2001.280.6.C1367] [PMID: 11350731]

[23]   Littlepage LE, Sternlicht MD, Rougier N, *et al.* Matrix metalloproteinases contribute distinct roles in neuroendocrine prostate carcinogenesis, metastasis, and angiogenesis progression. Cancer Res 2010; 70(6): 2224-34.
[http://dx.doi.org/10.1158/0008-5472.CAN-09-3515] [PMID: 20215503]

[24]   Maracle CX, Tas SW. Inhibitors of angiogenesis: ready for prime time? Best Pract Res Clin Rheumatol 2014; 28(4): 637-49.
[http://dx.doi.org/10.1016/j.berh.2014.10.012] [PMID: 25481555]

[25]   Blancas AA, Wong LE, Glaser DE, McCloskey KE. Specialized tip/stalk-like and phalanx-like endothelial cells from embryonic stem cells. Stem Cells Dev 2013; 22(9): 1398-407.
[http://dx.doi.org/10.1089/scd.2012.0376] [PMID: 23249281]

[26]   Pandya NM, Dhalla NS, Santani DD. Angiogenesis--a new target for future therapy. Vascul Pharmacol 2006; 44(5): 265-74.
[http://dx.doi.org/10.1016/j.vph.2006.01.005] [PMID: 16545987]

[27]   Bergers G, Song S. The role of pericytes in blood-vessel formation and maintenance. Neuro-oncol 2005; 7(4): 452-64.
[http://dx.doi.org/10.1215/S1152851705000232] [PMID: 16212810]

[28]   Izzedine H, Ederhy S, Goldwasser F, *et al.* Management of hypertension in angiogenesis inhibitor-treated patients. Ann Oncol 2009; 20(5): 807-15.
[http://dx.doi.org/10.1093/annonc/mdn713] [PMID: 19150949]

[29]   Brown JM, Giaccia AJ. The unique physiology of solid tumors: opportunities (and problems) for cancer therapy. Cancer Res 1998; 58(7): 1408-16.
[PMID: 9537241]

[30]   Folkman J, Watson K, Ingber D, Hanahan D. Induction of angiogenesis during the transition from hyperplasia to neoplasia. Nature 1989; 339(6219): 58-61.
[http://dx.doi.org/10.1038/339058a0] [PMID: 2469964]

[31]   Graeber TG, Osmanian C, Jacks T, *et al.* Hypoxia-mediated selection of cells with diminished apoptotic potential in solid tumours. Nature 1996; 379(6560): 88-91.
[http://dx.doi.org/10.1038/379088a0] [PMID: 8538748]

[32]   Jain RK, Tong RT, Munn LL. Effect of vascular normalization by antiangiogenic therapy on interstitial hypertension, peritumor edema, and lymphatic metastasis: insights from a mathematical model. Cancer Res 2007; 67(6): 2729-35.
[http://dx.doi.org/10.1158/0008-5472.CAN-06-4102] [PMID: 17363594]

[33]   De Bock K, Cauwenberghs S, Carmeliet P. Vessel abnormalization: another hallmark of cancer? Molecular mechanisms and therapeutic implications. Curr Opin Genet Dev 2011; 21(1): 73-9.
[http://dx.doi.org/10.1016/j.gde.2010.10.008] [PMID: 21106363]

[34]   Potente M, Gerhardt H, Carmeliet P. Basic and therapeutic aspects of angiogenesis. Cell 2011; 146(6): 873-87.
[http://dx.doi.org/10.1016/j.cell.2011.08.039] [PMID: 21925313]

[35]   Fukumura D, Jain RK. Tumor microvasculature and microenvironment: targets for anti-angiogenesis and normalization. Microvasc Res 2007; 74(2-3): 72-84.
[http://dx.doi.org/10.1016/j.mvr.2007.05.003] [PMID: 17560615]

[36]   Van de Veire S, Stalmans I, Heindryckx F, *et al.* Further pharmacological and genetic evidence for the efficacy of PlGF inhibition in cancer and eye disease. Cell 2010; 141(1): 178-90.

[http://dx.doi.org/10.1016/j.cell.2010.02.039] [PMID: 20371353]

[37] Rolny C, Mazzone M, Tugues S, *et al.* HRG inhibits tumor growth and metastasis by inducing macrophage polarization and vessel normalization through downregulation of PlGF. Cancer Cell 2011; 19(1): 31-44.
[http://dx.doi.org/10.1016/j.ccr.2010.11.009] [PMID: 21215706]

[38] Augustin HG, Koh GY, Thurston G, Alitalo K. Control of vascular morphogenesis and homeostasis through the angiopoietin-Tie system. Nat Rev Mol Cell Biol 2009; 10(3): 165-77.
[http://dx.doi.org/10.1038/nrm2639] [PMID: 19234476]

[39] Desgrosellier JS, Cheresh DA. Integrins in cancer: biological implications and therapeutic opportunities. Nat Rev Cancer 2010; 10(1): 9-22.
[http://dx.doi.org/10.1038/nrc2748] [PMID: 20029421]

[40] Kashiwagi S, Tsukada K, Xu L, *et al.* Perivascular nitric oxide gradients normalize tumor vasculature. Nat Med 2008; 14(3): 255-7.
[http://dx.doi.org/10.1038/nm1730] [PMID: 18278052]

[41] Izumi Y, Xu L, di Tomaso E, Fukumura D, Jain RK. Tumour biology: herceptin acts as an anti-angiogenic cocktail. Nature 2002; 416(6878): 279-80.
[http://dx.doi.org/10.1038/416279b] [PMID: 11907566]

[42] Ellis LM, Hicklin DJ. Pathways mediating resistance to vascular endothelial growth factor-targeted therapy. Clin Cancer Res 2008; 14(20): 6371-5.
[http://dx.doi.org/10.1158/1078-0432.CCR-07-5287] [PMID: 18927275]

[43] Heath VL, Bicknell R. Anticancer strategies involving the vasculature. Nat Rev Clin Oncol 2009; 6(7): 395-404.
[http://dx.doi.org/10.1038/nrclinonc.2009.52] [PMID: 19424102]

[44] Bagri A, Berry L, Gunter B, *et al.* Effects of anti-VEGF treatment duration on tumor growth, tumor regrowth, and treatment efficacy. Clin Cancer Res 2010; 16(15): 3887-900.
[http://dx.doi.org/10.1158/1078-0432.CCR-09-3100] [PMID: 20554752]

[45] Jain RK. Normalization of tumor vasculature: an emerging concept in antiangiogenic therapy. Science 2005; 307(5706): 58-62.
[http://dx.doi.org/10.1126/science.1104819] [PMID: 15637262]

[46] Chauhan VP, Stylianopoulos T, Martin JD, *et al.* Normalization of tumour blood vessels improves the delivery of nanomedicines in a size-dependent manner. Nat Nanotechnol 2012; 7(6): 383-8.
[http://dx.doi.org/10.1038/nnano.2012.45] [PMID: 22484912]

[47] Yang JC, Haworth L, Sherry RM, *et al.* A randomized trial of bevacizumab, an anti-vascular endothelial growth factor antibody, for metastatic renal cancer. N Engl J Med 2003; 349(5): 427-34.
[http://dx.doi.org/10.1056/NEJMoa021491] [PMID: 12890841]

[48] Vredenburgh JJ, Desjardins A, Herndon JE II, *et al.* Bevacizumab plus irinotecan in recurrent glioblastoma multiforme. J Clin Oncol 2007; 25(30): 4722-9.
[http://dx.doi.org/10.1200/JCO.2007.12.2440] [PMID: 17947719]

[49] Miller KD, Chap LI, Holmes FA, *et al.* Randomized phase III trial of capecitabine compared with bevacizumab plus capecitabine in patients with previously treated metastatic breast cancer. J Clin Oncol 2005; 23(4): 792-9.
[http://dx.doi.org/10.1200/JCO.2005.05.098] [PMID: 15681523]

[50] Kamba T, McDonald DM. Mechanisms of adverse effects of anti-VEGF therapy for cancer. Br J Cancer 2007; 96(12): 1788-95.
[http://dx.doi.org/10.1038/sj.bjc.6603813] [PMID: 17519900]

[51] Ebos JM, Kerbel RS. Antiangiogenic therapy: impact on invasion, disease progression, and metastasis. Nat Rev Clin Oncol 2011; 8(4): 210-21.
[http://dx.doi.org/10.1038/nrclinonc.2011.21] [PMID: 21364524]

[52]   Quesada AR, Medina MA, Alba E. Playing only one instrument may be not enough: limitations and future of the antiangiogenic treatment of cancer. BioEssays 2007; 29(11): 1159-68.
[http://dx.doi.org/10.1002/bies.20655] [PMID: 17935210]

[53]   Sato-Dahlman M, Wirth K, Yamamoto M. Role of Gene Therapy in Pancreatic Cancer-A Review. Cancers (Basel) 2018; 10(4): 10.
[http://dx.doi.org/10.3390/cancers10040103] [PMID: 29614005]

[54]   Ginn SL, Alexander IE, Edelstein ML, Abedi MR, Wixon J. Gene therapy clinical trials worldwide to 2012 - an update. J Gene Med 2013; 15(2): 65-77.
[http://dx.doi.org/10.1002/jgm.2698] [PMID: 23355455]

[55]   Edelstein ML, Abedi MR, Wixon J. Gene therapy clinical trials worldwide to 2007--an update. J Gene Med 2007; 9(10): 833-42.
[http://dx.doi.org/10.1002/jgm.1100] [PMID: 17721874]

[56]   Ortiz R, Melguizo C, Prados J, *et al.* New gene therapy strategies for cancer treatment: a review of recent patents. Recent Patents Anticancer Drug Discov 2012; 7(3): 297-312.
[http://dx.doi.org/10.2174/157489212801820093] [PMID: 22339358]

[57]   Cao S, Cripps A, Wei MQ. New strategies for cancer gene therapy: progress and opportunities. Clin Exp Pharmacol Physiol 2010; 37(1): 108-14.
[http://dx.doi.org/10.1111/j.1440-1681.2009.05268.x] [PMID: 19671071]

[58]   Tseng SJ, Liao ZX, Kao SH, *et al.* Highly specific *in vivo* gene delivery for p53-mediated apoptosis and genetic photodynamic therapies of tumour. Nat Commun 2015; 6: 6456.
[http://dx.doi.org/10.1038/ncomms7456] [PMID: 25739372]

[59]   Gogiraju R, Steinbrecher J, Lehnart S, Kessel M, Dobbelstein M, Schaefer K. Importance of tumor suppressor gene p53-mediated endothelial cell apoptosis for cardiac angiogenesis and hypertrophy. Eur Heart J 2013; •••: 34.
[http://dx.doi.org/10.1093/eurheartj/eht308.1616]

[60]   Tazawa H, Kagawa S, Fujiwara T. Advances in adenovirus-mediated p53 cancer gene therapy. Expert Opin Biol Ther 2013; 13(11): 1569-83.
[http://dx.doi.org/10.1517/14712598.2013.845662] [PMID: 24107178]

[61]   Chen H, Kuliszewski M, Rudenko D, Leong-Poi H. Pre-clinical evaluation of pro-angiogenic gene therapy by ultrasound-targeted microbubble destruction of vascular endothelial growth factor minicircle dna in an model of severe peripheral arterial disease in watanabe heritable hyperlipidemic rabbits. Can J Cardiol 2015; 31: S282.
[http://dx.doi.org/10.1016/j.cjca.2015.07.587]

[62]   Persano L, Crescenzi M, Indraccolo S. Anti-angiogenic gene therapy of cancer: current status and future prospects. Mol Aspects Med 2007; 28(1): 87-114.
[http://dx.doi.org/10.1016/j.mam.2006.12.005] [PMID: 17306361]

[63]   Feng X. Angiogenesis and antiangiogenesis therapies: spear and shield of pharmacotherapy. J Pharma Care Health Sys 2014; p. 1.

[64]   Albini A, Tosetti F, Li VW, Noonan DM, Li WW. Cancer prevention by targeting angiogenesis. Nat Rev Clin Oncol 2012; 9(9): 498-509.
[http://dx.doi.org/10.1038/nrclinonc.2012.120] [PMID: 22850752]

[65]   Ichihara E, Kiura K, Tanimoto M. Targeting angiogenesis in cancer therapy. Acta Med Okayama 2011; 65(6): 353-62.
[PMID: 22189475]

[66]   O'Reilly MS, Holmgren L, Shing Y, *et al.* Angiostatin: a novel angiogenesis inhibitor that mediates the suppression of metastases by a Lewis lung carcinoma. Cell 1994; 79(2): 315-28.
[http://dx.doi.org/10.1016/0092-8674(94)90200-3] [PMID: 7525077]

[67]   Wahl ML, Moser TL, Pizzo SV. Angiostatin and anti-angiogenic therapy in human disease. Recent Prog Horm Res 2004; 59: 73-104.
[http://dx.doi.org/10.1210/rp.59.1.73] [PMID: 14749498]

[68]   Kubo S, Takagi-Kimura M, Kasahara N. Combinatorial anti-angiogenic gene therapy in a human malignant mesothelioma model. Oncol Rep 2015; 34(2): 633-8.
[http://dx.doi.org/10.3892/or.2015.4058] [PMID: 26082103]

[69]   Hutzen B, Bid HK, Houghton PJ, *et al.* Treatment of medulloblastoma with oncolytic measles viruses expressing the angiogenesis inhibitors endostatin and angiostatin. BMC Cancer 2014; 14: 206.
[http://dx.doi.org/10.1186/1471-2407-14-206] [PMID: 24646176]

[70]   Zhang G, Jin G, Nie X, *et al.* Enhanced antitumor efficacy of an oncolytic herpes simplex virus expressing an endostatin-angiostatin fusion gene in human glioblastoma stem cell xenografts. PLoS One 2014; 9(4)e95872
[http://dx.doi.org/10.1371/journal.pone.0095872] [PMID: 24755877]

[71]   Sun X, Vale M, Jiang X, Gupta R, Krissansen GW. Antisense HIF-1alpha prevents acquired tumor resistance to angiostatin gene therapy. Cancer Gene Ther 2010; 17(8): 532-40.
[http://dx.doi.org/10.1038/cgt.2010.7] [PMID: 20348876]

[72]   Kuo CH, Chang BI, Lee FT, *et al.* Development of Recombinant Adeno-Associated Virus Serotype 2/8 Carrying Kringle Domains of Human Plasminogen for Sustained Expression and Cancer Therapy. Hum Gene Ther 2015; 26(9): 603-13.
[http://dx.doi.org/10.1089/hum.2013.220] [PMID: 25950911]

[73]   Chu Y, Liu H, Lou G, Zhang Q, Wu C. Human placenta mesenchymal stem cells expressing exogenous kringle1-5 protein by fiber-modified adenovirus suppress angiogenesis. Cancer Gene Ther 2014; 21(5): 200-8.
[http://dx.doi.org/10.1038/cgt.2014.19] [PMID: 24853622]

[74]   Maeshima Y, Colorado PC, Torre A, *et al.* Distinct antitumor properties of a type IV collagen domain derived from basement membrane. J Biol Chem 2000; 275(28): 21340-8.
[http://dx.doi.org/10.1074/jbc.M001956200] [PMID: 10766752]

[75]   Yang YP, Xu CX, Hou GS, Xin JX, Wang W, Liu XX. Effects of eukaryotic expression plasmid encoding human tumstatin gene on endothelial cells *in vitro*. Chin Med J (Engl) 2010; 123(16): 2269-73.
[PMID: 20819678]

[76]   Borza CM, Pozzi A, Borza DB, *et al.* Integrin alpha3beta1, a novel receptor for alpha3(IV) noncollagenous domain and a trans-dominant Inhibitor for integrin alphavbeta3. J Biol Chem 2006; 281(30): 20932-9.
[http://dx.doi.org/10.1074/jbc.M601147200] [PMID: 16731529]

[77]   Hwang-Bo J, Park JH, Chung IS. Tumstatin induces apoptosis mediated by Fas signaling pathway in oral squamous cell carcinoma SCC-VII cells. Oncol Lett 2015; 10(2): 1016-22.
[http://dx.doi.org/10.3892/ol.2015.3261] [PMID: 26622617]

[78]   Goto T, Ishikawa H, Matsumoto K, *et al.* Tum-1, a tumstatin fragment, gene delivery into hepatocellular carcinoma suppresses tumor growth through inhibiting angiogenesis. Int J Oncol 2008; 33(1): 33-40.
[http://dx.doi.org/10.3892/ijo.33.1.33] [PMID: 18575748]

[79]   Zhang X, Xu W, Qian H, Zhu W, Zhang R. Mesenchymal stem cells modified to express lentivirus TNF-α Tumstatin(45-132) inhibit the growth of prostate cancer. J Cell Mol Med 2011; 15(2): 433-44.
[http://dx.doi.org/10.1111/j.1582-4934.2009.00920.x] [PMID: 19799647]

[80]   Thevenard J, Ramont L, Mir LM, *et al.* A new anti-tumor strategy based on *in vivo* tumstatin overexpression after plasmid electrotransfer in muscle. Biochem Biophys Res Commun 2013; 432(4): 549-52.

[http://dx.doi.org/10.1016/j.bbrc.2013.02.074] [PMID: 23454380]

[81]   Gu Q, Sun C, Luo J, Zhang T, Wang L. Inhibition of angiogenesis by a synthetic fusion protein VTF derived from vasostatin and tumstatin. Anticancer Drugs 2014; 25(9): 1044-51.
[http://dx.doi.org/10.1097/CAD.0000000000000134] [PMID: 24942148]

[82]   Zhang X, Qi DD, Zhang TT, *et al.* Antitumor activity of adenoviral vector containing T42 and 4xT42 peptide gene through inducing apoptosis of tumor cells and suppressing angiogenesis. Mol Med Rep 2015; 11(3): 2083-91.
[http://dx.doi.org/10.3892/mmr.2014.2910] [PMID: 25384346]

[83]   O'Reilly MS, Boehm T, Shing Y, *et al.* Endostatin: an endogenous inhibitor of angiogenesis and tumor growth. Cell 1997; 88(2): 277-85.
[http://dx.doi.org/10.1016/S0092-8674(00)81848-6] [PMID: 9008168]

[84]   Sasaki T, Fukai N, Mann K, Göhring W, Olsen BR, Timpl R. Structure, function and tissue forms of the C-terminal globular domain of collagen XVIII containing the angiogenesis inhibitor endostatin. EMBO J 1998; 17(15): 4249-56.
[http://dx.doi.org/10.1093/emboj/17.15.4249] [PMID: 9687493]

[85]   Rong B, Yang S, Li W, Zhang W, Ming Z. Systematic review and meta-analysis of Endostar (rh-endostatin) combined with chemotherapy *versus* chemotherapy alone for treating advanced non-small cell lung cancer. World J Surg Oncol 2012; 10: 170.
[http://dx.doi.org/10.1186/1477-7819-10-170] [PMID: 22917490]

[86]   Huiqi G, Jing Z, Peng F, Yong L, Baozhong S. *In vivo* study of the effect of combining endostatin gene therapy with 32P-colloid on hepatocarcinoma and its functioning mechanism. J BUON 2015; 20(4): 1042-7.
[PMID: 26416054]

[87]   Yan F, Zheng Y, Huang L. Adenovirus-mediated combined anti-angiogenic and pro-apoptotic gene therapy enhances antitumor efficacy in hepatocellular carcinoma. Oncol Lett 2013; 5(1): 348-54.
[http://dx.doi.org/10.3892/ol.2012.987] [PMID: 23255947]

[88]   Xu Y, Xie Z, Zhou Y, *et al.* Experimental endostatin-GFP gene transfection into human retinal vascular endothelial cells using ultrasound-targeted cationic microbubble destruction. Mol Vis 2015; 21: 930-8.
[PMID: 26321867]

[89]   Zhou Y, Gu H, Xu Y, *et al.* Targeted antiangiogenesis gene therapy using targeted cationic microbubbles conjugated with CD105 antibody compared with untargeted cationic and neutral microbubbles. Theranostics 2015; 5(4): 399-417.
[http://dx.doi.org/10.7150/thno.10351] [PMID: 25699099]

[90]   Li XP, Zhang HL, Wang HJ, *et al.* Ad-endostatin treatment combined with low-dose irradiation in a murine lung cancer model. Oncol Rep 2014; 32(2): 650-8.
[http://dx.doi.org/10.3892/or.2014.3253] [PMID: 24927253]

[91]   Duda DG, Sunamura M, Lozonschi L, *et al.* Direct *in vitro* evidence and *in vivo* analysis of the antiangiogenesis effects of interleukin 12. Cancer Res 2000; 60(4): 1111-6.
[PMID: 10706132]

[92]   Dias S, Boyd R, Balkwill F. IL-12 regulates VEGF and MMPs in a murine breast cancer model. Int J Cancer 1998; 78(3): 361-5.
[http://dx.doi.org/10.1002/(SICI)1097-0215(19981029)78:3<361::AID-IJC17>3.0.CO;2-9] [PMID: 9766572]

[93]   Akiyama Y, Maruyama K, Watanabe M, Yamaguchi K. Retroviral-mediated IL-12 gene transduction into human CD34+ cell-derived dendritic cells. Int J Oncol 2002; 21(3): 509-14.
[http://dx.doi.org/10.3892/ijo.21.3.509] [PMID: 12168093]

[94]   Nguyen K, Koppolu B, Smith G, Ravindranathan S, Zaharoff D. Interleukin-12 elicits various

responses of splenocytes from different mouse strains. J Immunol 2015; 194: S49.

[95]   Hurteau JA, Blessing JA, DeCesare SL, Creasman WT. Evaluation of recombinant human interleukin-12 in patients with recurrent or refractory ovarian cancer: a gynecologic oncology group study. Gynecol Oncol 2001; 82(1): 7-10.
        [http://dx.doi.org/10.1006/gyno.2001.6255] [PMID: 11426954]

[96]   Gollob JA, Mier JW, Veenstra K, *et al.* Phase I trial of twice-weekly intravenous interleukin 12 in patients with metastatic renal cell cancer or malignant melanoma: ability to maintain IFN-gamma induction is associated with clinical response. Clin Cancer Res 2000; 6(5): 1678-92.
        [PMID: 10815886]

[97]   Daud A, Takamura KT, Diep T, Heller R, Pierce RH. Long-term overall survival from a phase I trial using intratumoral plasmid interleukin-12 with electroporation in patients with melanoma. J Transl Med 2015; 13: O3.
        [http://dx.doi.org/10.1186/1479-5876-13-S1-O3]

[98]   Daud A, Algazi A, Ashworth M, *et al.* Intratumoral electroporation of plasmid interleukin-12: efficacy and biomarker analyses from a phase 2 study in melanoma (OMS-I100). J Transl Med 2015; 13: O11.
        [http://dx.doi.org/10.1186/1479-5876-13-S1-O11]

[99]   Lampreht U, Kamensek U, Stimac M, *et al.* Gene Electrotransfer of Canine Interleukin 12 into Canine Melanoma Cell Lines. J Membr Biol 2015; 248(5): 909-17.
        [http://dx.doi.org/10.1007/s00232-015-9800-2] [PMID: 25840833]

[100]   Kramer MG, Masner M, Casales E, Moreno M, Smerdou C, Chabalgoity JA. Neoadjuvant administration of Semliki Forest virus expressing interleukin-12 combined with attenuated Salmonella eradicates breast cancer metastasis and achieves long-term survival in immunocompetent mice. BMC Cancer 2015; 15: 620.
        [http://dx.doi.org/10.1186/s12885-015-1618-x] [PMID: 26347489]

[101]   Poutou J, Bunuales M, Gonzalez-Aparicio M, *et al.* Safety and antitumor effect of oncolytic and helper-dependent adenoviruses expressing interleukin-12 variants in a hamster pancreatic cancer model. Gene Ther 2015; 22(9): 696-706.
        [http://dx.doi.org/10.1038/gt.2015.45] [PMID: 25938192]

[102]   Freytag SO, Zhang Y, Siddiqui F. Preclinical toxicology of oncolytic adenovirus-mediated cytotoxic and interleukin-12 gene therapy for prostate cancer. Mol Ther Oncolytics 2015; 2: 2.
        [http://dx.doi.org/10.1038/mto.2015.6] [PMID: 26767191]

[103]   Cutrera J, King G, Jones P, *et al.* Safe and effective treatment of spontaneous neoplasms with interleukin 12 electro-chemo-gene therapy. J Cell Mol Med 2015; 19(3): 664-75.
        [http://dx.doi.org/10.1111/jcmm.12382] [PMID: 25628149]

[104]   Date K, Matsumoto K, Shimura H, Tanaka M, Nakamura T. HGF/NK4 is a specific antagonist for pleiotrophic actions of hepatocyte growth factor. FEBS Lett 1997; 420(1): 1-6.
        [http://dx.doi.org/10.1016/S0014-5793(97)01475-0] [PMID: 9450538]

[105]   Kubota T, Matsumura A, Taiyoh H, *et al.* Interruption of the HGF paracrine loop by NK4, an HGF antagonist, reduces VEGF expression of CT26 cells. Oncol Rep 2013; 30(2): 567-72.
        [http://dx.doi.org/10.3892/or.2013.2509] [PMID: 23722408]

[106]   Suzuki Y, Sakai K, Ueki J, *et al.* Inhibition of Met/HGF receptor and angiogenesis by NK4 leads to suppression of tumor growth and migration in malignant pleural mesothelioma. Int J Cancer 2010; 127(8): 1948-57.
        [http://dx.doi.org/10.1002/ijc.25197] [PMID: 20104519]

[107]   Nakamura T, Sakai K, Nakamura T, Matsumoto K. Anti-cancer approach with NK4: Bivalent action and mechanisms. Anticancer Agents Med Chem 2010; 10(1): 36-46.
        [http://dx.doi.org/10.2174/1871520611009010036] [PMID: 20015005]

[108]   Kishi Y, Kuba K, Nakamura T, *et al.* Systemic NK4 gene therapy inhibits tumor growth and

metastasis of melanoma and lung carcinoma in syngeneic mouse tumor models. Cancer Sci 2009; 100(7): 1351-8.
[http://dx.doi.org/10.1111/j.1349-7006.2009.01184.x] [PMID: 19438869]

[109] Matsumoto G, Omi Y, Lee U, Kubota E, Tabata Y. NK4 gene therapy combined with cisplatin inhibits tumour growth and metastasis of squamous cell carcinoma. Anticancer Res 2011; 31(1): 105-11.
[PMID: 21273587]

[110] Taiyoh H, Kubota T, Fujiwara H, *et al.* NK4 gene expression enhances 5-fluorouracil-induced apoptosis of murine colon cancer cells. Anticancer Res 2011; 31(6): 2217-24.
[PMID: 21737644]

[111] Zhu Y, Cheng M, Yang Z, *et al.* Mesenchymal stem cell-based NK4 gene therapy in nude mice bearing gastric cancer xenografts. Drug Des Devel Ther 2014; 8: 2449-62.
[http://dx.doi.org/10.2147/DDDT.S71466] [PMID: 25525335]

[112] Tada Y, Hiroshima K, Shimada H, *et al.* A clinical protocol to inhibit the HGF/c-Met pathway for malignant mesothelioma with an intrapleural injection of adenoviruses expressing the NK4 gene. Springerplus 2015; 4: 358.
[http://dx.doi.org/10.1186/s40064-015-1123-3] [PMID: 26191485]

[113] Danhier F, Le Breton A, Préat V. RGD-based strategies to target alpha(v) beta(3) integrin in cancer therapy and diagnosis. Mol Pharm 2012; 9(11): 2961-73.
[http://dx.doi.org/10.1021/mp3002733] [PMID: 22967287]

[114] Trochon-Joseph V, Martel-Renoir D, Mir LM, *et al.* Evidence of antiangiogenic and antimetastatic activities of the recombinant disintegrin domain of metargidin. Cancer Res 2004; 64(6): 2062-9.
[http://dx.doi.org/10.1158/0008-5472.CAN-03-3272] [PMID: 15026344]

[115] Daugimont L, Vandermeulen G, Defresne F, *et al.* Antitumoral and antimetastatic effect of antiangiogenic plasmids in B16 melanoma: Higher efficiency of the recombinant disintegrin domain of ADAM 15. Eur J Pharm Biopharm 2011; 78(3): 314-9.
[http://dx.doi.org/10.1016/j.ejpb.2011.02.001] [PMID: 21316447]

[116] Spanggaard I, Snoj M, Cavalcanti A, *et al.* Gene electrotransfer of plasmid antiangiogenic metargidin peptide (AMEP) in disseminated melanoma: safety and efficacy results of a phase I first-in-man study. Hum Gene Ther Clin Dev 2013; 24(3): 99-107.
[http://dx.doi.org/10.1089/humc.2012.240] [PMID: 23980876]

[117] Bosnjak M, Prosen L, Dolinsek T, *et al.* Biological properties of melanoma and endothelial cells after plasmid AMEP gene electrotransfer depend on integrin quantity on cells. J Membr Biol 2013; 246(11): 803-19.
[http://dx.doi.org/10.1007/s00232-013-9550-y] [PMID: 23649038]

[118] Bosnjak M, Dolinsek T, Cemazar M, *et al.* Gene electrotransfer of plasmid AMEP, an integrin-targeted therapy, has antitumor and antiangiogenic action in murine B16 melanoma. Gene Ther 2015; 22(7): 578-90.
[http://dx.doi.org/10.1038/gt.2015.26] [PMID: 25781650]

[119] ten Dijke P, Goumans MJ, Pardali E. Endoglin in angiogenesis and vascular diseases. Angiogenesis 2008; 11(1): 79-89.
[http://dx.doi.org/10.1007/s10456-008-9101-9] [PMID: 18283546]

[120] Nassiri F, Cusimano MD, Scheithauer BW, *et al.* Endoglin (CD105): a review of its role in angiogenesis and tumor diagnosis, progression and therapy. Anticancer Res 2011; 31(6): 2283-90.
[PMID: 21737653]

[121] Muñoz R, Arias Y, Ferreras JM, *et al. In vitro* and *in vivo* effects of an anti-mouse endoglin (CD105)-immunotoxin on the early stages of mouse B16MEL4A5 melanoma tumours. Cancer Immunol Immunother 2013; 62(3): 541-51.
[http://dx.doi.org/10.1007/s00262-012-1357-7] [PMID: 23076642]

[122] Uneda S, Toi H, Tsujie T, *et al.* Anti-endoglin monoclonal antibodies are effective for suppressing metastasis and the primary tumors by targeting tumor vasculature. Int J Cancer 2009; 125(6): 1446-53.
[http://dx.doi.org/10.1002/ijc.24482] [PMID: 19533687]

[123] Dolinsek T, Markelc B, Sersa G, *et al.* Multiple delivery of siRNA against endoglin into murine mammary adenocarcinoma prevents angiogenesis and delays tumor growth. PLoS One 2013; 8(3)e58723
[http://dx.doi.org/10.1371/journal.pone.0058723] [PMID: 23593103]

[124] Xu Y, Hou J, Liu Z, *et al.* Gene therapy with tumor-specific promoter mediated suicide gene plus IL-12 gene enhanced tumor inhibition and prolonged host survival in a murine model of Lewis lung carcinoma. J Transl Med 2011; 9: 39.
[http://dx.doi.org/10.1186/1479-5876-9-39] [PMID: 21481255]

[125] Stimac M, Dolinsek T, Lampreht U, Cemazar M, Sersa G. Gene electrotransfer of plasmid with tissue specific promoter encoding shRNA against endoglin exerts antitumor efficacy against murine TS/A tumors by vascular targeted effects. PLoS One 2015; 10(4)e0124913
[http://dx.doi.org/10.1371/journal.pone.0124913] [PMID: 25909447]

[126] Dolinsek T, Sersa G, Cemazar M. Melanoma cell viability is reduced after endoglin silencing with gene electrotransfer. 1st World Congress on Electroporation and Pulsed Electric Fields in Biology, Medicine and Food & Environmental Technologies. 325-8.
[http://dx.doi.org/10.1007/978-981-287-817-5_72]

[127] Loges S, Schmidt T, Carmeliet P. Mechanisms of resistance to anti-angiogenic therapy and development of third-generation anti-angiogenic drug candidates. Genes Cancer 2010; 1(1): 12-25.
[http://dx.doi.org/10.1177/1947601909356574] [PMID: 21779425]

[128] Auguste P, Lemiere S, Larrieu-Lahargue F, Bikfalvi A. Molecular mechanisms of tumor vascularization. Crit Rev Oncol Hematol 2005; 54(1): 53-61.
[http://dx.doi.org/10.1016/j.critrevonc.2004.11.006] [PMID: 15780907]

[129] Bergers G, Hanahan D. Modes of resistance to anti-angiogenic therapy. Nat Rev Cancer 2008; 8(8): 592-603.
[http://dx.doi.org/10.1038/nrc2442] [PMID: 18650835]

[130] Carey R, Holland J, Whang H, Neter E, Bryant B. Clostridial oncolysis in man. Eur J Cancer 1967; 3: 37-46.
[http://dx.doi.org/10.1016/0014-2964(67)90060-6]

[131] Dang LH, Bettegowda C, Huso DL, Kinzler KW, Vogelstein B. Combination bacteriolytic therapy for the treatment of experimental tumors. Proc Natl Acad Sci USA 2001; 98(26): 15155-60.
[http://dx.doi.org/10.1073/pnas.251543698] [PMID: 11724950]

[132] Wei MQ, Ellem KA, Dunn P, West MJ, Bai CX, Vogelstein B. Facultative or obligate anaerobic bacteria have the potential for multimodality therapy of solid tumours. Eur J Cancer 2007; 43(3): 490-6.
[http://dx.doi.org/10.1016/j.ejca.2006.10.005] [PMID: 17113280]

[133] Cheong I, Huang X, Bettegowda C, *et al.* A bacterial protein enhances the release and efficacy of liposomal cancer drugs. Science 2006; 314(5803): 1308-11.
[http://dx.doi.org/10.1126/science.1130651] [PMID: 17124324]

[134] Bermudes D, Zheng LM, King IC. Live bacteria as anticancer agents and tumor-selective protein delivery vectors. Curr Opin Drug Discov Devel 2002; 5(2): 194-9.
[PMID: 11926125]

[135] Jia LJ, Xu HM, Ma DY, *et al.* Enhanced therapeutic effect by combination of tumor-targeting Salmonella and endostatin in murine melanoma model. Cancer Biol Ther 2005; 4(8): 840-5.
[http://dx.doi.org/10.4161/cbt.4.8.1891] [PMID: 16210914]

[136] Li X, Fu GF, Fan YR, *et al.* Bifidobacterium adolescentis as a delivery system of endostatin for cancer

gene therapy: selective inhibitor of angiogenesis and hypoxic tumor growth. Cancer Gene Ther 2003; 10(2): 105-11.
[http://dx.doi.org/10.1038/sj.cgt.7700530] [PMID: 12536198]

[137] Xu YF, Zhu LP, Hu B, *et al.* A new expression plasmid in Bifidobacterium longum as a delivery system of endostatin for cancer gene therapy. Cancer Gene Ther 2007; 14(2): 151-7.
[http://dx.doi.org/10.1038/sj.cgt.7701003] [PMID: 17068487]

[138] Fu GF, Li X, Hou YY, Fan YR, Liu WH, Xu GX. Bifidobacterium longum as an oral delivery system of endostatin for gene therapy on solid liver cancer. Cancer Gene Ther 2005; 12(2): 133-40.
[http://dx.doi.org/10.1038/sj.cgt.7700758] [PMID: 15565182]

[139] Niethammer AG, Xiang R, Becker JC, *et al.* A DNA vaccine against VEGF receptor 2 prevents effective angiogenesis and inhibits tumor growth. Nat Med 2002; 8(12): 1369-75.
[http://dx.doi.org/10.1038/nm1202-794] [PMID: 12415261]

[140] Gardlik R, Behuliak M, Palffy R, Celec P, Li CJ. Gene therapy for cancer: bacteria-mediated anti-angiogenesis therapy. Gene Ther 2011; 18(5): 425-31.
[http://dx.doi.org/10.1038/gt.2010.176] [PMID: 21228886]

[141] Hu B, Kou L, Li C, *et al.* Bifidobacterium longum as a delivery system of TRAIL and endostatin cooperates with chemotherapeutic drugs to inhibit hypoxic tumor growth. Cancer Gene Ther 2009; 16(8): 655-63.
[http://dx.doi.org/10.1038/cgt.2009.7] [PMID: 19229287]

[142] Signori E, Iurescia S, Massi E, *et al.* DNA vaccination strategies for anti-tumour effective gene therapy protocols. Cancer Immunol Immunother 2010; 59(10): 1583-91.
[http://dx.doi.org/10.1007/s00262-010-0853-x] [PMID: 20390416]

[143] Palena C, Schlom J. Vaccines against human carcinomas: strategies to improve antitumor immune responses. J Biomed Biotechnol 2010; 2010380697
[http://dx.doi.org/10.1155/2010/380697] [PMID: 20300434]

[144] Fioretti D, Iurescia S, Fazio VM, Rinaldi M. DNA vaccines: developing new strategies against cancer. J Biomed Biotechnol 2010; 2010174378
[http://dx.doi.org/10.1155/2010/174378] [PMID: 20368780]

[145] Gravekamp C, Paterson Y. Harnessing Listeria monocytogenes to target tumors. Cancer Biol Ther 2010; 9(4): 257-65.
[http://dx.doi.org/10.4161/cbt.9.4.11216] [PMID: 20139702]

[146] Reisfeld RA, Niethammer AG, Luo Y, Xiang R. DNA vaccines designed to inhibit tumor growth by suppression of angiogenesis. Int Arch Allergy Immunol 2004; 133(3): 295-304.
[http://dx.doi.org/10.1159/000077009] [PMID: 14988601]

[147] Maciag PC, Seavey MM, Pan ZK, Ferrone S, Paterson Y. Cancer immunotherapy targeting the high molecular weight melanoma-associated antigen protein results in a broad antitumor response and reduction of pericytes in the tumor vasculature. Cancer Res 2008; 68(19): 8066-75.
[http://dx.doi.org/10.1158/0008-5472.CAN-08-0287] [PMID: 18829565]

[148] Seavey MM, Maciag PC, Al-Rawi N, Sewell D, Paterson Y. An anti-vascular endothelial growth factor receptor 2/fetal liver kinase-1 Listeria monocytogenes anti-angiogenesis cancer vaccine for the treatment of primary and metastatic Her-2/neu+ breast tumors in a mouse model. J Immunol 2009; 182(9): 5537-46.
[http://dx.doi.org/10.4049/jimmunol.0803742] [PMID: 19380802]

[149] Daudel D, Weidinger G, Spreng S. Use of attenuated bacteria as delivery vectors for DNA vaccines. Expert Rev Vaccines 2007; 6(1): 97-110.
[http://dx.doi.org/10.1586/14760584.6.1.97] [PMID: 17280482]

[150] Wada S, Tsunoda T, Baba T, *et al.* Rationale for antiangiogenic cancer therapy with vaccination using epitope peptides derived from human vascular endothelial growth factor receptor 2. Cancer Res 2005;

65(11): 4939-46.
[http://dx.doi.org/10.1158/0008-5472.CAN-04-3759] [PMID: 15930316]

[151]   Hu B, Wei Y, Tian L, *et al.* Active antitumor immunity elicited by vaccine based on recombinant form of epidermal growth factor receptor. J Immunother 2005; 28(3): 236-44.
[http://dx.doi.org/10.1097/01.cji.0000161394.11831.3f] [PMID: 15838380]

[152]   Nair SK, Morse M, Boczkowski D, *et al.* Induction of tumor-specific cytotoxic T lymphocytes in cancer patients by autologous tumor RNA-transfected dendritic cells. Ann Surg 2002; 235(4): 540-9.
[http://dx.doi.org/10.1097/00000658-200204000-00013] [PMID: 11923611]

[153]   Lai MD, Yen MC, Lin CM, *et al.* The effects of DNA formulation and administration route on cancer therapeutic efficacy with xenogenic EGFR DNA vaccine in a lung cancer animal model. Genet Vaccines Ther 2009; 7: 2.
[http://dx.doi.org/10.1186/1479-0556-7-2] [PMID: 19178753]

[154]   Lee CH, Wu CL, Shiau AL. Endostatin gene therapy delivered by Salmonella choleraesuis in murine tumor models. J Gene Med 2004; 6(12): 1382-93.
[http://dx.doi.org/10.1002/jgm.626] [PMID: 15468191]

[155]   Yoon WS, Choi WC, Sin JI, Park YK. Antitumor therapeutic effects of *Salmonella typhimurium* containing Flt3 Ligand expression plasmids in melanoma-bearing mouse. Biotechnol Lett 2007; 29(4): 511-6.
[http://dx.doi.org/10.1007/s10529-006-9270-9] [PMID: 17235489]

[156]   Agorio C, Schreiber F, Sheppard M, *et al.* Live attenuated Salmonella as a vector for oral cytokine gene therapy in melanoma. J Gene Med 2007; 9(5): 416-23.
[http://dx.doi.org/10.1002/jgm.1023] [PMID: 17410612]

[157]   Lee CH, Wu CL, Shiau AL. Systemic administration of attenuated Salmonella choleraesuis carrying thrombospondin-1 gene leads to tumor-specific transgene expression, delayed tumor growth and prolonged survival in the murine melanoma model. Cancer Gene Ther 2005; 12(2): 175-84.
[http://dx.doi.org/10.1038/sj.cgt.7700777] [PMID: 15375381]

[158]   Castagliuolo I, Beggiao E, Brun P, *et al.* Engineered E. coli delivers therapeutic genes to the colonic mucosa. Gene Ther 2005; 12(13): 1070-8.
[http://dx.doi.org/10.1038/sj.gt.3302493] [PMID: 15815705]

[159]   Larsen MD, Griesenbach U, Goussard S, *et al.* Bactofection of lung epithelial cells *in vitro* and *in vivo* using a genetically modified Escherichia coli. Gene Ther 2008; 15(6): 434-42.
[http://dx.doi.org/10.1038/sj.gt.3303090] [PMID: 18317498]

[160]   Aigner A. Transkingdom RNA interference (tkRNAi) as a new delivery tool for therapeutic RNA. Expert Opin Biol Ther 2009; 9(12): 1533-42.
[http://dx.doi.org/10.1517/14712590903307354] [PMID: 19769540]

[161]   Jiang Z, Zhao P, Zhou Z, Liu J, Qin L, Wang H. Using attenuated Salmonella typhi as tumor targeting vector for MDR1 siRNA delivery. Cancer Biol Ther 2007; 6(4): 555-60.
[http://dx.doi.org/10.4161/cbt.6.4.3850] [PMID: 17374987]

[162]   Xiang S, Fruehauf J, Li CJ. Short hairpin RNA-expressing bacteria elicit RNA interference in mammals. Nat Biotechnol 2006; 24(6): 697-702.
[http://dx.doi.org/10.1038/nbt1211] [PMID: 16699500]

[163]   Zhang L, Gao L, Zhao L, *et al.* Intratumoral delivery and suppression of prostate tumor growth by attenuated Salmonella enterica serovar typhimurium carrying plasmid-based small interfering RNAs. Cancer Res 2007; 67(12): 5859-64.
[http://dx.doi.org/10.1158/0008-5472.CAN-07-0098] [PMID: 17575154]

[164]   Yang N, Zhu X, Chen L, Li S, Ren D. Oral administration of attenuated S. typhimurium carrying shRNA-expressing vectors as a cancer therapeutic. Cancer Biol Ther 2008; 7(1): 145-51.
[http://dx.doi.org/10.4161/cbt.7.1.5195] [PMID: 18059172]

[165] Easwaran V, Lee SH, Inge L, *et al.* beta-Catenin regulates vascular endothelial growth factor expression in colon cancer. Cancer Res 2003; 63(12): 3145-53.
[PMID: 12810642]

[166] Wei D, Le X, Zheng L, *et al.* Stat3 activation regulates the expression of vascular endothelial growth factor and human pancreatic cancer angiogenesis and metastasis. Oncogene 2003; 22(3): 319-29.
[http://dx.doi.org/10.1038/sj.onc.1206122] [PMID: 12545153]

[167] Jia RB, Zhang P, Zhou YX, *et al.* VEGF-targeted RNA interference suppresses angiogenesis and tumor growth of retinoblastoma. Ophthalmic Res 2007; 39(2): 108-15.
[http://dx.doi.org/10.1159/000099247] [PMID: 17284938]

[168] Kim WJ, Chang CW, Lee M, Kim SW. Efficient siRNA delivery using water soluble lipopolymer for anti-angiogenic gene therapy. J Control Release 2007; 118(3): 357-63.
[http://dx.doi.org/10.1016/j.jconrel.2006.12.026] [PMID: 17313987]

[169] Hadj-Slimane R, Lepelletier Y, Lopez N, Garbay C, Raynaud F. Short interfering RNA (siRNA), a novel therapeutic tool acting on angiogenesis. Biochimie 2007; 89(10): 1234-44.
[http://dx.doi.org/10.1016/j.biochi.2007.06.012] [PMID: 17707573]

[170] Xiang R, Lode HN, Chao TH, *et al.* An autologous oral DNA vaccine protects against murine melanoma. Proc Natl Acad Sci USA 2000; 97(10): 5492-7.
[http://dx.doi.org/10.1073/pnas.090097697] [PMID: 10779556]

[171] Petrovan RJ, Kaplan CD, Reisfeld RA, Curtiss LK. DNA vaccination against VEGF receptor 2 reduces atherosclerosis in LDL receptor-deficient mice. Arterioscler Thromb Vasc Biol 2007; 27(5): 1095-100.
[http://dx.doi.org/10.1161/ATVBAHA.106.139246] [PMID: 17303776]

[172] Hauer AD, van Puijvelde GH, Peterse N, *et al.* Vaccination against VEGFR2 attenuates initiation and progression of atherosclerosis. Arterioscler Thromb Vasc Biol 2007; 27(9): 2050-7.
[http://dx.doi.org/10.1161/ATVBAHA.107.143743] [PMID: 17600223]

[173] Kim B, Suvas S, Sarangi PP, Lee S, Reisfeld RA, Rouse BT. Vascular endothelial growth factor receptor 2-based DNA immunization delays development of herpetic stromal keratitis by antiangiogenic effects. J Immunol 2006; 177(6): 4122-31.
[http://dx.doi.org/10.4049/jimmunol.177.6.4122] [PMID: 16951377]

[174] Lu XL, Jiang XB, Liu RE, Zhang SM. The enhanced anti-angiogenic and antitumor effects of combining flk1-based DNA vaccine and IP-10. Vaccine 2008; 26(42): 5352-7.
[http://dx.doi.org/10.1016/j.vaccine.2008.08.012] [PMID: 18723067]

[175] Luo Y, Zhou H, Mizutani M, Mizutani N, Reisfeld RA, Xiang R. Transcription factor Fos-related antigen 1 is an effective target for a breast cancer vaccine. Proc Natl Acad Sci USA 2003; 100(15): 8850-5.
[http://dx.doi.org/10.1073/pnas.1033132100] [PMID: 12857959]

[176] Xiang R, Mizutani N, Luo Y, *et al.* A DNA vaccine targeting survivin combines apoptosis with suppression of angiogenesis in lung tumor eradication. Cancer Res 2005; 65(2): 553-61.
[PMID: 15695399]

[177] Lee SH, Mizutani N, Mizutani M, *et al.* Endoglin (CD105) is a target for an oral DNA vaccine against breast cancer. Cancer Immunol Immunother 2006; 55(12): 1565-74.
[http://dx.doi.org/10.1007/s00262-006-0155-5] [PMID: 16565828]

[178] Epaulard O, Toussaint B, Quenee L, *et al.* Anti-tumor immunotherapy *via* antigen delivery from a live attenuated genetically engineered Pseudomonas aeruginosa type III secretion system-based vector. Mol Ther 2006; 14(5): 656-61.
[http://dx.doi.org/10.1016/j.ymthe.2006.06.011] [PMID: 17010670]

[179] Pálffy R, Gardlík R, Hodosy J, *et al.* Bacteria in gene therapy: bactofection *versus* alternative gene therapy. Gene Ther 2006; 13(2): 101-5.

[http://dx.doi.org/10.1038/sj.gt.3302635] [PMID: 16163379]

[180] Sasaki T, Fujimori M, Hamaji Y, *et al.* Genetically engineered Bifidobacterium longum for tumor-targeting enzyme-prodrug therapy of autochthonous mammary tumors in rats. Cancer Sci 2006; 97(7): 649-57.
[http://dx.doi.org/10.1111/j.1349-7006.2006.00221.x] [PMID: 16827806]

[181] Schmidt W, Fabricius EM, Schneeweiss U. The tumour-Clostridium phenomenon: 50 years of developmental research (Review). Int J Oncol 2006; 29(6): 1479-92. [Review].
[http://dx.doi.org/10.3892/ijo.29.6.1479] [PMID: 17088987]

[182] Wei MQ, Ren R, Good D, Anné J. Clostridial spores as live 'Trojan horse' vectors for cancer gene therapy: comparison with viral delivery systems. Genet Vaccines Ther 2008; 6: 8.
[http://dx.doi.org/10.1186/1479-0556-6-8] [PMID: 18279524]

[183] Li Z, Fallon J, Mandeli J, Wetmur J, Woo SL. A genetically enhanced anaerobic bacterium for oncopathic therapy of pancreatic cancer. J Natl Cancer Inst 2008; 100(19): 1389-400.
[http://dx.doi.org/10.1093/jnci/djn308] [PMID: 18812551]

[184] Loessner H, Endmann A, Leschner S, *et al.* Remote control of tumour-targeted Salmonella enterica serovar Typhimurium by the use of L-arabinose as inducer of bacterial gene expression *in vivo*. Cell Microbiol 2007; 9(6): 1529-37.
[http://dx.doi.org/10.1111/j.1462-5822.2007.00890.x] [PMID: 17298393]

[185] Stritzker J, Weibel S, Hill PJ, Oelschlaeger TA, Goebel W, Szalay AA. Tumor-specific colonization, tissue distribution, and gene induction by probiotic Escherichia coli Nissle 1917 in live mice. Int J Med Microbiol 2007; 297(3): 151-62.
[http://dx.doi.org/10.1016/j.ijmm.2007.01.008] [PMID: 17448724]

[186] Mengesha A, Dubois L, Lambin P, *et al.* Development of a flexible and potent hypoxia-inducible promoter for tumor-targeted gene expression in attenuated Salmonella. Cancer Biol Ther 2006; 5(9): 1120-8.
[http://dx.doi.org/10.4161/cbt.5.9.2951] [PMID: 16855381]

[187] Ryan RM, Green J, Williams PJ, *et al.* Bacterial delivery of a novel cytolysin to hypoxic areas of solid tumors. Gene Ther 2009; 16(3): 329-39.
[http://dx.doi.org/10.1038/gt.2008.188] [PMID: 19177133]

[188] Arrach N, Zhao M, Porwollik S, Hoffman RM, McClelland M. Salmonella promoters preferentially activated inside tumors. Cancer Res 2008; 68(12): 4827-32.
[http://dx.doi.org/10.1158/0008-5472.CAN-08-0552] [PMID: 18559530]

[189] Westphal K, Leschner S, Jablonska J, Loessner H, Weiss S. Containment of tumor-colonizing bacteria by host neutrophils. Cancer Res 2008; 68(8): 2952-60.
[http://dx.doi.org/10.1158/0008-5472.CAN-07-2984] [PMID: 18413765]

[190] Stritzker J, Pilgrim S, Szalay AA, Goebel W. Prodrug converting enzyme gene delivery by L. monocytogenes. BMC Cancer 2008; 8: 94.
[http://dx.doi.org/10.1186/1471-2407-8-94] [PMID: 18402662]

[191] Loeffler M, Le'Negrate G, Krajewska M, Reed JC. Attenuated Salmonella engineered to produce human cytokine LIGHT inhibit tumor growth. Proc Natl Acad Sci USA 2007; 104(31): 12879-83.
[http://dx.doi.org/10.1073/pnas.0701959104] [PMID: 17652173]

[192] Loeffler M, Le'Negrate G, Krajewska M, Reed JC. IL-18-producing Salmonella inhibit tumor growth. Cancer Gene Ther 2008; 15(12): 787-94.
[http://dx.doi.org/10.1038/cgt.2008.48] [PMID: 18654612]

[193] Loeffler M, Le'Negrate G, Krajewska M, Reed JC. *Salmonella typhimurium* engineered to produce CCL21 inhibit tumor growth. Cancer Immunol Immunother 2009; 58(5): 769-75.
[http://dx.doi.org/10.1007/s00262-008-0555-9] [PMID: 18633610]

[194] al-Ramadi BK, Fernandez-Cabezudo MJ, El-Hasasna H, Al-Salam S, Bashir G, Chouaib S. Potent

anti-tumor activity of systemically-administered IL2-expressing Salmonella correlates with decreased angiogenesis and enhanced tumor apoptosis. Clin Immunol 2009; 130(1): 89-97.
[http://dx.doi.org/10.1016/j.clim.2008.08.021] [PMID: 18849195]

[195] Nemunaitis J, Cunningham C, Senzer N, *et al.* Pilot trial of genetically modified, attenuated Salmonella expressing the E. coli cytosine deaminase gene in refractory cancer patients. Cancer Gene Ther 2003; 10(10): 737-44.
[http://dx.doi.org/10.1038/sj.cgt.7700634] [PMID: 14502226]

[196] Toso JF, Gill VJ, Hwu P, *et al.* Phase I study of the intravenous administration of attenuated *Salmonella typhimurium* to patients with metastatic melanoma. J Clin Oncol 2002; 20(1): 142-52.
[http://dx.doi.org/10.1200/JCO.2002.20.1.142] [PMID: 11773163]

[197] Yu YA, Shabahang S, Timiryasova TM, *et al.* Visualization of tumors and metastases in live animals with bacteria and vaccinia virus encoding light-emitting proteins. Nat Biotechnol 2004; 22(3): 313-20.
[http://dx.doi.org/10.1038/nbt937] [PMID: 14990953]

[198] Agrawal N, Bettegowda C, Cheong I, *et al.* Bacteriolytic therapy can generate a potent immune response against experimental tumors. Proc Natl Acad Sci USA 2004; 101(42): 15172-7.
[http://dx.doi.org/10.1073/pnas.0406242101] [PMID: 15471990]

[199] Ramlau R, Gorbunova V, Ciuleanu TE, *et al.* Aflibercept and Docetaxel *versus* Docetaxel alone after platinum failure in patients with advanced or metastatic non-small-cell lung cancer: a randomized, controlled phase III trial. J Clin Oncol 2012; 30(29): 3640-7.
[http://dx.doi.org/10.1200/JCO.2012.42.6932] [PMID: 22965962]

[200] Tortorici MA, Cohen EE, Pithavala YK, *et al.* Pharmacokinetics of single-agent axitinib across multiple solid tumor types. Cancer Chemother Pharmacol 2014; 74(6): 1279-89.
[http://dx.doi.org/10.1007/s00280-014-2606-6] [PMID: 25336084]

[201] Pujade-Lauraine E, Hilpert F, Weber B, *et al.* Bevacizumab combined with chemotherapy for platinum-resistant recurrent ovarian cancer: The AURELIA open-label randomized phase III trial. J Clin Oncol 2014; 32(13): 1302-8.
[http://dx.doi.org/10.1200/JCO.2013.51.4489] [PMID: 24637997]

[202] Schwandt A, von Gruenigen VE, Wenham RM, *et al.* Randomized phase II trial of sorafenib alone or in combination with carboplatin/paclitaxel in women with recurrent platinum sensitive epithelial ovarian, peritoneal, or fallopian tube cancer. Invest New Drugs 2014; 32(4): 729-38.
[http://dx.doi.org/10.1007/s10637-014-0078-5] [PMID: 24619298]

[203] Heinemann V, von Weikersthal LF, Decker T, *et al.* FOLFIRI plus cetuximab *versus* FOLFIRI plus bevacizumab as first-line treatment for patients with metastatic colorectal cancer (FIRE-3): a randomised, open-label, phase 3 trial. Lancet Oncol 2014; 15(10): 1065-75.
[http://dx.doi.org/10.1016/S1470-2045(14)70330-4] [PMID: 25088940]

[204] Van Cutsem E, Tabernero J, Lakomy R, *et al.* Addition of aflibercept to fluorouracil, leucovorin, and irinotecan improves survival in a phase III randomized trial in patients with metastatic colorectal cancer previously treated with an oxaliplatin-based regimen. J Clin Oncol 2012; 30(28): 3499-506.
[http://dx.doi.org/10.1200/JCO.2012.42.8201] [PMID: 22949147]

[205] Ramalingam S, Mack P, Vokes E, *et al.* Cediranib (AZD2171) for the treatment of recurrent small cell lung cancer (SCLC): A California Consortium phase II study (NCI# 7097). J Clin Oncol 2008; 26: 8078-8.
[http://dx.doi.org/10.1200/jco.2008.26.15_suppl.8078]

[206] Cheng A, Kang Y, Lin D, *et al.* Phase III trial of sunitinib (Su) *versus* sorafenib (So) in advanced hepatocellular carcinoma (HCC). J Clin Oncol 2011; 29: 4000-0.
[http://dx.doi.org/10.1200/jco.2011.29.15_suppl.4000]

[207] Zhu AX, Rosmorduc O, Evans TR, *et al.* SEARCH: a phase III, randomized, double-blind, placebo-controlled trial of sorafenib plus erlotinib in patients with advanced hepatocellular carcinoma. J Clin Oncol 2015; 33(6): 559-66.

[http://dx.doi.org/10.1200/JCO.2013.53.7746] [PMID: 25547503]

[208] Rini BI, Bellmunt J, Clancy J, *et al.* Randomized phase III trial of temsirolimus and bevacizumab *versus* interferon alfa and bevacizumab in metastatic renal cell carcinoma: INTORACT trial. J Clin Oncol 2014; 32(8): 752-9.
[http://dx.doi.org/10.1200/JCO.2013.50.5305] [PMID: 24297945]

[209] Sternberg CN, Davis ID, Mardiak J, *et al.* Pazopanib in locally advanced or metastatic renal cell carcinoma: results of a randomized phase III trial. J Clin Oncol 2010; 28(6): 1061-8.
[http://dx.doi.org/10.1200/JCO.2009.23.9764] [PMID: 20100962]

[210] Tannock IF, Fizazi K, Ivanov S, *et al.* Aflibercept *versus* placebo in combination with docetaxel and prednisone for treatment of men with metastatic castration-resistant prostate cancer (VENICE): a phase 3, double-blind randomised trial. Lancet Oncol 2013; 14(8): 760-8.
[http://dx.doi.org/10.1016/S1470-2045(13)70184-0] [PMID: 23742877]

[211] Brassard M, Rondeau G. Role of vandetanib in the management of medullary thyroid cancer. Biologics 2012; 6: 59-66.
[http://dx.doi.org/10.2147/BTT.S24220] [PMID: 22500115]

[212] Moore MJ, Goldstein D, Hamm J, *et al.* Erlotinib plus gemcitabine compared with gemcitabine alone in patients with advanced pancreatic cancer: a phase III trial of the National Cancer Institute of Canada Clinical Trials Group. J Clin Oncol 2007; 25(15): 1960-6.
[http://dx.doi.org/10.1200/JCO.2006.07.9525] [PMID: 17452677]

[213] Cui C, Mao L, Chi Z, *et al.* A phase II, randomized, double-blind, placebo-controlled multicenter trial of Endostar in patients with metastatic melanoma. Mol Ther 2013; 21(7): 1456-63.
[http://dx.doi.org/10.1038/mt.2013.79] [PMID: 23670576]

[214] Kluger HM, Dudek AZ, McCann C, *et al.* A phase 2 trial of dasatinib in advanced melanoma. Cancer 2011; 117(10): 2202-8.
[http://dx.doi.org/10.1002/cncr.25766] [PMID: 21523734]

[215] Lordick F, Kang YK, Chung HC, *et al.* Capecitabine and cisplatin with or without cetuximab for patients with previously untreated advanced gastric cancer (EXPAND): a randomised, open-label phase 3 trial. Lancet Oncol 2013; 14(6): 490-9.
[http://dx.doi.org/10.1016/S1470-2045(13)70102-5] [PMID: 23594786]

[216] Yuhua L, Kunyuan G, Hui C, *et al.* Oral cytokine gene therapy against murine tumor using attenuated *Salmonella typhimurium*. Int J Cancer 2001; 94(3): 438-43.
[http://dx.doi.org/10.1002/ijc.1489] [PMID: 11745427]

CHAPTER 4

Novel Anti-angiogenic Strategies in Cancer Drug Development

Hoorieh Soleimanjahi* and **Ala Habibian**

Department of Virology, Faculty of Medical Sciences, Tarbiat Modares University, Tehran, Iran

Abstract: Cancer, which is a complex disease of various types, is the most important health problem in modern life. Several conventional methods such as chemotherapy, radiotherapy and surgery have been adapted to fight against tumors. Nevertheless, recent studies revealed that tumors may acquire resistance against a variety of therapies based on the physiological state known as microenvironment. Tumor microenvironment is formed by different types of normal, inflammatory and immune cells, as well as blood vessels, which are efficient nutrient providers for the different types of tumors. Vascular endothelial growth factor (VEGF) is a tumor growth inducer that plays a crucial role in angiogenesis; besides, it contributes to the development of resistance against common therapies.

Anti-angiogenesis therapy has emerged as an approach to overcome the challenges of tumor therapy. It has been suggested that a combination of new strategies and conventional therapies may help in more efficient inhibition of tumor growth. Various approaches were designed to restrict the expansion of tumors. For instance, angiogenesis mechanisms trigger VEGF to inhibit tumor growth. Also, VEGF activation can be repressed by suppression of some signaling pathways such as RAS, MAPK, and PI3KAKT.

Besides the mentioned strategies, mesenchymal stem cells (MSCs) were introduced as a vehicle to deliver anti-angiogenic agents to tumors. In fact, some limitations that exist with anti-angiogenesis agents such as short endurance as the most important one, led to their application along with MSCs. Another way to suppress angiogenesis and tumor expansion is the application of MSCs-derived exosomes. These nanovesicles could down-regulate VEGF function by some special class of RNAs called miRs, as an anti-angiogenic strategy in cancer therapy. Another strategy that was recently applied in this context is using oncolytic viruses.

Different kinds of virus families may be utilized as oncolytic viruses to selectively replicate in tumor cells. Reovirus, adenovirus, herpes simplex virus, measles virus, and vesicular stomatitis virus are examples of oncolytic viruses. Oncolytic characteristics of some viruses such as reovirus, make them potentially beneficial agents for curing tumors. Since reovirus is a benign virus for humans, its oncolytic properties are demon-

---

* **Corresponding author Hoorieh Soleimanjahi:** Department of Virology, Faculty of Medical Sciences, Tarbiat Modares University, Tehran, Iran. P.O.Box: 14115-331; E-mail: soleim_h@modares.ac.ir

Atta-ur-Rahman & M. Iqbal Choudhary (Eds.)

strated more importantly in clinical settings. This kind of oncolytic virus may inhibit angiogenesis by Reolysin. In fact, interferon-γ-inducible protein 10 (IP-10), a member of the C-X- C chemokine family, which is also called CXCL10, is a target for Reolysin to induce anti-angiogenic activity. This anti-angiogenic chemokine is active both in wild type and Ras mutant cells.

This chapter demonstrates the potential activity of anti-angiogenesis agents in the prevention of tumor growth and cancer progression, with a particular focus on powerful regulators that were demonstrated to play crucial roles in cancer suppression by re-engineering tumor microenvironment.

Keywords: Angiogenesis, Anti-Angiogenesis, Apoptosis, Cancer therapy, Exosome, Mesenchymal Stem Cell, Micro-Environment, Oncolytic Virus, Targeting, VEGF.

INTRODUCTION

Angiogenesis is followed by tumor cell growth and a network of new blood vessels around the tumor. This process is required for the provision of nutrients and oxygen for the growth of tumor cells as well as the removal of their waste products. Also, angiogenesis is the gateway for the entry of metastatic tumor cells into the circulatory system [1, 2].

Tumor progression and metastasis result from tumor microenvironment (TME), which is involved in stromal cells as well as tumor cells [3]. In other words, tumor angiogenesis is controlled by TME and the interaction between different types of interfering cells [4, 5]. Tumors comprise of stromal cells and tumor cells; the former commonly include macrophages, fibroblasts, and endothelial cells [2, 6]. The great attention paid to the complexity of sprouting angiogenesis is due to the imbalance between angiogenic inducers and angiogenic suppressors, which leads to the development of new vessels from endothelial cells. Angiogenesis process initiates by the production of proteases, which are proteolytic enzymes that are able to disrupt the function of extracellular matrix and proliferation and migration of endothelial cells. Angiogenesis continues by vascular tubes formation and blood vessel maturation [7 - 9].

Angiogenesis is an essential step not only in tissue regeneration but also in tumorigenesis. There are three kinds of endothelial cell phenotypes distinguished in sprouting angiogenesis: i) Tip cells located at the foreside of the sprout of vessels. This type of cell is the motive and direct angiogenesis incitement; ii) Stalk cells which are immobilized and located behind the tip cells. Stalk cells are proliferative and support the sprout; and iii) Phalanx cells that are neither immobile nor proliferative and participate in cell connections and cell-to-cell communication [10, 11] (Fig. **1**).

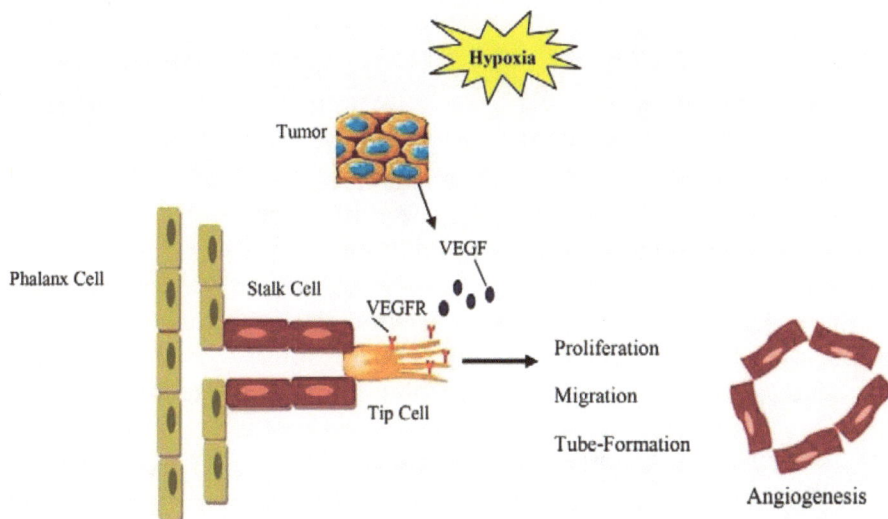

Fig. (1). A schematic representation of different phenotypes of endothelial cells. Tip cells are followed by stalk cells and extend in response to angiogenic stimuli such as hypoxia. Angiogenesis is done through proliferation, migration, and tube formation of endothelial cells. Phalanx cells remain quiescent during this process.

Angiogenesis Stimulator Factors and Receptors

Many tumors produce growth factors as angiogenesis stimulators while others may influence on circumambient cells to generate factors such as vascular endothelial growth factor (VEGF), tumor necrosis factor α (TNF-α), transforming growth factor α and β (TGF-α and β), basic fibroblast growth factor (β-FGF) and PROK2 which all are angiogenic factors [8, 12]. Additionally, some cytokines such as interleukin 22 (IL-22) and IL-17 that are expressed by TH17 cells, may play a crucial role in angiogenesis [4, 7, 13]. Since VEGF plays a crucial role in sprouting and proliferation of endothelial cells, it contributes to the development of resistance towards common therapies and facilitates cancer development [14].

As shown in Fig. (**2**), there is a well-known family of proteins that promote vessels and act as modulators. Five members of this family are VEGFA (as the major one), VEGFB, VEGFC, and VEGFD and placental growth factor (PIGF). These vascular endothelial growth factors can bind to tyrosine kinase receptors named VEGFR1 (VEGF receptor 1/ FLT-1), VEGFR2 (also known as KDR in humans and Flk-1 in the mouse) and VEGFR3 (also named Flt-4). VEGFB interacts with VEGFR1, while VEGFA interacts with both VEGFR1 and VEGFR2. Generally, the kinase activity of VEGFR2 is more marked than

VEGFR1, albeit the affinity for VEGFR1 is higher. VEGFC and VEGFD both interact with VEGFR2 and VEFGR3 [2, 12, 15].

Angiogenesis Inhibition

There are several therapeutic strategies for VEGF signaling pathway (VSP) inhibition in order to control the angiogenesis and tumor growth (15). Angiogenesis inhibitors are categorized as direct and indirect inhibitors. In indirect inhibition, the prevention of proliferation and migration of vascular endothelial cells is a common response to inhibitors. Moreover, indirect pathways inhibit angiogenesis by proteolysis or blocking the activity of pro-angiogenesis agents. VEGFs act as T cell immune-suppressors, play a key role in angiogenesis and are essential for the growth and survival of tumors. Thus, molecules that interfere with the VEGF/VEGFR axis may inhibit tumor propagation.

Table 1. Anti-angiogenic drugs approved for cancer therapy.

Angiogenic inhibitor	Inhibiting Target	Feature	Clinical study	References
Exogenous Drugs				
Bevacizumab (Avastin)	VEGFA	Monoclonal antibody	various cancers (colorectal, lung, breast, glioblastoma,, kidney, and ovarian)	[26, 27]
Ramucirumab (Cyramza)	VEGFR2	Monoclonal antibody	metastatic colorectal cancer, non-small cell lung cancer, gastric or gastroesophageal junction adenocarcinoma	[28, 29]
Aflibercept (Zaltrap)	VEGFA, VEGFB, PIGF	Chimeric protein	metastatic colorectal cancer	[30]
Sorafenib (Nexavar)	VEGFR2, VEGFR3, PDGFR, RAF, KIT	Tyrosine kinase inhibitor	Leukemia, glioblastoma, lymphoma, melanoma, gastro-intestinal stromal tumor, kidney, liver, breast, prostate, lung, ovarian, colorectal, thyroid, head and neck, gastric, pancreatic cancer	[31]
Pazopanib (Votrient)	VEGFRs, PDGFRs, FGFR1, KIT	Tyrosine kinase inhibitor	Melanoma, glioblastoma, kidney, breast, lung, cervical, liver, thyroid, prostate, colorectal cancer	[32, 33]
Rivoceranib (Apatinib)	VEGFR2, PDGFR, IGF-IR, Dtk	Tyrosine kinase inhibitor	Hepatocellular carcinoma, gastric and non-small cell lung cancers	[34]
Axitinib (Inlyta)	VEGFRs, PDGFRβ, KIT	Tyrosine kinase inhibitor	Melanoma, kidney, lung, thyroid, pancreatic, colorectal and breast cancers	[35]

(Table 1) cont.....

Angiogenic inhibitor	Inhibiting Target	Feature	Clinical study	References
Regorafenib (Stivarga)	VEGFRs, PDGFRs, FGFRs, RET, KIT	Tyrosine kinase inhibitor	Metastatic colorectal cancer, gastro-intestinal stromal tumor and hepatocellular carcinoma	[36]
Sunitinib (Sutent)	VEGFRs, PDGFRs, KIT, FLT3	Tyrosine kinase inhibitor	Melanoma, glioblastoma, myeloma, lymphoma, gastro-intestinal stromal tumor, kidney, breast, prostate, lung, liver, ovarian, colorectal, thyroid, head and neck, gastric, bladder, cervical and pancreatic cancers	[37]
Vandetanib (Caprelsa)	VEGFRs, EGFR, RET	Tyrosine kinase inhibitor	Glioma, neuroblastoma, lung, kidney, thyroid, head and neck, prostate, ovarian, breast, colorectal, medullary thyroid cancers	[38]
Cediranib (Recentin)	VEGFRs, PDGFRβ, KIT	Tyrosine kinase inhibitor	Gastro-intestinal stromal tumor, glioblastoma, melanoma, kidney, breast, liver, ovarian, head and neck, prostate, colorectal and non-small cell lung cancers	[39, 40]
Brivanib	VEGFR1-3, FGFR1-3	Tyrosine kinase inhibitor	Colorectal cancer and hepatocellular carcinoma	[41]
Endogenous Drugs				
Angiostatin	VEGF, FGF	Plasminogen fragment	Various cancers (glioma, liver, lung, ovarian, colorectal and breast cancers)	[21]
Endostatin	VEGFA, FGF	Collagen XVIII fragment	non-small-cell lung cancer, breast cancer	[42, 43]

Numerous angiogenesis inhibitors have been tested in preclinical and clinical studies [8, 15 - 19].

Some of the Food and Drug Administration (FDA)-approved antiangiogenic drugs are described in Table **1** . Bevacizumab is the first antiangiogenic drug that was approved in 2004. Bevacizumab is a monoclonal antibody that targets VEGFA and does not allow VEGFR2 binding to VEGFA. Another approved monoclonal antibody-derived drug is ramucirumab, which targets the extracellular domain of VEGFR2. VEGFA, VEGFB, and PIGF are targeted by a recombinant fusion VEGF protein known as aflibercept [1, 6, 20]. There are some multi-target small molecules, which are tyrosine kinase inhibitors and act as inhibitors of VEGFRs (*e.g.* apatinib, axitinib, cabozantinib, lenvatinib, nintedanib, pazopanib, regorafenib, sorafenib, sunitinib, and vandetanib) [15, 20].

Moreover, there are several endogenous angiogenesis inhibitors such as angiostatin, alphastatin, arrestin, caplostatin, endostatin, kininostatin, and vasostatin that are generated from large proteins. Among these, angiostatin and endostatin have the broadest spectrum of applications and were approved by FDA [21 - 25].

Role of Angiogenesis and Anti-Angiogenesis Signaling Pathways

Anti-angiogenesis therapy was firstly introduced in 1971 by Professor Folkman. Although drugs such as bevacizumab are well tolerated and generally safe, some side effects were observed following their application. Phosphatidylinositol3-kinase (PI3K)/AKT pathway is activated in a large number of human cancers.

There is a relation between the PI3K pathway and angiogenesis, and hypoxia-inducible factor1 (HIF1α) is stabilized by hypoxia and increased VEGF in tumor cells. Actually, the receptors of VEGF, for instance, VEGFR2 as the best characterized one, are transduced intracellular signals due to diverse modulators such as PI3K/AKT, to develop angiogenesis. Additionally, in common epithelial cells, following VEGF binding to its receptor, RAS and PI3K pathways are activated. RAS is a family of GTPases that mediate angiogenesis through a mechanism independent of PI3K. VEGF is an inducer of the release of nitric oxide (NO) as a vasodilator in vascular structures. This procedure is carried out by endothelial nitric oxide synthase (eNOS) and prostacyclin (PGI2) upregulation and leads to activation of downstream pathways known as mitogen-activated protein kinase (MAPK) and PI3K. It should be noted that MAPK pathway only affects angiogenesis induction, while PI3K controls both angiogenesis and vasculature permeability. Consequently, NO generation is mitigated by the suppression of VEGF by its inhibitors. In this situation, vasoconstriction is induced and blood pressure rises.

As described above, hypertension, and other symptoms such as stomatitis, proteinuria, diarrhea and other gastrointestinal symptoms, epistaxis, anorexia, upper respiratory infections, dyspnea, headache, fatigue, and exfoliative dermatitis are the most common adverse effects observed following application of these VEGF inhibitors. So, monotherapy by using these inhibitors, is not a perfect approach [8, 15, 20, 44 - 47].

Targeting Angiogenesis for Cancer Therapy by Mesenchymal Stem Cells

At present, Mesenchymal Stem Cells (MSCs) are recruited for tumor suppression. The name of MSCs was first coined by Caplan around 30 years ago. MSCs are isolated from different types of tissues, for instance, umbilical cord blood, bone marrow, and adipose tissue, which are particular sources of MSCs. Also, MSCs may be isolated from the amniotic fluid, placenta, fetal liver, and peripheral blood. All these tissues share special cell markers involved in CD73, CD90, CD105, CD29 and lack of CD14, CD11b, CD34, CD45, CD79α, and HLA-DR markers [48 - 51].

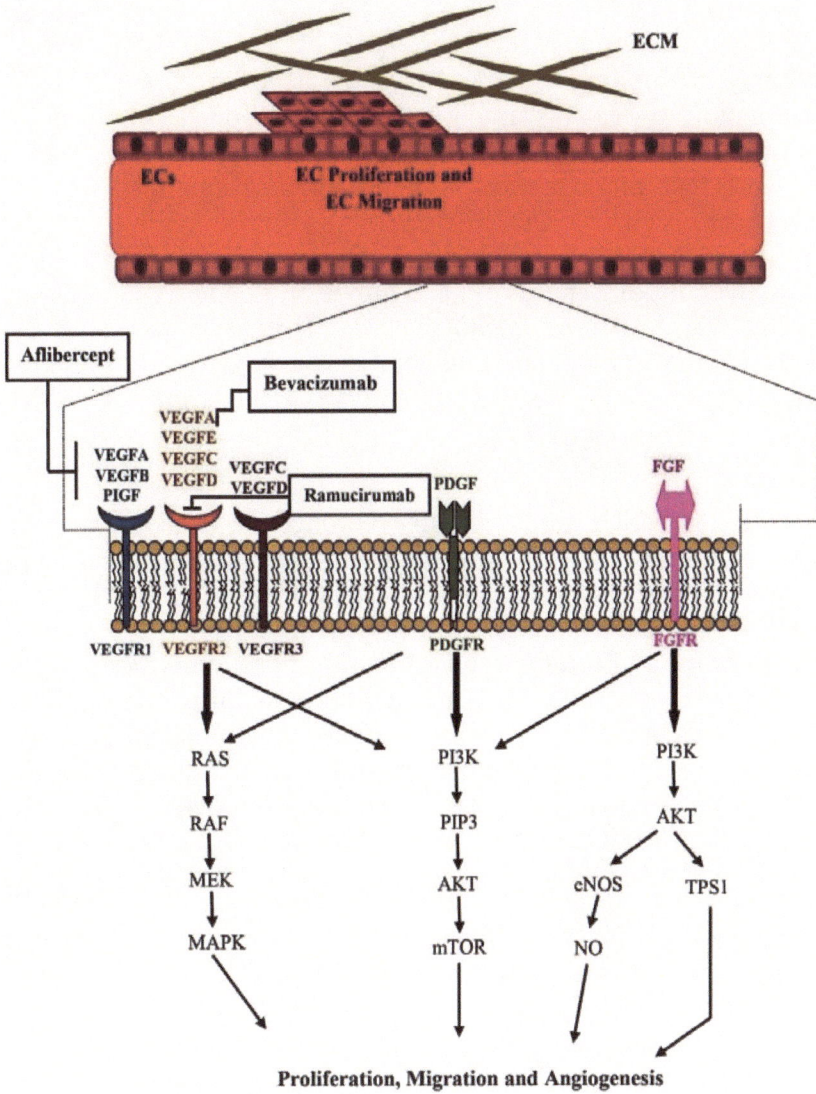

Fig. (2). A schematic presentation of the interaction between VEGFs, PDGF, and FGF and their receptors and angiogenesis signaling pathways. Also, some angiogenesis inhibitors are indicated. EC: Endothelial Cell; ECM: Extra Cellular Matrix

MSCs are known as non-hematopoietic progenitor cells with regenerative properties. Also, adherence to plastic surface and ability to differentiate into adipogenic, osteogenic, and chondrogenic lineage cells are other MSCs properties. They are identified by their cell homing, self-renewal and multi-potent properties and known as safe therapeutic candidates for wound healing and tumor treatment. Additionally, MSCs may play a vector role to deliver anti-tumor agents into cancerous cells. However, the effect of MSCs on tumor development is still controversial [50 - 54].

MSCs may play a supportive or suppressive role in tumor cells. Tumor suppressive function of MSCs was observed in some types of cancers such as liver tumors (hepatoma), breast cancer, and skin cancer. Indeed, several shreds of evidence support that angiogenesis is inhibited and apoptosis is developed following treatment with MSCs. In addition, some signaling pathways are regulated by these kinds of cells in tumor microenvironments [54 - 56]. Consequently, diversity of tumor types and tumor microenvironments, variability of donors, MSCs tissue source, MSCs heterogeneity, and variations in MSCs isolation methods, may explain contradictory effects reported for these cells [54, 57].

Evidence for Anti Tumoral Potency of MSCs

As mentioned earlier, MSCs are commonly recruited for tissue regeneration and wound healing and repair due to their migratory activity toward inflammatory signals released by the injured tissue. In addition, various cytokines with immunomodulatory functions are plentifully generated in tumor milieu and they induce MSCs migration into tumor cells. Most of these cytokines such as IL10, TGF-β, and prostaglandin E2 (PGE2), along with inducible nitric oxide synthase (iNOS) are able to suppress allogeneic T-cell response by inhibition of T cell proliferation. Also, low expression of the major histocompatibility complex class 1 (MHC-I) molecules known in humans as human leukocyte antigen 1 (HLA-I) molecules, and lack of MHC class II, are the major reason for MSCs escape from immunogenic surveillance [48, 50, 56, 58, 59].

MSCs as a source of therapeutic cells are more appropriate than other sources of stromal cells. Among MSCs, adipose-derived MSCs (ADSCs) are the best source not only because of the ease of access but also because their isolation is absolutely less invasive compared to other sources. Moreover, some abundant factors such as insulin-like growth factor-1 (IGF-1), VEGF-D and IL-8 are present in ADSCs but not in bone marrow MSCs (BM-MSCs); nonetheless, other factors like VEGFA, bFGF, and angiogenin are present at comparable levels [56, 60 - 62].

Role of MSCs as an Angiogenic Agent

The anti-tumoral effects of MSCs were observed in several studies. It was revealed that the reduction of the tumor size depends on the concentration of MSCs injected. Following the application of high-dose MSCs, reactive oxygen species (ROS) are produced and they prevent vasculature development while at low concentrations of MSCs, proangiogenic factors are secreted to promote angiogenesis [55, 56, 63, 64]. Several studies demonstrated that angiogenesis was inhibited by the connection between endothelial cells (EC) and MSCs. This combination can prevent vessel network expansion around tumor sites in some types of tumors such as glioblastoma multiforme and Kaposi's sarcoma [55, 65 - 68]. However, other studies revealed that MSCs play a dual role in different types of cancers and cause cancer metastasis. It was shown that these cells may also promote angiogenesis and tumor development [69, 70].

Although MSCs have pros and cons in cancer therapy, they can be used as a targeted vector to deliver various anti-tumor drugs, anti-angiogenesis agents and oncolytic viruses in tumor therapy [56, 71 - 74]. Some anti-angiogenesis drugs such as endostatin and derivatives, angiostatin, thrombospondins and IL-12 were delivered by MSCs to inhibit vasculature expansion [75, 76].

In general, engineered MSCs may be considered a novel targeted therapeutic approach to deliver anti-angiogenesis agents into tumor site in order to cure cancer. By employing this strategy, angiogenesis pathways such as VEGF/VEGFR, FGF/FGFR, and Notch signaling pathway, as well as cytokines, would be targeted by modified MSCs, which would lead to the inhibition of angiogenesis through tumor microenvironments [55 - 57, 77].

MSCs are considered a vehicle for genes, drugs, and oncolytic virus. These functions depend on a variety of MSCs specificities, including the facility of achievement, *in vitro* expanding with the paracrine release of small molecules, and low immunogenicity (Fig. **3**). Nevertheless, MSCs application has encountered some problems such as the requirement of cells with stable phenotypes and the time-consuming nature of the process. Additionally, cellular rejection, configuration of iatrogenic tumor, and the effect of toxicity in MSCs transplantation, still remain unsolved and deserve further studies [78 - 80].

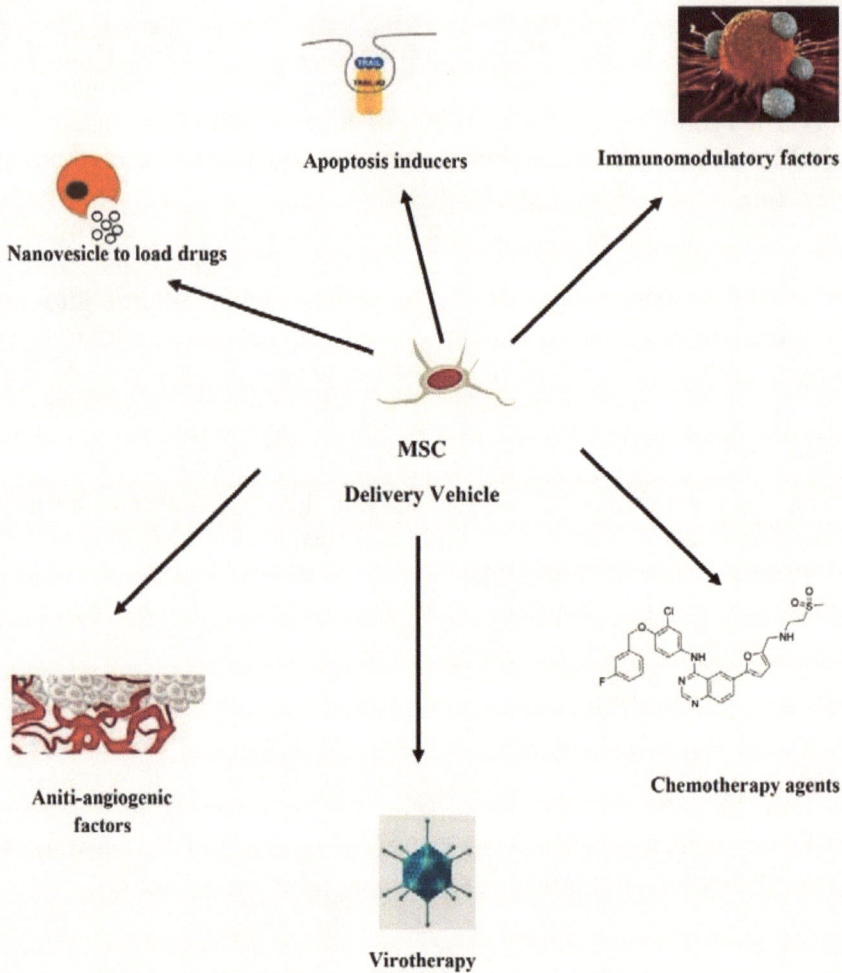

Fig. (3). Different strategies for delivery of various agents by Mesenchymal Stem Cell (MSC)

Emerging Extracellular Vesicles

The above mentioned characteristics of MSCs led to the introduction of significant factors derived from these cells known as extracellular vesicles, including microvesicles (0.1-1mm) and exosome (30-100nm) with cell-to-cell communication potency and paracrine factors that can help in tissue repair and immune modulation. The most important vesicle derived from MSCs, are nanoparticles called exosome with small size, ease of production and storage, and low immunogenicity. They were introduced as cell-free therapy to substitute MSCs [80 - 83]. Exosomes are extracellular endosomal nanoparticles produced by complicated processes during the formation of the multivesicular body. Exosomes are also achieved from conditioned media of a variety of cell types, especially MSCs [84, 85]. Some evidence suggested that stromal and tumoral cells exchange biological information and have interactions through these extracellular vesicles [86, 87]. Evaluation by electron microscopy revealed that exosomes are composed of a phospholipid bilayer and other biomolecules, including lipids, proteins, and nucleic acids. Exosomes have over-expressed levels of sphingomyelin, cholesterol, phosphatidylserine, and saturated fatty acids in comparison with cell membranes. Proteins in exosome are divided into three categories, including endosomal, nuclear, and plasma proteins, which are associated with secretion and biogenesis pathways of the exosome. Furthermore, some other proteins from different cell types such as TSG101, Alix, Rab-GTPase, Heat Shock Proteins (HSP 70 and 90), integrins, tetraspanins (CD9, CD63, CD81, and CD82) and MHC-II were specified in exosomes [88 - 90]. The roles of some of the above-mentioned components were identified in tumor microenvironments. For instance, elevated basal expression of HSP in cancer cells is supposed to facilitate the maintenance of protein homeostasis under high-stress conditions in the cancer microenvironment [91]. Moreover, exosomes carry genetic material such as mRNA, long non-coding RNA, microRNA (miRNA) as small non-coding RNAs (~22nt) and even double-stranded DNA [92, 93].

Exosomes can modulate physiological intracellular actions*via*signaling molecules present on their surface or secretion of mediators into the extracellular spaces [94].

Role of Exosome Contents

Recent studies specified that exosomes may be released by different types of cells such as stem cells, endothelial cells, tumor cell lines, platelets, lymphocytes, and dendritic cells [95-98]. Components of exosome originated from different cells are not similar in physiological and pathological aspects, thus, they exert different functions. It was revealed that MSCs-derived exosomes have different functions from tumoral cells-derived ones [90, 92]. Recently, it was definitely claimed that exosomal miRNAs play as a biomarker for the diagnosis and treatment of different types of cancers. These small molecules can act as a vehicle and be transferred from a cell to another in order to deliver the cargo to regulate targets [95, 99, 100].

By investigating the role of miRNAs in the tumor microenvironment, a dichotomy of their function was remained open to debate. Some evidence revealed that exosome-loaded miRNAs act as tumor suppressors, while their progressive role in tumor growth was also indicated [101, 102].

Several studies showed pivotal roles of MSCs-derived miRNAs such as miR-16, in down-regulation of VEGF expression *in vitro* and *in vivo* to induce anti-angiogenesis in breast cancer [101, 103, 104]. Another study indicated that a group of miRNAs (let-7a, miR-23b, miR-27a/b, miR-21, let-7, and miR-320b) act as anti-angiogenesis agents in breast cancer by cell-to-cell communication [105].

Additionally, two miRNAs (miR-340 and miR-365) extracted from BMSCs-derived exosomes, were assessed to suppress angiogenesis in multiple myeloma (MM) disease. It was confirmed that hepatocyte growth factor (HGF) has a vital role in angiogenesis regulation together with cMET. Since these two factors are highly expressed and activated in endothelial cells of MM patients in comparison with normal individuals, angiogenesis is negatively controlled by miR-340 and cMET expression is prevented by these miRNAs [106].

MSCs–derived exosomes also play a critical role in autoimmune diseases mediated by miRNAs. In Rheumatoid arthritis (RA), miR-150-5p was proven to control angiogenesis by targeting VEGF and matrix metalloproteinase 14 (MMP 14) to inhibit angiogenesis and decrease the migration of fibroblast-like synoviocyte as a crucial cell in the pathogenesis of inflammatory diseases [107].

On the other hand, some studies revealed the progressive role of cancer stem cells-derived exosomes and miRNAs in pathogenesis and angiogenesis of cancer. For instance, c-MYB protein was targeted by miR-130a derived from gastric cancer cells, and it affected angiogenesis and tumor growth [108]. Also, Chen and his colleague confirmed that miR-130a is able to regulate angiogenesis by modulating the expression of GAX and HOXA5 signaling pathways. These are two important anti-angiogenic molecules so that HOXA5 decreases the expression of angiogenic genes such as VEGFR2, hypoxia-inducible factor-1α, ephrin A1 and cyclooxygenase 2 [109].

Taken together, beside wound healing and hepatic regeneration activities, several kinds of diseases such as graft-*versus*-host disease, myocardial injury, renal injury, limb ischemia and above-mentioned types of cancers were improved by the application of MSCs-derived exosomes. Contrarily, it was indicated that these nanoparticles support angiogenesis in tumor growth [110 - 114].

These components may act as a double-bladed sword and were reported as an oncogene that promotes tumor metastasis by inducing epithelial–mesenchymal transition (EMT). Therefore, these molecules may play a major role in angiogenesis by secretion of VEGFA [115].

Virotherapy and Oncolytic Viruses

A novel therapy that was introduced during recent years is virotherapy which employs oncolytic virus (OV) to cure cancers in the early 20th century. Indeed, viruses may play a role as a vehicle to transport biological molecules to the target cells [116]. Moreover, engineered MSCs or exosomes may be used as a vector to deliver these viruses to a certain target to trigger oncogenic factors. In this procedure, the virus selectively proliferates in tumor cells and destroys them while causing no injury to the normal cells and tissues [117, 118]. In actual fact, some defective conditions, such as increased cell proliferation, suppression of immune factors in TME, and dysfunction of the immune response against viral infection, may occur in tumor cells. Consequently, oncolytic viruses can effectively reawake immune responses against tumoral cells in TME [119 - 121]. Oncolytic viruses must have some special characteristics to be used as cancer therapeutic agents (Fig. **4**). Oncolytic viruses must be non-pathogenic and engineered for expressing immune-attenuated factors or selective killing of cancer cells intrinsically [122, 123].

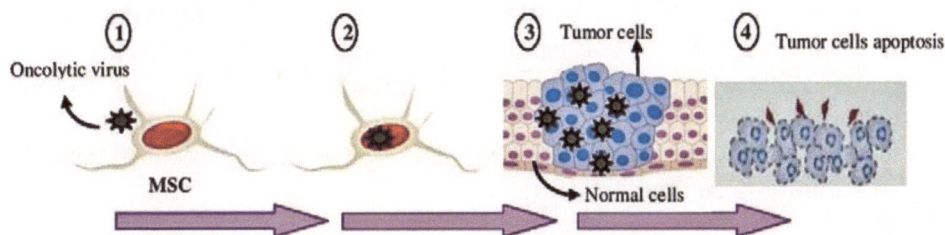

Fig. (4). Apoptosis and necrosis of the tumor cells. Stages 1 and 2 distinguishing and up-taking oncolytic virus (OV) by mesenchymal stem cells (MSCs). Stage 3, virus replication in tumor cells. Stage 4, killing the infected cells typically by induction of apoptosis.

By using oncolytic viruses pattern recognition receptors (PRRs) located on the cell surface or in the host cells, distinguished viral pathogen-associated molecular patterns (PAMPs) and some signaling pathways are activated by the generation of different inflammatory cytokines and chemokines. Thus, the oncolytic virus operates as a vaccine against cancer cells [124, 125].

Oncolytic viruses are categorized into two classes. The first group has an autonomous preference for tumor cells and is not pathogenic for humans such as reovirus, parvoviruses, Newcastle disease virus, Seneca Valley virus and myxoma virus while the second group includes herpes simplex virus, adenovirus, measles virus, vesicular stomatitis virus, poliovirus, and vaccinia virus, manipulated or engineered to become tumor-specific [126 - 128].

It is notable that oncolytic virus must be protected from the immune system through the transmission into cancer cells. MSCs are also able to efficiently transfer oncolytic virus into the tumor site [126, 129, 130]. Recently, another delivery strategy known as ultrasound cavitation, was introduced to carry oncolytic viruses into solid tumors in order to increase tumor permeability and effectively treat cancer [131, 132].

Oncolytic Herpes Simplex Virus

The modified herpes simplex virus type 1 or talimogene laherparepvec (T-Vec) is preferentially triggered cancer cells. T-Vec was the first oncolytic virus approved by the FDA in 2015 and is the only oncolytic virus approved to be applied in the United States and Europe [121, 131, 133].

Moreover, another type of Oncolytic herpes simplex virus was recruited as a kind of manipulated therapeutic agent against cancer cells. This oncolytic virus was armed with some anti-angiogenesis factors such as endostatin, IL-12, and angiostatin in different studies. The anti-angiogenic polypeptide, angiostatin, and an important immunoregulatory cytokine with strong anti-angiogenic effect, IL-12, were expressed by oncolytic herpes simplex virus to improve anti-angiogenesis achievement in glioblastoma model [134, 135]. Furthermore, oncolytic herpes virus was armed with a fused gene, angiostatin-endostatin, as a new strategy to develop anti-angiogenesis for effective enhancement of anti-tumor activity in a glioblastoma model [136].

Oncolytic Reovirus

Reovirus, which does not produce serious conditions in humans, was used as an oncolytic virus to induce death in cancer cells by its anti-angiogenesis properties. Three serotypes of reovirus, serotype 1 strain Lang (T1L), serotype 2 strain Jones (T2J) and serotype 3 strain Dearing (T3D) are circulated among humans [137]. Several phase I and II clinical trials revealed that T3D is the safest strain for virotherapy [138]. The immuno-oncology reoviral agent known as reolysin, upregulates expression of anti-angiogenesis factor, CXC chemokine ligand 10 (CXCL-10) also named interferon-γ-inducible protein 10 (IP-10), and induces it. CXCL-10 inhibits metastasis and cell proliferation. Previous studies demonstrated that both reolysin and CXCL-10 prevent tube formation in endothelial cells by inhibiting VEGF-induction. Moreover, reolysin is an antagonist of hypoxia inducible factor (HIF)-1α and downregulates its expression. Consequently, oncolytic reovirus is able to decrease the level of HIF-1α and inhibit VEGF activity [139, 140].

Oncolytic Adenovirus

Adenovirus- Soluble Flt-1 (Ad-sflt-1) was constructed as an engineered oncolytic adenovirus by inserting anti-angionenic gene, sflt-1, into an E1B-55-kDa-deleted oncolytic adenovirus (ZD55). sFlt-1 is known to play a fundamental role in anti-angiogenesis as an endogenous factor to inhibit VEGF. By producing the mentioned construct, sFlt-1 was expressed in this engineered vector to inhibit angiogenesis in different cancer cells such as colorectal cancer cells (SW620), cervical cancer cells (HeLa) and hepatocarcinoma (BEL7404) [141].

MSCs Loading Oncolytic Viruses

Oncolytic viruses are capable of infecting different kinds of host cells. They selectively replicate in cancer cells and trigger some anti-cancer responses *in vitro* and *in vivo* without causing significant pathogenicity in normal cells. This progression occurs at 2-4 hours for more than 1-2 days, depending on virus titer and cell type. Previous studies showed that oncolytic virus therapy alone is not effective because antiviral antibodies circulating in host blood neutralize the OVs before reaching the target site. Additionally, it is conceivable that macrophages recognize OV and destroy them. The main problem in this kind of therapy is OVs delivery to target cells and the interaction between OVs and the immune system. To overcome this problem, an innovative approach focused on the use of cell carriers. In order to enhance the oncolytic effect, AD-MSCs were applied as a delivery system [139, 142].

Although the delivery of OVs by MSCs was shown to be effective, the efficacy of intravenous delivery of MSCs has been controversial. The MSCs may show diversity in proliferation, migration, intracellular spread, apoptosis induction, and angiogenesis or anti-angiogenesis effect [70].

CONCLUSION AND FUTURE PERSPECTIVE

Improvements of the consequences require better prevention, rapid access to diagnosis, and improved treatment and care for individuals diagnosed with cancer. We need rapid diagnosis and more uniform treatment, as well as the prevention of cancer. Nowadays, medicine is becoming more personalized to the individual, offering higher cure rates and fewer side effects. A range of novel therapeutic approaches has emerged recently and some of them were reviewed in this chapter. Although they would be safe and efficient to treat cancers, several studies indicated that combination therapies such as chemotherapy or radiotherapy and the oncolytic virus may be more effective and could reach maximum efficiency

[143 - 146].

Modulating tumor angiogenesis by inhibiting VEGF derivatives expression may be a potential strategy for cancer prevention and therapy. Importantly, normalization of tumor vasculature is the main developing concept in antiangiogenic therapy.

CONSENT FOR PUBLICATION

Not applicable.

CONFLICT OF INTEREST

The authors confirm that the contents of this chapter have no conflict of interest.

ACKNOWLEDGEMENTS

We would like to thank the research deputy of Tarbiat Modares University for kind assistant and support. We thank Dr Rezaee R, Pharm D., PhD, ERT (European Registered Toxicologist), Associate Editor of Toxicology Reports, for his assistance with editing, that greatly improved the manuscript.

REFERENCES

[1]   Hida K, Maishi N, Annan DA, Hida Y. Contribution of tumor endothelial cells in cancer progression. Int J Mol Sci 2018; 19(5): 1272-83.
[http://dx.doi.org/10.3390/ijms19051272] [PMID: 29695087]

[2]   Lopes-Bastos BM, Jiang WG, Cai J. Tumour–endothelial cell communications: Important and indispensable mediators of tumour angiogenesis. Anticancer Res 2016; 36(3): 1119-26.
[PMID: 26977007]

[3]   Maishi N, Hida K. Tumor endothelial cells accelerate tumor metastasis. Cancer Sci 2017; 108(10): 1921-6.
[http://dx.doi.org/10.1111/cas.13336] [PMID: 28763139]

[4]   Protopsaltis NJ, Liang W, Nudleman E, Ferrara N. Interleukin-22 promotes tumor angiogenesis. Angiogenesis 2019; 22(2): 311-23.
[http://dx.doi.org/10.1007/s10456-018-9658-x] [PMID: 30539314]

[5]   Xie C, Ji N, Tang Z, Li J, Chen Q. The role of extracellular vesicles from different origin in the microenvironment of head and neck cancers. Mol Cancer 2019; 18(1): 83-97.
[http://dx.doi.org/10.1186/s12943-019-0985-3] [PMID: 30954079]

[6]   Salazar N, Zabel BA. Support of Tumor Endothelial Cells by Chemokine Receptors. Front Immunol 2019; 10: 147-55.
[http://dx.doi.org/10.3389/fimmu.2019.00147] [PMID: 30800123]

[7]   Wang R, Lou X, Feng G, *et al.* IL-17A-stimulated endothelial fatty acid β-oxidation promotes tumor angiogenesis. Life Sci 2019; 229: 46-56.
[http://dx.doi.org/10.1016/j.lfs.2019.05.030] [PMID: 31085243]

[8]   Rajabi M, Mousa SA. The role of angiogenesis in cancer treatment. Biomedicines 2017; 5(2): 34-45.
[http://dx.doi.org/10.3390/biomedicines5020034] [PMID: 28635679]

[9]　Huang Z, Zhang M, Chen G, *et al.* Bladder cancer cells interact with vascular endothelial cells triggering EGFR signals to promote tumor progression. Int J Oncol 2019; 54(5): 1555-66.
[http://dx.doi.org/10.3892/ijo.2019.4729] [PMID: 30816487]

[10]　Li S, Xu H-X, Wu C-T, *et al.* Angiogenesis in pancreatic cancer: current research status and clinical implications. Angiogenesis 2019; 22(1): 15-36.
[http://dx.doi.org/10.1007/s10456-018-9645-2] [PMID: 30168025]

[11]　Kühn C, Checa S. Computational modeling to quantify the contributions of VEGFR1, VEGFR2, and lateral inhibition in sprouting angiogenesis. Front Physiol 2019; 10: 288.
[http://dx.doi.org/10.3389/fphys.2019.00288] [PMID: 30971939]

[12]　Lodish H. Molecular Cell Biology.1033-141. New York, US.: WH Freeman, Macmillian Learning 2016; pp.

[13]　Pan B, Shen J, Cao J, *et al.* Interleukin-17 promotes angiogenesis by stimulating VEGF production of cancer cells*via*the STAT3/GIV signaling pathway in non-small-cell lung cancer. Sci Rep 2015; 5: 16053.
[http://dx.doi.org/10.1038/srep16053] [PMID: 26524953]

[14]　Zhang Q, Lu S, Li T, *et al.* ACE2 inhibits breast cancer angiogenesis*via*suppressing the VEGFa/VEGFR2/ERK pathway. J Exp Clin Cancer Res 2019; 38(1): 173-84.
[http://dx.doi.org/10.1186/s13046-019-1156-5] [PMID: 31023337]

[15]　Pandey AK, Singhi EK, Arroyo JP, *et al.* Mechanisms of VEGF (vascular endothelial growth factor) inhibitor–associated hypertension and vascular disease. Hypertension 2018; 71(2): e1-8.
[http://dx.doi.org/10.1161/HYPERTENSIONAHA.117.10271] [PMID: 29279311]

[16]　Apte RS, Chen DS, Ferrara N. VEGF in signaling and disease: beyond discovery and development. Cell 2019; 176(6): 1248-64.
[http://dx.doi.org/10.1016/j.cell.2019.01.021] [PMID: 30849371]

[17]　Gardner V, Madu CO, Lu Y. Anti-VEGF Therapy in Cancer: A Double-Edged Sword.Physiologic and Pathologic Angiogenesis Signaling Mechanisms and Targeted Therapy. . London, UK: InTechOpen 2017; pp. 385-410.

[18]　Yang J, Yan J, Liu B. Targeting VEGF/VEGFR to modulate antitumor immunity. Front Immunol 2018; 9: 978.
[http://dx.doi.org/10.3389/fimmu.2018.00978] [PMID: 29774034]

[19]　El-Kenawi AE, El-Remessy AB. Angiogenesis inhibitors in cancer therapy: mechanistic perspective on classification and treatment rationales. Br J Pharmacol 2013; 170(4): 712-29.
[http://dx.doi.org/10.1111/bph.12344] [PMID: 23962094]

[20]　Kanat O, Ertas H. Existing anti-angiogenic therapeutic strategies for patients with metastatic colorectal cancer progressing following first-line bevacizumab-based therapy. World J Clin Oncol 2019; 10(2): 52-61.
[http://dx.doi.org/10.5306/wjco.v10.i2.52] [PMID: 30815371]

[21]　Doll JA, Soff GA. Angiostatin Cytokines and Cancer. Springer 2005; pp. 175-204.
[http://dx.doi.org/10.1007/0-387-24361-5_8]

[22]　Chamani R, Asghari SM, Alizadeh AM, *et al.* Engineering of a disulfide loop instead of a Zn binding loop restores the anti-proliferative, anti-angiogenic and anti-tumor activities of the N-terminal fragment of endostatin: Mechanistic and therapeutic insights. Vascul Pharmacol 2015; 72: 73-82.
[http://dx.doi.org/10.1016/j.vph.2015.07.006] [PMID: 26187352]

[23]　Pike SE, Yao L, Jones KD, *et al.* Vasostatin, a calreticulin fragment, inhibits angiogenesis and suppresses tumor growth. J Exp Med 1998; 188(12): 2349-56.
[http://dx.doi.org/10.1084/jem.188.12.2349] [PMID: 9858521]

[24]　Satchi-Fainaro R, Mamluk R, Wang L, *et al.* Inhibition of vessel permeability by TNP-470 and its

polymer conjugate, caplostatin. Cancer Cell 2005; 7(3): 251-61.
[http://dx.doi.org/10.1016/j.ccr.2005.02.007] [PMID: 15766663]

[25] Saadat P, Soleimanjahi H, Asghari SM, Fazeli M, Razavinikoo H, Karimi H. Co-administration of anti-angiogenic peptide and DNA vaccine in cervical cancer tumor model. Int J Cancer Manag 2017; 10(3): e4723-30.
[http://dx.doi.org/10.5812/ijcm.4723]

[26] Chellappan DK, Leng KH, Jia LJ, *et al.* The role of bevacizumab on tumour angiogenesis and in the management of gynaecological cancers: A review. Biomed Pharmacother 2018; 102: 1127-44.
[http://dx.doi.org/10.1016/j.biopha.2018.03.061] [PMID: 29710531]

[27] Gampenrieder SP, Westphal T, Greil R. Antiangiogenic therapy in breast cancer. Memo 2017; 10(4): 194-201.
[http://dx.doi.org/10.1007/s12254-017-0362-0] [PMID: 29250196]

[28] Tabernero J, Hozak RR, Yoshino T, *et al.* Analysis of angiogenesis biomarkers for ramucirumab efficacy in patients with metastatic colorectal cancer from RAISE, a global, randomized, double-blind, phase III study. Ann Oncol 2018; 29(3): 602-9.
[http://dx.doi.org/10.1093/annonc/mdx767] [PMID: 29228087]

[29] Javle M, Smyth EC, Chau I. Ramucirumab: successfully targeting angiogenesis in gastric cancer. Clin Cancer Res 2014; 20(23): 5875-81.
[http://dx.doi.org/10.1158/1078-0432.CCR-14-1071] [PMID: 25281695]

[30] Giordano G, Febbraro A, Venditti M, *et al.* Targeting angiogenesis and tumor microenvironment in metastatic colorectal cancer: role of aflibercept. Gastroenterol Res Pract 2014; 2014: 526178-91.
[http://dx.doi.org/10.1155/2014/526178] [PMID: 25136356]

[31] Llovet JM, Ricci S, Mazzaferro V, *et al.* Sorafenib in advanced hepatocellular carcinoma. N Engl J Med 2008; 359(4): 378-90.
[http://dx.doi.org/10.1056/NEJMoa0708857] [PMID: 18650514]

[32] Chellappan DK, Chellian J, Ng ZY, *et al.* The role of pazopanib on tumour angiogenesis and in the management of cancers: A review. Biomed Pharmacother 2017; 96: 768-81.
[http://dx.doi.org/10.1016/j.biopha.2017.10.058] [PMID: 29054093]

[33] Bellmunt J, Esteban E, del Muro XG, Sepúlveda JM, Maroto P, Gallardo E, *et al.* Pazopanib as Second-line Antiangiogenic Treatment in Metastatic Renal Cell Carcinoma After Tyrosine Kinase Inhibitor (TKI) Failure: A Phase 2 Trial Exploring Immune-related Biomarkers for Testing in the Post-immunotherapy/TKI Era. Eur Urol Oncol 2019; S2588-9311.(19): 30117-20.

[34] Liang Q, Kong L, Du Y, Zhu X, Tian J. Antitumorigenic and antiangiogenic efficacy of apatinib in liver cancer evaluated by multimodality molecular imaging. Exp Mol Med 2019; 51(7): 76-86.
[http://dx.doi.org/10.1038/s12276-019-0274-7] [PMID: 31285418]

[35] Bellesoeur A, Carton E, Alexandre J, Goldwasser F, Huillard O. Axitinib in the treatment of renal cell carcinoma: design, development, and place in therapy. Drug Des Devel Ther 2017; 11: 2801-11.
[http://dx.doi.org/10.2147/DDDT.S109640] [PMID: 29033542]

[36] Fondevila F, Méndez-Blanco C, Fernández-Palanca P, González-Gallego J, Mauriz JL. Anti-tumoral activity of single and combined regorafenib treatments in preclinical models of liver and gastrointestinal cancers. Exp Mol Med 2019; 51(9): 1-15.
[http://dx.doi.org/10.1038/s12276-019-0308-1] [PMID: 31551425]

[37] Hao Z, Sadek I. Sunitinib: the antiangiogenic effects and beyond. OncoTargets Ther 2016; 9: 5495-505.
[http://dx.doi.org/10.2147/OTT.S112242] [PMID: 27660467]

[38] Ferrari SM, Bocci G, Di Desidero T, *et al.* Vandetanib has antineoplastic activity in anaplastic thyroid cancer, *in vitro* and *in vivo*. Oncol Rep 2018; 39(5): 2306-14.
[http://dx.doi.org/10.3892/or.2018.6305] [PMID: 29517106]

[39]   Orbegoso C, Marquina G, George A, Banerjee S. The role of Cediranib in ovarian cancer. Expert Opin Pharmacother 2017; 18(15): 1637-48.
[http://dx.doi.org/10.1080/14656566.2017.1383384] [PMID: 28933580]

[40]   Zhou C, Taylor S, Tugwood J, *et al.* Dynamics of circulating vascular endothelial growth factor-A predict benefit from antiangiogenic cediranib in metastatic or recurrent cervical cancer patients. Br J Clin Pharmacol 2019; 85(8): 1781-9.
[http://dx.doi.org/10.1111/bcp.13965] [PMID: 30980733]

[41]   Huynh H, Ngo VC, Fargnoli J, *et al.* Brivanib alaninate, a dual inhibitor of vascular endothelial growth factor receptor and fibroblast growth factor receptor tyrosine kinases, induces growth inhibition in mouse models of human hepatocellular carcinoma. Clin Cancer Res 2008; 14(19): 6146-53.
[http://dx.doi.org/10.1158/1078-0432.CCR-08-0509] [PMID: 18829493]

[42]   Chamani R, Soleimanjahi H, Asghari SM, Karimi H, Kianmehr Z, Ardestani SK. Re-engineering of the Immunosuppressive Tumor Microenvironment by Antiangiogenic Therapy. Int J Pept Res Ther 2019; 1-8.

[43]   Folkman J. Antiangiogenesis in cancer therapy--endostatin and its mechanisms of action. Exp Cell Res 2006; 312(5): 594-607.
[http://dx.doi.org/10.1016/j.yexcr.2005.11.015] [PMID: 16376330]

[44]   Liang J, Cheng Q, Huang J, *et al.* Monitoring tumour microenvironment changes during anti-angiogenesis therapy using functional MRI. Angiogenesis 2019; 22(3): 457-70.
[http://dx.doi.org/10.1007/s10456-019-09670-4] [PMID: 31147887]

[45]   Kamba T, McDonald DM. Mechanisms of adverse effects of anti-VEGF therapy for cancer. Br J Cancer 2007; 96(12): 1788-95.
[http://dx.doi.org/10.1038/sj.bjc.6603813] [PMID: 17519900]

[46]   Di Lorenzo A, Lin MI, Murata T, *et al.* eNOS-derived nitric oxide regulates endothelial barrier function through VE-cadherin and Rho GTPases. J Cell Sci 2013; 126(Pt 24): 5541-52.
[http://dx.doi.org/10.1242/jcs.115972] [PMID: 24046447]

[47]   Karar J, Maity A. PI3K/AKT/mTOR pathway in angiogenesis. Front Mol Neurosci 2011; 4: 51-8.
[http://dx.doi.org/10.3389/fnmol.2011.00051] [PMID: 22144946]

[48]   Caplan AI. Mesenchymal stem cells. J Orthop Res 1991; 9(5): 641-50.
[http://dx.doi.org/10.1002/jor.1100090504] [PMID: 1870029]

[49]   Zhao Q, Ren H, Han Z. Mesenchymal stem cells: Immunomodulatory capability and clinical potential in immune diseases. J Cell Immunother 2016; 2(1): 3-20.
[http://dx.doi.org/10.1016/j.jocit.2014.12.001]

[50]   Lazennec G, Lam PY. Recent discoveries concerning the tumor - mesenchymal stem cell interactions. Biochim Biophys Acta 2016; 1866(2): 290-9.
[PMID: 27750042]

[51]   Sohni A, Verfaillie CM. Mesenchymal stem cells migration homing and tracking. Stem Cells Int 2013; 2013: 130763-70.
[http://dx.doi.org/10.1155/2013/130763] [PMID: 24194766]

[52]   Chulpanova DS, Kitaeva KV, Tazetdinova LG, James V, Rizvanov AA, Solovyeva VV. Application of mesenchymal stem cells for therapeutic agent delivery in anti-tumor treatment. Front Pharmacol 2018; 9: 259-68.
[http://dx.doi.org/10.3389/fphar.2018.00259] [PMID: 29615915]

[53]   Li Y, Wu Q, Wang Y, Li L, Bu H, Bao J. Senescence of mesenchymal stem cells (Review). Int J Mol Med 2017; 39(4): 775-82.
[http://dx.doi.org/10.3892/ijmm.2017.2912] [PMID: 28290609]

[54]   Klopp AH, Gupta A, Spaeth E, Andreeff M, Marini F III. Concise review: Dissecting a discrepancy in

the literature: do mesenchymal stem cells support or suppress tumor growth? Stem Cells 2011; 29(1): 11-9.
[http://dx.doi.org/10.1002/stem.559] [PMID: 21280155]

[55]   Kwon S, Yoo KH, Sym SJ, Khang D. Mesenchymal stem cell therapy assisted by nanotechnology: a possible combinational treatment for brain tumor and central nerve regeneration. Int J Nanomedicine 2019; 14: 5925-42.
[http://dx.doi.org/10.2147/IJN.S217923] [PMID: 31534331]

[56]   Javan MR, Khosrojerdi A, Moazzeni SM. New Insights Into Implementation of Mesenchymal Stem Cells in Cancer Therapy: Prospects for Anti-angiogenesis Treatment. Front Oncol 2019; 9: 840-56.
[http://dx.doi.org/10.3389/fonc.2019.00840] [PMID: 31555593]

[57]   Dwyer RM, Khan S, Barry FP, O'Brien T, Kerin MJ. Advances in mesenchymal stem cell-mediated gene therapy for cancer. Stem Cell Res Ther 2010; 1(3): 25-31.
[http://dx.doi.org/10.1186/scrt25] [PMID: 20699014]

[58]   Wang Y, Huang J, Gong L, Yu D, An C, Bunpetch V, *et al.* The Plasticity of Mesenchymal Stem Cells in Regulating Surface HLA-I. iScience 2019; 15: 66-78.

[59]   Longoni A, Knežević L, Schepers K, Weinans H, Rosenberg AJWP, Gawlitta D. The impact of immune response on endochondral bone regeneration. NPJ Regen Med 2018; 3(1): 22-32.
[http://dx.doi.org/10.1038/s41536-018-0060-5] [PMID: 30510772]

[60]   Konala VBR, Mamidi MK, Bhonde R, Das AK, Pochampally R, Pal R. The current landscape of the mesenchymal stromal cell secretome: A new paradigm for cell-free regeneration. Cytotherapy 2016; 18(1): 13-24.
[http://dx.doi.org/10.1016/j.jcyt.2015.10.008] [PMID: 26631828]

[61]   Miana VV, González EAP. Adipose tissue stem cells in regenerative medicine. Ecancermedicalscience 2018; 12: 822-35.
[http://dx.doi.org/10.3332/ecancer.2018.822] [PMID: 29662535]

[62]   Francis SL, Duchi S, Onofrillo C, Di Bella C, Choong PFM. Adipose-derived mesenchymal stem cells in the use of cartilage tissue engineering: the need for a rapid isolation procedure. Stem Cells Int 2018; 2018: 8947548-56.
[http://dx.doi.org/10.1155/2018/8947548] [PMID: 29765427]

[63]   Lee MW, Ryu S, Kim DS, *et al.* Mesenchymal stem cells in suppression or progression of hematologic malignancy: current status and challenges. Leukemia 2019; 33(3): 597-611.
[http://dx.doi.org/10.1038/s41375-018-0373-9] [PMID: 30705410]

[64]   Yang C, Lei D, Ouyang W, *et al.* Conditioned media from human adipose tissue-derived mesenchymal stem cells and umbilical cord-derived mesenchymal stem cells efficiently induced the apoptosis and differentiation in human glioma cell lines *in vitro.* BioMed Res Int 2014; 2014: 109389-402.
[http://dx.doi.org/10.1155/2014/109389] [PMID: 24971310]

[65]   Pacioni S, D'Alessandris QG, Giannetti S, *et al.* Human mesenchymal stromal cells inhibit tumor growth in orthotopic glioblastoma xenografts. Stem Cell Res Ther 2017; 8(1): 53-67.
[http://dx.doi.org/10.1186/s13287-017-0516-3] [PMID: 28279193]

[66]   Otsu K, Das S, Houser SD, Quadri SK, Bhattacharya S, Bhattacharya J. Concentration-dependent inhibition of angiogenesis by mesenchymal stem cells. Blood 2009; 113(18): 4197-205.
[http://dx.doi.org/10.1182/blood-2008-09-176198] [PMID: 19036701]

[67]   Kéramidas M, De Fraipont F, Karageorgis A, Moisan A, Persoons V, Richard M-J, *et al.* The dual effect of mesenchymal stem cells on tumour growth and tumour angiogenesis. Stem cell Res Thera 2013; 4(2): 41-52.

[68]   Menge T, Gerber M, Wataha K, *et al.* Human mesenchymal stem cells inhibit endothelial proliferation and angiogenesis*via*cell-cell contact through modulation of the VE-Cadherin/β-catenin signaling pathway. Stem Cells Dev 2013; 22(1): 148-57.

[http://dx.doi.org/10.1089/scd.2012.0165] [PMID: 22734943]

[69]   Suzuki K, Sun R, Origuchi M, *et al.* Mesenchymal stromal cells promote tumor growth through the enhancement of neovascularization. Mol Med 2011; 17(7-8): 579-87.
[http://dx.doi.org/10.2119/molmed.2010.00157] [PMID: 21424106]

[70]   Karnoub AE, Dash AB, Vo AP, *et al.* Mesenchymal stem cells within tumour stroma promote breast cancer metastasis. Nature 2007; 449(7162): 557-63.
[http://dx.doi.org/10.1038/nature06188] [PMID: 17914389]

[71]   Mader EK, Butler G, Dowdy SC, *et al.* Optimizing patient derived mesenchymal stem cells as virus carriers for a phase I clinical trial in ovarian cancer. J Transl Med 2013; 11(1): 20-33.
[http://dx.doi.org/10.1186/1479-5876-11-20] [PMID: 23347343]

[72]   Sage EK, Thakrar RM, Janes SM. Genetically modified mesenchymal stromal cells in cancer therapy. Cytotherapy 2016; 18(11): 1435-45.
[http://dx.doi.org/10.1016/j.jcyt.2016.09.003] [PMID: 27745603]

[73]   Wang S, Miao Z, Yang Q, Wang Y, Zhang J. The Dynamic Roles of Mesenchymal Stem Cells in Colon Cancer. Can J Gastroenterol Hepatol 2018; 2018: 7628763-71.
[http://dx.doi.org/10.1155/2018/7628763] [PMID: 30533404]

[74]   Banijamali RS, Soleimanjahi H, Soudi S, *et al.* Kinetics of oncolytic reovirus T3D replication and growth pattern in mesenchymal stem cells. Cell J 2020; 22(3): 283-92.
[PMID: 31863653]

[75]   Zheng L, Zhang D, Chen X, Yang L, Wei Y, Zhao X. Antitumor activities of human placenta-derived mesenchymal stem cells expressing endostatin on ovarian cancer. PLoS One 2012; 7(7): e39119-28.
[http://dx.doi.org/10.1371/journal.pone.0039119] [PMID: 22911684]

[76]   Li T, Kang G, Wang T, Huang H. Tumor angiogenesis and anti-angiogenic gene therapy for cancer. Oncol Lett 2018; 16(1): 687-702.
[http://dx.doi.org/10.3892/ol.2018.8733] [PMID: 29963134]

[77]   Al-Abd AM, Alamoudi AJ, Abdel-Naim AB, Neamatallah TA, Ashour OM. Anti-angiogenic agents for the treatment of solid tumors: Potential pathways, therapy and current strategies - A review. J Adv Res 2017; 8(6): 591-605.
[http://dx.doi.org/10.1016/j.jare.2017.06.006] [PMID: 28808589]

[78]   Hu Y-L, Huang B, Zhang T-Y, *et al.* Mesenchymal stem cells as a novel carrier for targeted delivery of gene in cancer therapy based on nonviral transfection. Mol Pharm 2012; 9(9): 2698-709.
[http://dx.doi.org/10.1021/mp300254s] [PMID: 22862421]

[79]   Kim J, Hall RR, Lesniak MS, Ahmed AU. Stem cell-based cell carrier for targeted oncolytic virotherapy: translational opportunity and open questions. Viruses 2015; 7(12): 6200-17.
[http://dx.doi.org/10.3390/v7122921] [PMID: 26633462]

[80]   Lou G, Chen Z, Zheng M, Liu Y. Mesenchymal stem cell-derived exosomes as a new therapeutic strategy for liver diseases. Exp Mol Med 2017; 49(6): e346-55.
[http://dx.doi.org/10.1038/emm.2017.63] [PMID: 28620221]

[81]   Willis GR, Mitsialis SA, Kourembanas S. "Good things come in small packages": application of exosome-based therapeutics in neonatal lung injury. Pediatr Res 2018; 83(1-2): 298-307.
[http://dx.doi.org/10.1038/pr.2017.256] [PMID: 28985201]

[82]   Kim DK, Nishida H, An SY, Shetty AK, Bartosh TJ, Prockop DJ. Chromatographically isolated CD63+CD81+ extracellular vesicles from mesenchymal stromal cells rescue cognitive impairments after TBI. Proc Natl Acad Sci USA 2016; 113(1): 170-5.
[http://dx.doi.org/10.1073/pnas.1522297113] [PMID: 26699510]

[83]   Phinney DG, Pittenger MF. Concise review: MSC☐derived exosomes for cell☐free therapy. Stem Cells 2017; 35(4): 851-8.
[http://dx.doi.org/10.1002/stem.2575] [PMID: 28294454]

[84]   Alcayaga-Miranda F, Varas-Godoy M, Khoury M. Harnessing the angiogenic potential of stem cell-derived exosomes for vascular regeneration. Stem Cells Int 2016; 20163409169
[http://dx.doi.org/10.1155/2016/3409169] [PMID: 27127516]

[85]   Tamkovich S, Tutanov O, Laktionov P. Exosomes: Generation, structure, transport, biological activity, and diagnostic application. Biochemistry (Moscow). Supplement Series A: Membr Cell Biol 2016; 10(3): 163-73.

[86]   Wu J, Qu Z, Fei ZW, Wu JH, Jiang CP. Role of stem cell-derived exosomes in cancer. Oncol Lett 2017; 13(5): 2855-66.
[http://dx.doi.org/10.3892/ol.2017.5824] [PMID: 28521391]

[87]   Tao H, Han Z, Han ZC, Li Z. Proangiogenic features of mesenchymal stem cells and their therapeutic applications. Stem Cells Int 2016; 20161314709
[http://dx.doi.org/10.1155/2016/1314709] [PMID: 26880933]

[88]   Colombo M, Raposo G, Théry C. Biogenesis, secretion, and intercellular interactions of exosomes and other extracellular vesicles. Annu Rev Cell Dev Biol 2014; 30: 255-89.
[http://dx.doi.org/10.1146/annurev-cellbio-101512-122326] [PMID: 25288114]

[89]   Crescitelli R, Lässer C, Szabó TG, et al. Distinct RNA profiles in subpopulations of extracellular vesicles: apoptotic bodies, microvesicles and exosomes. J Extracell Vesicles 2013; 2(1): 20677-87.
[http://dx.doi.org/10.3402/jev.v2i0.20677] [PMID: 24223256]

[90]   Guo W, Gao Y, Li N, et al. Exosomes: New players in cancer (Review). Oncol Rep 2017; 38(2): 665-75.
[http://dx.doi.org/10.3892/or.2017.5714] [PMID: 28627679]

[91]   Soleimanjahi H, Abdoli A. Role of Chaperone Mediated Autophagy in Viral Infections Chaperokine Activity of Heat Shock Proteins. Springer 2019; pp. 147-54.
[http://dx.doi.org/10.1007/978-3-030-02254-9_7]

[92]   Xu W, Yang Z, Lu N. From pathogenesis to clinical application: insights into exosomes as transfer vectors in cancer. J Exp Clin Cancer Res 2016; 35(1): 156-67.
[http://dx.doi.org/10.1186/s13046-016-0429-5] [PMID: 27686593]

[93]   Kowal J, Tkach M, Théry C. Biogenesis and secretion of exosomes. Curr Opin Cell Biol 2014; 29: 116-25.
[http://dx.doi.org/10.1016/j.ceb.2014.05.004] [PMID: 24959705]

[94]   Wu CY, Du SL, Zhang J, Liang AL, Liu YJ. Exosomes and breast cancer: a comprehensive review of novel therapeutic strategies from diagnosis to treatment. Cancer Gene Ther 2017; 24(1): 6-12.
[http://dx.doi.org/10.1038/cgt.2016.69] [PMID: 27982016]

[95]   Bhome R, Del Vecchio F, Lee G-H, et al. Exosomal microRNAs (exomiRs): Small molecules with a big role in cancer. Cancer Lett 2018; 420: 228-35.
[http://dx.doi.org/10.1016/j.canlet.2018.02.002] [PMID: 29425686]

[96]   Li Q-L, Bu N, Yu Y-C, Hua W, Xin X-Y. Ex vivo experiments of human ovarian cancer ascites-derived exosomes presented by dendritic cells derived from umbilical cord blood for immunotherapy treatment. Clin Med Oncol 2008; 2: 461-7.
[http://dx.doi.org/10.4137/CMO.S776] [PMID: 21892318]

[97]   Zeng Y, Yao X, Liu X, et al. Anti-angiogenesis triggers exosomes release from endothelial cells to promote tumor vasculogenesis. J Extracell Vesicles 2019; 8(1)1629865
[http://dx.doi.org/10.1080/20013078.2019.1629865] [PMID: 31258881]

[98]   Fernandes Ribeiro M, Zhu H. W Millard R, Fan G-C. Exosomes function in pro-and anti-angiogenesis. Curr Angiogenes 2013; 2(1): 54-9.
[PMID: 25374792]

[99]   Sun Z, Shi K, Yang S, et al. Effect of exosomal miRNA on cancer biology and clinical applications.

Mol Cancer 2018; 17(1): 147-65.
[http://dx.doi.org/10.1186/s12943-018-0897-7] [PMID: 30309355]

[100] Chen M, Xu R, Rai A, *et al.* Distinct shed microvesicle and exosome microRNA signatures reveal diagnostic markers for colorectal cancer. PLoS One 2019; 14(1)e0210003
[http://dx.doi.org/10.1371/journal.pone.0210003] [PMID: 30608951]

[101] Lee J-K, Park S-R, Jung B-K, *et al.* Exosomes derived from mesenchymal stem cells suppress angiogenesis by down-regulating VEGF expression in breast cancer cells. PLoS One 2013; 8(12)e84256
[http://dx.doi.org/10.1371/journal.pone.0084256] [PMID: 24391924]

[102] Vakhshiteh F, Atyabi F, Ostad SN. Mesenchymal stem cell exosomes: a two-edged sword in cancer therapy. Int J Nanomedicine 2019; 14: 2847-59.
[http://dx.doi.org/10.2147/IJN.S200036] [PMID: 31114198]

[103] Jang J-Y, Lee J-K, Jeon Y-K, Kim C-W. Exosome derived from epigallocatechin gallate treated breast cancer cells suppresses tumor growth by inhibiting tumor-associated macrophage infiltration and M2 polarization. BMC Cancer 2013; 13(1): 421-32.
[http://dx.doi.org/10.1186/1471-2407-13-421] [PMID: 24044575]

[104] Qu W, Fei M, Xu B. Role of exosome microRNA in breast cancer. Cancer Transl Med 2017; 3(5): 167-73.
[http://dx.doi.org/10.4103/ctm.ctm_14_17]

[105] Hannafon BN, Carpenter KJ, Berry WL, Janknecht R, Dooley WC, Ding W-Q. Exosome-mediated microRNA signaling from breast cancer cells is altered by the anti-angiogenesis agent docosahexaenoic acid (DHA). Mol Cancer 2015; 14(1): 133-45.
[http://dx.doi.org/10.1186/s12943-015-0400-7] [PMID: 26178901]

[106] Umezu T, Imanishi S, Azuma K, *et al.* Replenishing exosomes from older bone marrow stromal cells with miR-340 inhibits myeloma-related angiogenesis. Blood Adv 2017; 1(13): 812-23.
[http://dx.doi.org/10.1182/bloodadvances.2016003251] [PMID: 29296725]

[107] Chen Z, Wang H, Xia Y, Yan F, Lu Y. Therapeutic Potential of Mesenchymal Cell-Derived miRNA-150-5p-Expressing Exosomes in Rheumatoid Arthritis Mediated by the Modulation of MMP14 and VEGF. J Immunol 2018; 201(8): 2472-82.
[http://dx.doi.org/10.4049/jimmunol.1800304] [PMID: 30224512]

[108] Yang H, Zhang H, Ge S, *et al.* Exosome-derived miR-130a activates angiogenesis in gastric Cancer by targeting C-MYB in vascular endothelial cells. Mol Ther 2018; 26(10): 2466-75.
[http://dx.doi.org/10.1016/j.ymthe.2018.07.023] [PMID: 30120059]

[109] Chen Y, Gorski DH. Regulation of angiogenesis through a microRNA (miR-130a) that down-regulates antiangiogenic homeobox genes GAX and HOXA5. Blood 2008; 111(3): 1217-26.
[http://dx.doi.org/10.1182/blood-2007-07-104133] [PMID: 17957028]

[110] Zhang J, Guan J, Niu X, *et al.* Exosomes released from human induced pluripotent stem cells-derived MSCs facilitate cutaneous wound healing by promoting collagen synthesis and angiogenesis. J Transl Med 2015; 13(1): 49-62.
[http://dx.doi.org/10.1186/s12967-015-0417-0] [PMID: 25638205]

[111] Tan CY, Lai RC, Wong W, Dan YY, Lim S-K, Ho HK. Mesenchymal stem cell-derived exosomes promote hepatic regeneration in drug-induced liver injury models. Stem Cell Res Ther 2014; 5(3): 76-89.
[http://dx.doi.org/10.1186/scrt465] [PMID: 24915963]

[112] Hu GW, Li Q, Niu X, *et al.* Exosomes secreted by human-induced pluripotent stem cell-derived mesenchymal stem cells attenuate limb ischemia by promoting angiogenesis in mice. Stem Cell Res Ther 2015; 6(1): 10-24.
[http://dx.doi.org/10.1186/scrt546] [PMID: 26268554]

[113] Lai RC, Arslan F, Lee MM, *et al.* Exosome secreted by MSC reduces myocardial ischemia/reperfusion injury. Stem Cell Res (Amst) 2010; 4(3): 214-22.
[http://dx.doi.org/10.1016/j.scr.2009.12.003] [PMID: 20138817]

[114] Zhou J, Tan X, Tan Y, Li Q, Ma J, Wang G. Mesenchymal stem cell derived exosomes in Cancer progression, metastasis and drug delivery: a comprehensive review. J Cancer 2018; 9(17): 3129-37.
[http://dx.doi.org/10.7150/jca.25376] [PMID: 30210636]

[115] Lin J, Cao S, Wang Y, *et al.* Long non-coding RNA UBE2CP3 enhances HCC cell secretion of VEGFA and promotes angiogenesis by activating ERK1/2/HIF-1α/VEGFA signalling in hepatocellular carcinoma. J Exp Clin Cancer Res 2018; 37(1): 113-25.
[http://dx.doi.org/10.1186/s13046-018-0727-1] [PMID: 29866133]

[116] Rathore P, Swami G. Virosomes: a novel vaccination technology. Int J Pharm Sci Res 2012; 3(10): 3591-7.

[117] Marofi F, Vahedi G, Biglari A, Esmaeilzadeh A, Athari SS. Mesenchymal stromal/stem cells: a new era in the cell-based targeted gene therapy of cancer. Front Immunol 2017; 8: 1770-85.
[http://dx.doi.org/10.3389/fimmu.2017.01770] [PMID: 29326689]

[118] Zhang Q, Xiang W, Yi DY, *et al.* Current status and potential challenges of mesenchymal stem cell-based therapy for malignant gliomas. Stem Cell Res Ther 2018; 9(1): 228-36.
[http://dx.doi.org/10.1186/s13287-018-0977-z] [PMID: 30143053]

[119] Ilkow CS, Marguerie M, Batenchuk C, *et al.* Reciprocal cellular cross-talk within the tumor microenvironment promotes oncolytic virus activity. Nat Med 2015; 21(5): 530-6.
[http://dx.doi.org/10.1038/nm.3848] [PMID: 25894825]

[120] Fritz V, Fajas L. Metabolism and proliferation share common regulatory pathways in cancer cells. Oncogene 2010; 29(31): 4369-77.
[http://dx.doi.org/10.1038/onc.2010.182] [PMID: 20514019]

[121] Marchini A, Daeffler L, Pozdeev VI, Angelova A, Rommelaere J. Immune conversion of tumor microenvironment by oncolytic viruses: the protoparvovirus H-1PV case study. Front Immunol 2019; 10: 1848-64.
[http://dx.doi.org/10.3389/fimmu.2019.01848] [PMID: 31440242]

[122] Russell L, Peng K-W. The emerging role of oncolytic virus therapy against cancer. Linchuang Zhongliuxue Zazhi 2018; 7(2): 16-28.
[http://dx.doi.org/10.21037/cco.2018.04.04] [PMID: 29764161]

[123] Maroun J, Muñoz-Alía M, Ammayappan A, Schulze A, Peng K-W, Russell S. Designing and building oncolytic viruses. Future Virol 2017; 12(4): 193-213.
[http://dx.doi.org/10.2217/fvl-2016-0129] [PMID: 29387140]

[124] Russell L, Peng KW, Russell SJ, Diaz RM. Oncolytic Viruses: Priming Time for Cancer Immunotherapy. BioDrugs 2019; 33(5): 485-501.
[http://dx.doi.org/10.1007/s40259-019-00367-0] [PMID: 31321623]

[125] van Vloten JP, Workenhe ST, Wootton SK, Mossman KL, Bridle BW. Critical interactions between immunogenic cancer cell death, oncolytic viruses, and the immune system define the rational design of combination immunotherapies. J Immunol 2018; 200(2): 450-8.
[http://dx.doi.org/10.4049/jimmunol.1701021] [PMID: 29311387]

[126] Russell SJ, Peng K-W, Bell JC. Oncolytic virotherapy. Nat Biotechnol 2012; 30(7): 658-70.
[http://dx.doi.org/10.1038/nbt.2287] [PMID: 22781695]

[127] Atherton MJ, Lichty BD. Evolution of oncolytic viruses: novel strategies for cancer treatment. Immunotherapy 2013; 5(11): 1191-206.
[http://dx.doi.org/10.2217/imt.13.123] [PMID: 24188674]

[128] Chiocca EA, Rabkin SD. Oncolytic viruses and their application to cancer immunotherapy. Cancer

Immunol Res 2014; 2(4): 295-300.
[http://dx.doi.org/10.1158/2326-6066.CIR-14-0015] [PMID: 24764576]

[129] Gomes JPA, Assoni AF, Pelatti M, Coatti G, Okamoto OK, Zatz M. Assoni AF, Pelatti M, Coatti G, Okamoto OK, Zatz M. Deepening a simple question: Can MSCs be used to treat cancer? Anticancer Res 2017; 37(9): 4747-58.
[PMID: 28870893]

[130] Kazimirsky G, Jiang W, Slavin S, Ziv-Av A, Brodie C. Mesenchymal stem cells enhance the oncolytic effect of Newcastle disease virus in glioma cells and glioma stem cells*via*the secretion of TRAIL. Stem Cell Res Ther 2016; 7(1): 149-58.
[http://dx.doi.org/10.1186/s13287-016-0414-0] [PMID: 27724977]

[131] Harrington K, Freeman DJ, Kelly B, Harper J, Soria J-C. Optimizing oncolytic virotherapy in cancer treatment. Nat Rev Drug Discov 2019; 18(9): 689-706.
[http://dx.doi.org/10.1038/s41573-019-0029-0] [PMID: 31292532]

[132] Carlisle R, Choi J, Bazan-Peregrino M, *et al.* Enhanced tumor uptake and penetration of virotherapy using polymer stealthing and focused ultrasound. J Natl Cancer Inst 2013; 105(22): 1701-10.
[http://dx.doi.org/10.1093/jnci/djt305] [PMID: 24168971]

[133] Harrington KJ, Puzanov I, Hecht JR, *et al.* Clinical development of talimogene laherparepvec (T-VEC): a modified herpes simplex virus type-1-derived oncolytic immunotherapy. Expert Rev Anticancer Ther 2015; 15(12): 1389-403.
[http://dx.doi.org/10.1586/14737140.2015.1115725] [PMID: 26558498]

[134] Sokolowski NA, Rizos H, Diefenbach RJ. Oncolytic virotherapy using herpes simplex virus: how far have we come? Oncolytic Virother 2015; 4: 207-19.
[PMID: 27512683]

[135] Zhang W, Fulci G, Wakimoto H, *et al.* Combination of oncolytic herpes simplex viruses armed with angiostatin and IL-12 enhances antitumor efficacy in human glioblastoma models. Neoplasia 2013; 15(6): 591-9.
[http://dx.doi.org/10.1593/neo.13158] [PMID: 23730207]

[136] Zhang G, Jin G, Nie X, *et al.* Enhanced antitumor efficacy of an oncolytic herpes simplex virus expressing an endostatin-angiostatin fusion gene in human glioblastoma stem cell xenografts. PLoS One 2014; 9(4): e95872-81.
[http://dx.doi.org/10.1371/journal.pone.0095872] [PMID: 24755877]

[137] Fields B, Knipe D, Howley P. Fields virology. Philadelphia: Wolters Kluwer Health/Lippincott Williams & Wilkins 2013; p. 1307.

[138] Phillips MB, Stuart JD, Rodríguez Stewart RM, Berry JT, Mainou BA, Boehme KW. Current understanding of reovirus oncolysis mechanisms. Oncolytic Virother 2018; 7: 53-63.
[http://dx.doi.org/10.2147/OV.S143808] [PMID: 29942799]

[139] Sahin E, Egger ME, McMasters KM, Zhou HS. Development of oncolytic reovirus for cancer therapy. J Cancer Ther 2013; 4(06): 1100-15.
[http://dx.doi.org/10.4236/jct.2013.46127]

[140] Carew JS, Espitia CM, Zhao W, Mita MM, Mita AC, Nawrocki ST. Oncolytic reovirus inhibits angiogenesis through induction of CXCL10/IP-10 and abrogation of HIF activity in soft tissue sarcomas. Oncotarget 2017; 8(49): 86769-83.
[http://dx.doi.org/10.18632/oncotarget.21423] [PMID: 29156834]

[141] Zhang Z, Zou W, Wang J, *et al.* Suppression of tumor growth by oncolytic adenovirus-mediated delivery of an antiangiogenic gene, soluble Flt-1. Mol Ther 2005; 11(4): 553-62.
[http://dx.doi.org/10.1016/j.ymthe.2004.12.015] [PMID: 15771958]

[142] Ramírez M, García-Castro J, Melen GJ, González-Murillo Á, Franco-Luzón L. Patient-derived mesenchymal stem cells as delivery vehicles for oncolytic virotherapy: novel state-of-the-art

technology. Oncolytic Virother 2015; 4: 149-55.
[http://dx.doi.org/10.2147/OV.S66010] [PMID: 27512678]

[143]   Huang B, Sikorski R, Kirn DH, Thorne SH. Synergistic anti-tumor effects between oncolytic vaccinia virus and paclitaxel are mediated by the IFN response and HMGB1. Gene Ther 2011; 18(2): 164-72.
[http://dx.doi.org/10.1038/gt.2010.121] [PMID: 20739958]

[144]   Tilgase A, Olmane E, Nazarovs J, *et al.* Multimodality Treatment of a Colorectal Cancer Stage IV Patient with FOLFOX-4, Bevacizumab, Rigvir Oncolytic Virus, and Surgery. Case Rep Gastroenterol 2018; 12(2): 457-65.
[http://dx.doi.org/10.1159/000492210] [PMID: 30283278]

[145]   Heinemann L, Simpson GR, Boxall A, *et al.* Synergistic effects of oncolytic reovirus and docetaxel chemotherapy in prostate cancer. BMC Cancer 2011; 11(1): 221-9.
[http://dx.doi.org/10.1186/1471-2407-11-221] [PMID: 21645351]

[146]   Chaurasiya S, Chen NG, Warner SG. Oncolytic virotherapy *versus* cancer stem cells: A review of approaches and mechanisms. Cancers (Basel) 2018; 10(4): 124-42.
[http://dx.doi.org/10.3390/cancers10040124] [PMID: 29671772]

CHAPTER 5

Angiogenesis and Chromene-based Antiangiogenic Therapeutic Agents

Olívia Pontes[1,2], Ana Raquel-Cunha[1,2], Sofia Oliveira-Pinto[1,2], Fátima Baltazar[1,2], Olga Martinho[1,2,3] and Marta Costa[1,2,*]

[1] *Life and Health Sciences Research Institute (ICVS), University of Minho, Campus of Gualtar, Braga, Portugal*

[2] *ICVS/3Bs-PT Government Associate Laboratory, Braga/Guimarães, Portugal*

[3] *Molecular Oncology Research Center, Barretos Cancer Hospital, Barretos, São Paulo, Brazil*

Abstract: Tumor vascularization plays an essential role in cancer progression. Tumor vasculature provides oxygen and nutrients to cancer cells and removes waste products which is important for the rapid growth of tumors. Importantly, the tumor associated vessels are also used for tumor cell metastization, in which cancer cells invade distant organs. Therefore, inhibition of angiogenesis constitutes one of the elected targeted approaches for cancer treatment.

The first FDA approved antiangiogenic drug was bevacizumab, an antibody against vascular endothelial growth factor (VEGF) that has been used to treat metastatic tumors. However, despite the initial increase in survival rates, no major benefit in global survival was described and patients ended up relapsing due to acquired resistance. Further, monotherapy with this type of agents is not generally associated with improvement of survival, being antiangiogenic therapy a strategy that is worth pursuing as combination therapy. Thus, the efficacy of angiogenesis inhibitors is still a major challenge.

Several families of naturally occurring compounds have been described as antiangiogenic agents with promising results, such as stilbenes, chalcones, terpenoids, phenylethanoids and others. Due to their remarkable structure variety, plant polyphenols have been extensively studied and found to inhibit angiogenesis and metastasis through the regulation of multiple signaling pathways involved in cancer development. Chromenes and coumarins, such as crolibulin (EPC2407), have already been identified as vascular disrupting agents with promising antiangiogenic properties. The substitution pattern highly influences the activity and mode of action in various types of cancer. Specifically, chromenes are found to regulate the expression of VEGF, matrix metalloproteinases (MMPs) and receptor tyrosine kinases RTKs (*e.g.* EGFR) signaling pathways.

* Corresponding author Marta Costa: Life and Health Sciences Research Institute (ICVS), School of Health Sciences, University of Minho, Campus de Gualtar, Braga, Portugal; Tel: + 351 253 604837; E-mail: martafcosta@med.uminho.pt

This chapter focuses on the antiangiogenic properties of chromenes, coumarins and derivatives, highlighting the recent progress in drug development and clinical applications.

Keywords: Angiogenesis, Antiangiogenic agents, Cancer, Chromenes.

INTRODUCTION

Angiogenesis Overview

The importance of blood vessels in life is irrefutable as they are the first organ to be formed in the embryo and is the largest network in our body. Blood vessels can be either small, consisting of only endothelial cells, or larger, consisting of medium sized pericytes, smooth muscle cells and surrounded by mural cells [1]. Two essential mechanisms implement the development of the vascular network: vasculogenesis, which refers to the formation of blood vessels from endothelial progenitors; and angiogenesis, also known by neovascularization, which is the term given to the outgrowth of new capillaries from pre-existing ones, forming collateral bridges between arterial networks [2]. The latter term was first adopted by John Hunter in 1787 to describe this phenomenon [3], but it remained underexplored up until Judah Folkman proposed, in 1971, that tumor growth was angiogenesis dependent [4], this hypothesis is the start of a considerable generation of knowledge about angiogenesis, observed in the years ahead until nowadays.

The role of angiogenesis can be recognized both in normal physiology and disease. It is essential during the female reproductive cycle, to rebuild the uterus lining, to mature the egg during ovulation and during the fetal development, to build the placenta, allowing the communication between the mother and the fetus [5]. Additionally, angiogenesis is crucial for the repair and regeneration of tissues during the wound healing process [6]. In a healthy organism, angiogenesis is maintained due to a delicately balanced activity between "on" and "off" regulatory switches (Fig. **1**), being those angiogenic growth factors and endogenous angiogenesis inhibitors, respectively, which surround the endothelium [7].

Angiogenin	Angiostatin
Angiopoietin	Canstatin
Fibroblast growth factors	Endostatin
Granulocyte colony-stimulating factor	Interferon-αβγ
Hepatocyte growth factor	Interleukin 4, 12, 18
Interleukin-8	Tissue inhibitor metalloproteinases
Placent growth factor	Platelet factor-4
Platelet-derived endothelial growth factor	Prolactin 16kD fragment
Vascular endothelial growth factor	Trombospondin-1

Activators   **Inhibitors**

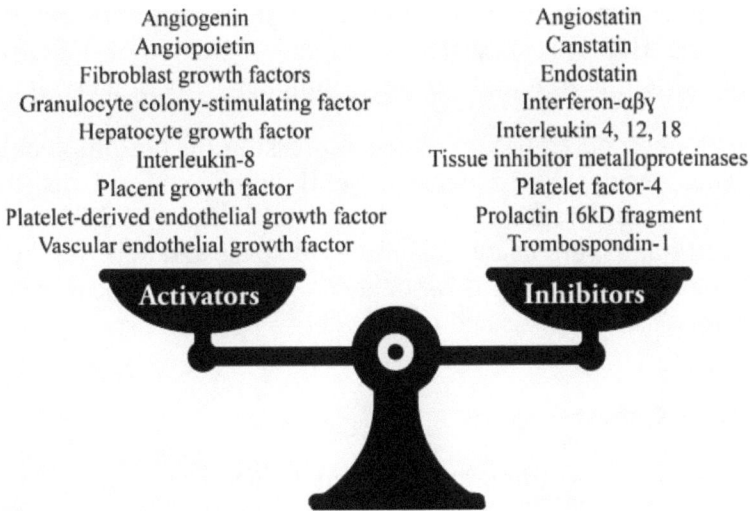

Fig. (1). Angiogenesis is maintained due to balanced activity between "on" and "off" regulatory switches. The balance is driven by activators and inhibitors, which can be growth factors (PDGF, VEGF, FGF, *etc*), cytokines (Interleukines) and endogenous modulators (metalloproteinases, angiostatin, *etc*).

From the several molecules controlling angiogenesis, vascular endothelial growth factor (VEGF), is one of the most specific and critical. VEGF is a mitogenic and chemotactic factor for endothelial cells, capable of stimulating capillary formation *in vivo*, regulating endothelial proliferation, permeability and survival [7]. Despite its importance, VEGF cannot alone direct blood vessel organization and maturation, therefore factors like angiopoietins are important partners. The presence of angiopoietin-1 enables the increase of the girth and stability of the endothelium, thus stimulating branching and remodeling of new blood vessels [8]. Other growth factors like fibroblast growth factor (FGF) and platelet derived growth factor (PDGF) have a role in activating angiogenesis. PDGF is central in maintaining the stability of capillary wall through the recruitment of pericytes to the newly formed vessels [9]. FGF, although not crucial for vascular development, stimulates protease synthesis, migration, proliferation and formation of a tube-like structure in the three-dimensional matrices [10].

Besides the activity of the angiogenesis activators, negative regulators are also needed for the growth of blood vessels (Fig. **1**). An example is angiostatin that can induce apoptosis and inhibit migration and the formation of tubules in endothelial cells [11].

Additionally, metabolic stresses like low oxygen tension, low extracellular pH and low glucose concentration, can trigger angiogenesis [12]. Hypoxia is an important stimulus for the expansion of the blood vessels network. Oxygen is delivered to the cells by simple diffusion, however, when tissues grow beyond the oxygenation limit, hypoxia triggers vessel growth by signaling through hypoxia-inducible transcription factors (HIFs) [13]. HIFs upregulate many angiogenic genes, including HIF-1α a key transcriptional regulator of VEGF, PDGF and angiopoietin, which, as referred above, stimulates neovascularization.

Unfortunately, upon deregulation of the expression of these molecules and their delicate balance, serious disorders can arise. If on the one hand, insufficient vessel growth and vessel regression can cause heart and brain ischemia, neurodegeneration, hypertension, respiratory distress and delaying healing, on the other hand, vessel overgrowth is associated with diseases like cancer, psoriasis, rheumatoid arthritis, blindness and obesity [1].

Angiogenesis in Cancer

As with normal tissues, tumors also need to acquire vascular supply to get nutrients and oxygen, as well as to evacuate metabolic wastes and carbon dioxide. This sustainability is assured by tumor-associated neovascularization, generated by angiogenesis [14].

During tumor progression, there are two known phases. The first phase, called avascular or dormant phase, observed in tumors with approximately 1-2 mm in diameter, is characterized by a steady state between proliferation and apoptosis of tumor cells. Due to the tumor's reduced size, oxygen and nutrients, as well as metabolic wastes, can still diffuse from and out of the tumor through pre-existent vasculature. This is the case of most human tumors that remain *in situ* for months to years, without inducing angiogenesis [15]. However, if there is continuous growth, the tumor becomes necrotic and hypoxic due to poor oxygenation, resulting from deficient vascularization. At this stage, an "angiogenic switch" is almost always activated, and remains on, enabling the tumor's growth, development and metastization (Fig. **2**). This angiogenic switch is considered not only a rate limiting step for tumor progression but also for the onset of malignancy occurring when the equilibrium between pro- and antiangiogenic factors is lost, either by raising of angiogenic inducers or by reduction of angiogenic inhibitors [16]. Specifically, the switch can be triggered by physiological stimuli, such as hypoxia, which induces the expression of angiogenic growth factors *via* HIF-1α [13].

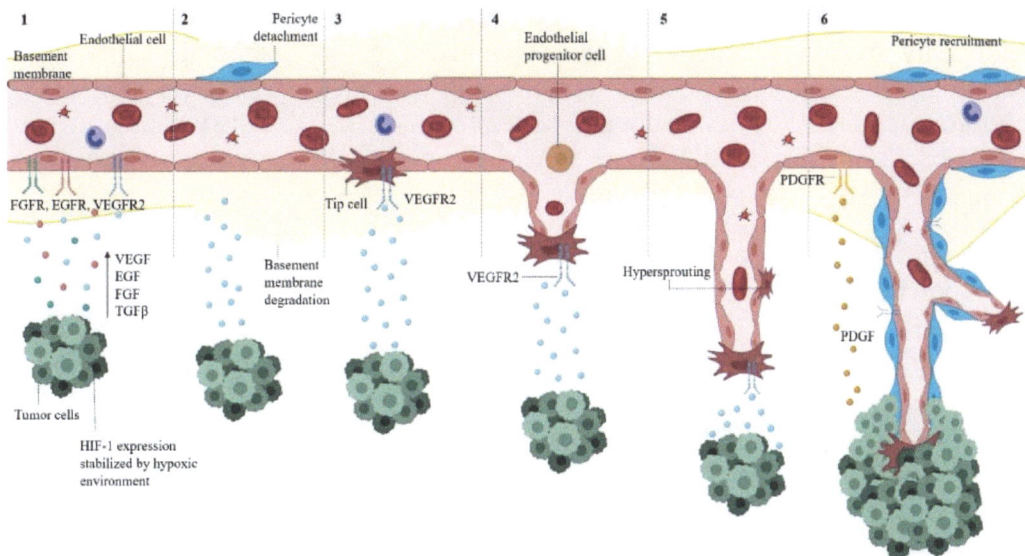

Fig. (2). Angiogenesis and cancer. Tumor angiogenesis is a multistep process that occurs in almost all tumors and that is mediated by endothelial cells (ECs). When a cell has acquired genetic alterations that allow unlimited growth and escape from apoptosis, a small tumor is formed (1). As soon as the tumor volume has reached a few cubic millimeters, oxygen and nutrient supply are insufficient, and the tumor cells undergo an angiogenesis switch. This results in the production and release of growth factors into the surrounding tissue. The secreted growth factors bind to receptors on ECs in nearby vessels. Pericytes that stabilize the vessel detach, and vessel dilation occurs (2). In addition, the activated ECs start to produce matrix metallopeptidases (MMPs) that degrade the basal membrane and the extracellular matrix (3). Subsequently, the ECs start to migrate (4) and proliferate (5) into the growth factor gradient, forming new vascular structures. Finally, matrix proteins are deposited, and the new vessel is stabilized by pericytes to form a functional and mature blood vessel. The tumor cells can continue to grow, and metastasis formation is facilitated since the tumor cells now have easy access to the circulation (6).

The HIF-1α subunit presents an oxygen degradation domain composed of two defined prolyl residues [17]. Hence, when tissues are under normoxia (a condition in which the levels of oxygen are normal), these residues are hydroxylated by prolyl hydroxylase domain protein 2 (PHD2) that uses oxygen to hydrolyze HIF [18]. This hydroxylation promotes the ubiquitination of HIFs by Von Hippel-Lindau (VHL) complex and consequently leads to degradation by the proteasome [19]. Under hypoxic conditions, PHD2 becomes inactive due to its enzymatic dependence on oxygen and so HIF-1α, which is not degraded, becomes stabilized [20]. Thus, when HIFs binds to hypoxia response elements [21], a DNA sequence motif present in the promoter of HIF target genes promotes the appearance of tumor masses [22, 23].

HIF expression can also be regulated through the activation of oncogenic pathways. For instance, several growth factors play a crucial role in the ERK signaling cascade that promotes an increase in mRNA translation into HIF-1α

protein [24]. Increased levels of activated HIF proteins can trigger the transcription of several genes involved in adaptive responses of the tumor cells against hypoxia conditions [24], such as glucose metabolism, cell proliferation, cell migration and angiogenesis [25]. VEGF, glucose transporter-1 (GLUT-1), erythropoietin (EPO), plasminogen activator-1 (PAI-1), transforming growth factor-$\beta1$ (TGF-$\beta1$) and PDGF are some examples of genes whose expression is regulated by HIF-1α [26].

Of the several vascular endothelial growth factors, VEGF-A is considered the most potent regulator of physiological and pathological angiogenesis, showing a binding affinity for VEGFR-1 and VEGFR-2 [27]. The binding between VEGF-A and its receptors promotes blood vessel formation [28] enabling the production of higher levels of this protein by the tumor [29]. Although VEGF-A can bind to two receptors, the role of both is different, being VEGFR-2 indispensable for the development of blood vessels [30].

Besides VEGF-A, VEGF-B also can bind and activate VEGFR-1, controlling extracellular matrix degradation, cell adhesion and migration [31]. VEGF-C and -D usually bind to VEGFR-3 that are largely expressed on lymphatic endothelial cells and so instigate lymphangiogenesis [32]. Additionally, these proteins can also contribute to tumor angiogenesis through binding to both VEGFR-2 and -3 [33, 34]. Finally, VEGF-E, a homologue protein of VEGF-A, shows an affinity for VEGFR-2 and it was identified as an angiogenic protein that is encoded by the poxvirus orf virus [35].

As already mentioned, under hypoxia conditions, the transcription of VEGF mRNA is promoted *via* HIF-1α. Nevertheless, the VEGF expression in tumor cells might be mediated by genetic events such as the loss of tumor suppressor genes, like p53 and PTEN [36], or by the activation of certain oncogenes, as RAS gene [37]. Thus, resistance to apoptosis as well as aberrant proliferation and angiogenesis are some examples of the effects caused by these events [38].

Antiangiogenic Therapies in Cancer

VEGF/VEGFR signaling is crucial for the development of tumors, in which protein overexpression stimulates angiogenesis. In the last decades, an increased effort has been made to develop more sophisticated and personalized therapies, to reduce the limitations of conventional therapies like chemotherapy or radiation. In this sense, targeting angiogenesis has been the focus of research for the last 4 decades [4]. Thus, mainly three approaches have been refined for targeting the VEGF signaling pathways: ligand binding agents that interrupt the binding of VEGF to its receptors; antibodies that bind to the receptor and prevent signaling;

and tyrosine kinase inhibitors (TKI) which block the kinase activity of the receptors [39] (Fig. **3**).

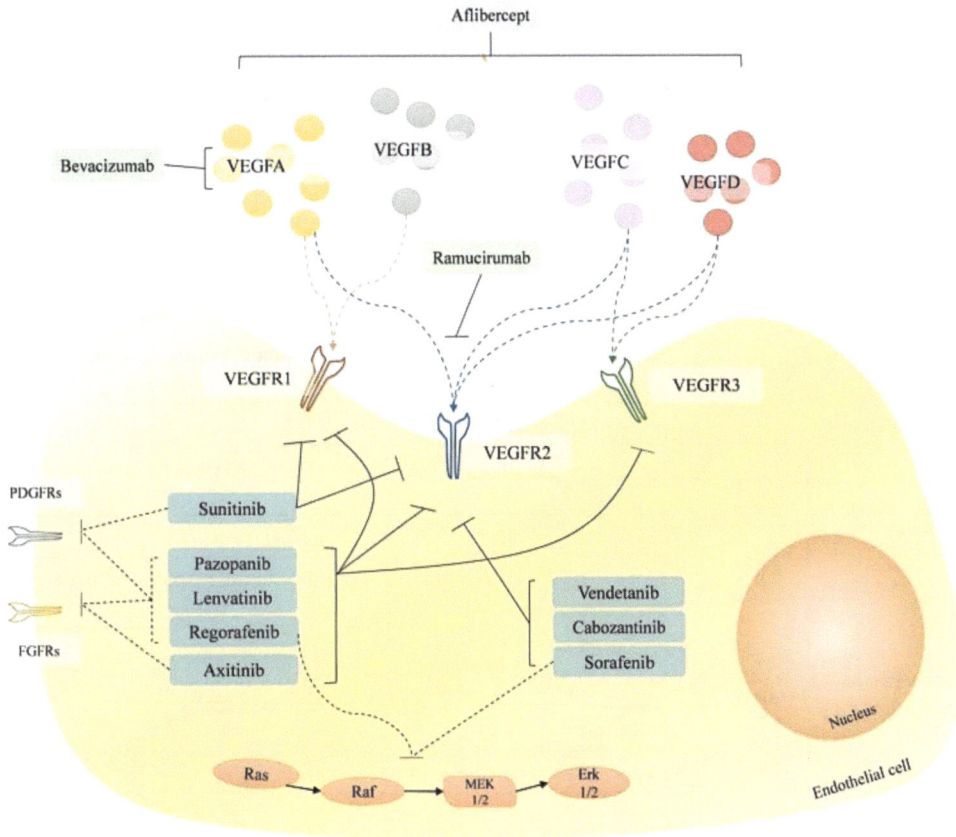

Fig. (3). Angiogenesis as a therapeutic target in cancer. Major molecular targets against angiogenesis and respective mechanisms of drugs action to fight cancer progression. Adapted from [67].

The development of ligand binding agents capable of inhibiting VEGF were, for many years, the years the predominant studies [40]. Promising results led to the design and development of the first antiangiogenic inhibitor – Bevacizumab – a recombinant humanized monoclonal antibody capable of blocking VEGF-A, inhibiting the formation of the complex VEGF-A/VEGFR-2 [41]. The efficacy of this drug in combination with chemotherapy showed to increase overall survival (OS) and/or progression-free survival (PFS) in several types of tumors like metastatic colorectal cancer (mCRC), as first and second line [42 - 44], ovarian cancer [45 - 47], non-small cell lung cancer (NSCLC) [48], among others [49 - 51]. Additionally, immunotherapy with bevacizumab and interferon alpha (IFNα) is currently used as standard therapy for metastatic renal cell carcinoma (RCC), as it prolongs PFS [52]. Although having approval by FDA to be used for the treatment of several cancers (summarized in Table **1**), such as breast, melanoma, and prostate cancer, bevacizumab has failed to increase survival, unbeknownst as to why [53]. With a slightly different approach, aflibercept, a novel VEGFR chimera, was designed to block multiple VEGF family members, VEGF, VEGF-B and P1GF, and inhibit in a broader way VEGF-2 activity [54, 55]. This drug was approved by the FDA for the combined treatment, with chemotherapy, of mCRC [56] and is a promising candidate for the treatment of hepatocellular carcinoma (HCC) [57].

Table 1. Vascular endothelial growth factor (VEGF)-targeted therapies approved by US Food and Drug Administration agency (FDA) used in the treatment of solid tumors.

	Mechanism	Drug	Malignancy
Monoclonal Antibody (mAb)	Anti-VEGF	Bevacizumab	mCRC, NSCLC, GBM, RCC, epithelial ovarian cancer, fallopian tube cancer, primary peritoneal cancer, cervical cancer
		Aflibercept	mCRC
	Anti- VEGFR	Ramucirumab	mCRC, NSCLC, gastric or gastroesophageal junction adenocarcinoma
Tyrosine Kinase Inhibitor (TKI)	Anti- VEGFR	Sorafenib	RCC, HCC, thyroid cancer
		Sunitinib	RCC, pancreatic neuroendocrine tumors, gastrointestinal stromal tumors
		Regorafenib	GIST, mCRC, HCC
		Pazopanib	RCC, soft tissue sarcoma
		Axitinib	RCC
		Vandetanib	medullary thyroid cancer
		Lenvatinib	thyroid cancer, RCC
		Cabozantinib	medullary thyroid cancer, RCC

mCRC- metastatic colorectal cancer, NSCLC- non-small cell lung cancer, GBM- glioblastoma, RCC- renal cell carcinoma, GIST- gastrointestinal stromal tumor, HCC- hepatocellular carcinoma.

Rather than directly targeting VEGF, others proposed the development of antiangiogenic therapies through inhibition of VEGF receptors and, consequently, its downstream targets, so that endothelial proliferation is suppressed, and vascular supply of nutrients and oxygen is disrupted [39]. Ramucirumab is a fully humanized monoclonal antibody, which specifically targets VEGFR-2 through the blockage of the interaction between the receptor and its VEGF ligands [58]. Its use in the clinic was approved in 2014 for the treatment of advanced gastric or gastro-esophageal junction adenocarcinoma and metastatic NSCLC, when in combination with chemotherapy [59 - 61].

Concerning antiangiogenic TKIs, several were approved to be used in the clinic in a monotherapy strategy for various types of cancer, due to promising results on the improvement of OS and PFS in phase III trials (summarized in Table **1**). The first antiangiogenic TKI to be developed was sorafenib, an inhibitor of VEGFR-2 and PDGFRβ, initially approved for the treatment of RCC [62], later for HCC [63] and more recently for differentiated thyroid cancer treatment [64, 65]. Sunitinib soon followed, as an inhibitor of VEGFR-1-2 and PDGFR-α/β, and was approved for the treatment of gastrointestinal stromal tumors, RCC and thyroid cancer [66].

The new generation of TKIs opened the way for the development of new drugs with better toxicity profiles, known as second generation TKIs. An example of this is regorafenib, an inhibitor of the activity of several kinases, including those involved in angiogenesis, such as VEGFR1-3 and PDGFRβ [67]. Also part of these group are the drugs pazopanib and axitinib (both VEGFR1-3 and PDGFRβ), cabozanitinib and vandetanib (VEGFR-2) and lenvatinib (VEGFR1-3 and PDGEFRα), used in the treatment of various cancers (Table **1**). These second-generation TKIs have the advantage of having a higher specific activity, which ultimately leads to greater pharmacological potency and fewer side effects [68].

Unfortunately, although promising, these antiangiogenic targeted therapies still have some limitations. On one hand, and besides an initial positive response to the treatment, most often the tumor ends up acquiring resistance to the treatment. This happens due to the ability of the tumor to circumvent the blocked independent pathway, usually VEGF/VEGFR-2, promoting angiogenesis anyway [69]. Thus, combined treatments with conventional therapies may be a way to surpass this problem [70]. However, this cannot always be done. On the other hand, antiangiogenic treatments still have associated side effects regarding their toxicity. In the whole, the continuous search for new drugs with low toxicity associated with high potency and the ability to inhibit events such as angiogenesis is greatly relevant. Thus, natural compounds might be a promising way to proceed, as they are accessible, have low toxicity and have been used throughout the centuries to treat various diseases [71].

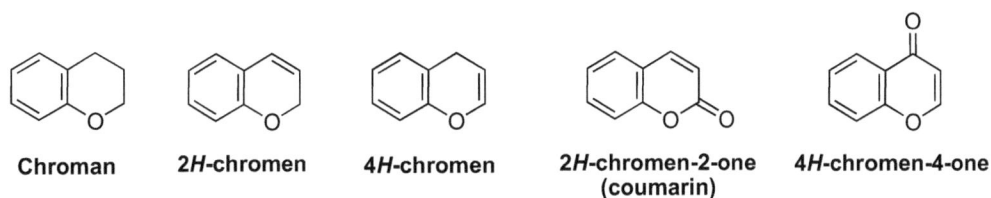

| **Chroman** | **2H-chromen** | **4H-chromen** | **2H-chromen-2-one (coumarin)** | **4H-chromen-4-one** |

Fig. (4). Representation of chromene-based scaffolds. Different chromenes according to the level of oxidation and saturation [71].

CHROMENE-BASED COMPOUNDS

The fusion of a benzene ring with a heterocyclic pyran ring results in a polycyclic compound named benzopyran [72, 73]. Chromene was the nomenclature adopted by the International Union of Pure and Applied Chemistry (IUPAC) to define these compounds (Fig. **4**). Owing to their wide natural occurrence, chromene derivatives were explored for many therapeutic applications. Numerous biological potentials were found including antitumor, anti-HIV therapy, antibacterial, antifungal, anti-inflammatory, anti-coagulant, antioxidant and antidepressant [74 - 77]. Due to their biological potential, this family of compounds inspired the synthesis of new derivatives in order to enhance the potential applications with better outcomes, as for cancer management. Crolibulin, a 4*H*-chromene, is described as a tubulin inhibitor and is currently in phase I/II of clinical trials for the treatment of anaplastic thyroid cancer patients [78]. The properties of this chromene include the induction of apoptosis and disruption of neovascular endothelial cells, with consequent impairment of blood flow to the tumor.

This class of compounds is present in several pharmaceutical preparations, for a wide range of diseases [79, 80]. Examples can be found in European countries that use coumarin-based drugs for therapeutic purposes, namely to treat lymphedema. In the past few years, several drugs containing the chromene scaffold were approved by the U.S. FDA (Fig. **5**). From the wide range of therapeutic applications, they were approved as antidiabetic and anti-inflammatory (troglitazone **1**), antiviral (velpatasvir **2**) and synthetic cannabinoids (nabilone **4** effective for fibromyalgia and multiple sclerosis and dronabinol **3** used in sleep apnea). More importantly, it was found that the combination of dronabinol **3** and velpatasvir **4** with sofosbuvir could treat hepatitis C. Also, coumarin-based pharmaceuticals were approved by the FDA and are currently being used in the treatment of asthma (cromoglicic acid **5** and pranlukast **6**), skin diseases such as psoriasis, eczema, and cutaneous lymphomas (methoxsalen **7**), blood clots (warfarin **8** and dicoumarol **9**) and bacterial infections (novobiocin **10**).

Natural Chromenes as Angiogenesis Inhibitors

Hematoxylin **11** (Fig. **6**) is a naturally occurring chromene isolated from the heartwood of *Haematoxylon campechianum* that demonstrated to have an inhibitory power against tyrosine kinases and *in vitro* antitumor activity [81]. Lin *et al.* showed that hematoxylin was a potent c-Src inhibitor and, by molecular docking, the computational simulation helped to unravel other recognized homoisoflavonoids as a new class of promising PTK inhibitors.

Scopoletin **12** (Fig. **6**) is one of the main constituents occurring in the stems of *Erycibe obtusifolia*, traditionally used for the treatment of various rheumatoid diseases. Scopoletin was already associated with a wide range of biological activities, such as anti-inflammatory, hypouricemic and antioxidant activities. Recently, scopoletin was investigated for its antiangiogenic potential on the chick chorioallantoic membrane (CAM) model, and revealed a dose-dependent reduction of blood vessel formation [82] inhibited proliferation and migration of HUVEC cells (human umbilical vein endothelial vascular cells) *in vitro* and interrupted autophosphorylation of VEGFR-2 and the downstream signaling pathways.

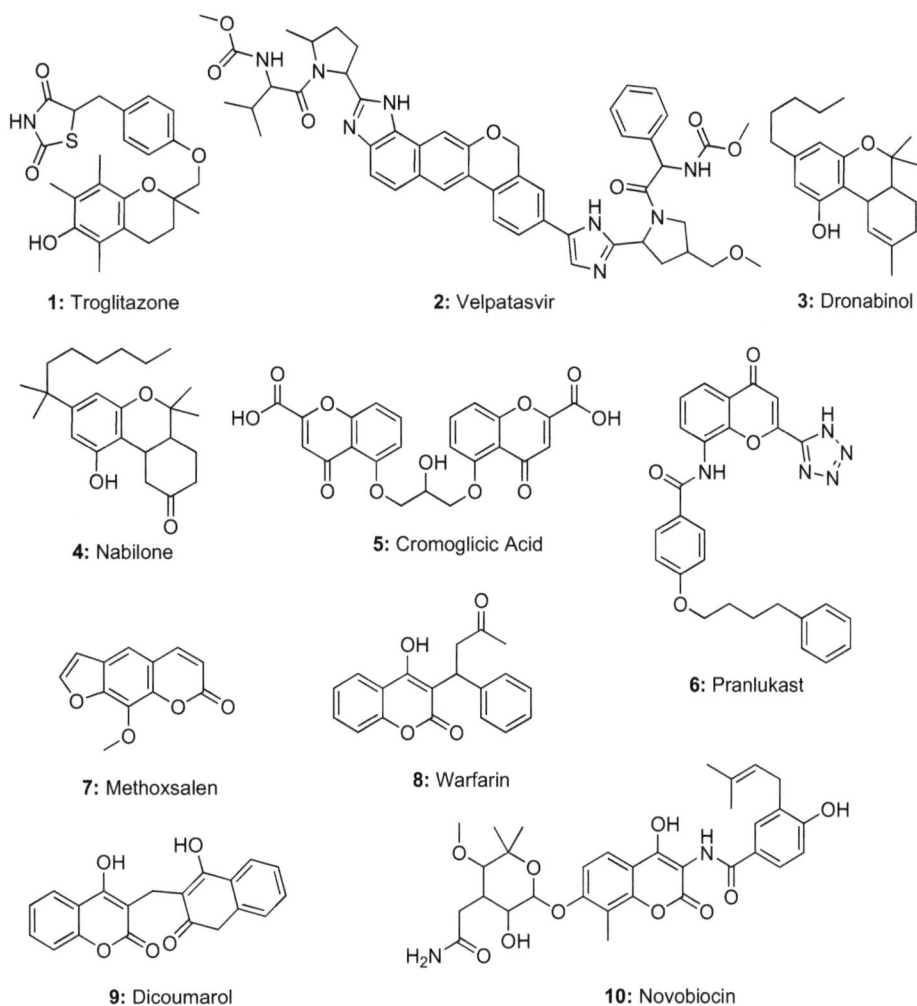

1: Troglitazone   **2: Velpatasvir**   **3: Dronabinol**

4: Nabilone   **5: Cromoglicic Acid**   **6: Pranlukast**

7: Methoxsalen   **8: Warfarin**

9: Dicoumarol   **10: Novobiocin**

Fig. (5). U.S. FDA approved molecules for therapeutic use. Several examples of chromene-based compounds with a wide range of medical applications.

Luteolin **13** (Fig. **6**) is a common dietary flavonoid found in fruits, vegetables, and medicinal herbs. This compound possesses a variety of antitumor properties, such as the inhibition of proliferation and the induction of apoptosis. It was also found that luteolin inhibited invasion and migration in hepatoma, lung and breast cancers. Recently, a study showed that luteolin could target VEGFR-2-regulated AKT/ERK/mTOR/P70S6K/MMPs pathway and, consequently, inhibit VEGF-stimulated endothelial cell proliferation, migration, invasion, tube formation, and tumor angiogenesis leading to the suppression of prostate tumor growth and tumor angiogenesis [83]. Luteolin also suppressed angiogenesis *ex vivo* by the CAM assay and *in vivo* in a human prostate xenograft mouse model.

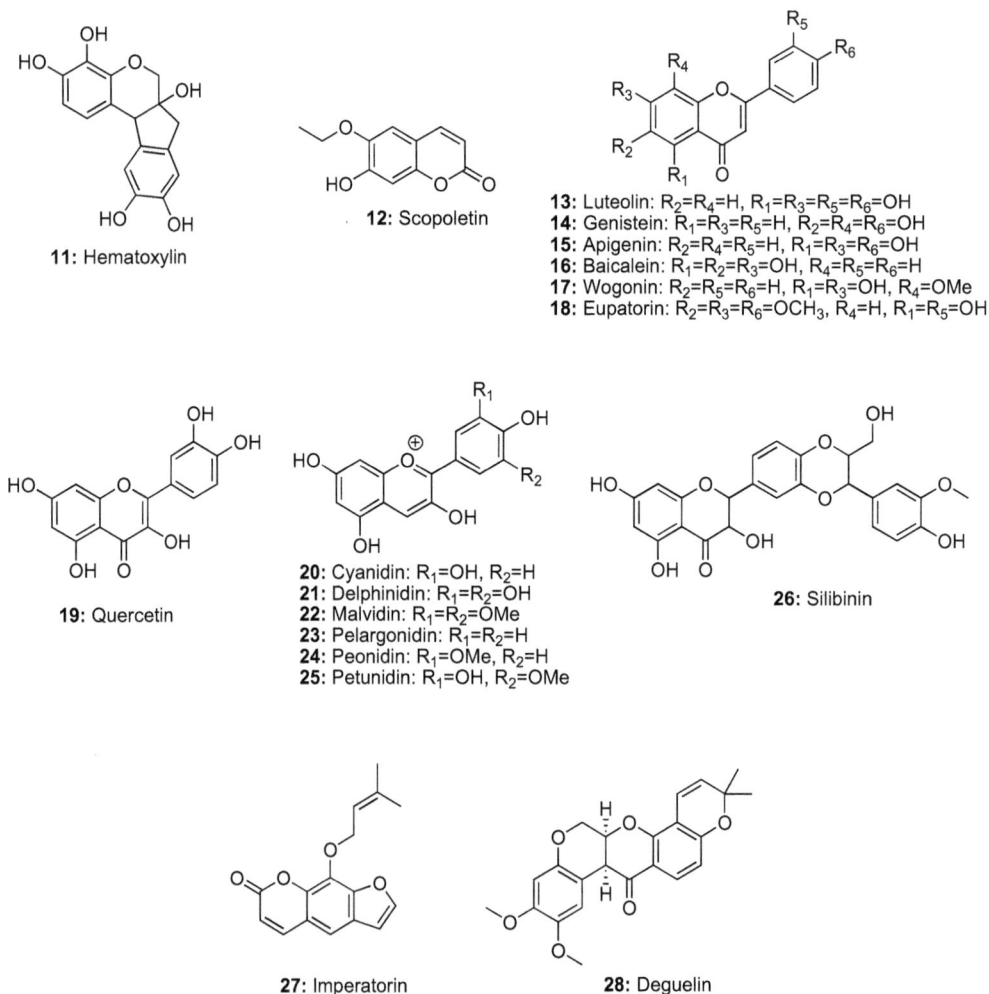

11: Hematoxylin

12: Scopoletin

13: Luteolin: $R_2=R_4=H$, $R_1=R_3=R_5=R_6=OH$
14: Genistein: $R_1=R_3=R_5=H$, $R_2=R_4=R_6=OH$
15: Apigenin: $R_2=R_4=R_5=H$, $R_1=R_3=R_6=OH$
16: Baicalein: $R_1=R_2=R_3=OH$, $R_4=R_5=R_6=H$
17: Wogonin: $R_2=R_5=R_6=H$, $R_1=R_3=OH$, $R_4=OMe$
18: Eupatorin: $R_2=R_3=R_6=OCH_3$, $R_4=H$, $R_1=R_5=OH$

19: Quercetin

20: Cyanidin: $R_1=OH$, $R_2=H$
21: Delphinidin: $R_1=R_2=OH$
22: Malvidin: $R_1=R_2=OMe$
23: Pelargonidin: $R_1=R_2=H$
24: Peonidin: $R_1=OMe$, $R_2=H$
25: Petunidin: $R_1=OH$, $R_2=OMe$

26: Silibinin

27: Imperatorin

28: Deguelin

Fig. (6). Naturally occurring chromenes. Several natural compounds bearing antiangiogenic properties.

Quercetin **19** (Fig. **6**) is found in various plant-based foods and attributed to a wide range of biological therapeutic applications as anti-inflammatory, antiviral, anti-thrombotic and others. The chemopreventive potential of quercetin has been associated with numerous mechanisms including antioxidant activity and ability to inhibit enzymes that trigger carcinogens, to change signal transduction pathways, and to interact with and regulate cell receptors and other proteins. In 2012, it was found that quercetin could inhibit proliferation, invasion, migration and tube formation of HUVEC *in vitro* by suppression of VEGFR-2-regulated AKT/mTOR/P70S6K activation. When tested in prostate tumor cells (PC-3), quercetin exhibited cytotoxicity and induced apoptosis. *In vivo*, quercetin blocks vascular density in CAM and inhibits cancer growth and angiogenesis in human prostate xenograft mouse model [84].

Genistein **14** (Fig. **6**) has recently attracted attention in the treatment and prophylaxis of cancer. This flavonoid is present in the *Leguminosae* plant family and widely used in Chinese medicine due to high content in flavonoids. Experiments with zebrafish demonstrated that genistein was able to inhibit angiogenesis through a decrease in VEGF expression [85]. In 2006, Piao *et al.* discovered alterations in the expression of more than 250 genes related to translation, metabolism, adhesion, apoptosis and various kinases in HUVEC cells when exposed to micromolar concentrations of this flavonoid [86]. Moreover, genistein revealed the ability to inhibit the activation of NF-κB and AKT signaling pathways in the intestinal epithelium [87] and a significant reduction of HIF-1α expression in retinal cells [88]. Recently, a study claimed a bivalent role for genistein in sprouting angiogenesis. Representative results indicated that genistein significantly promoted tube formation at low concentrations, as revealed by total length and anchorage junctions. In contrast, high genistein concentrations completely abrogated endothelial activity, reducing tube formation [89].

Lamy *et al.* found that anthocyanidins, polyphenols extensively present in pigmented fruits, exhibited promising antiangiogenic effects [90]. A wide range of anthocyanidins was tested (including cyaniding **20**, delphinidin **21**, malvidin **22**, pelargonidin **23**, peonidin **24** and petunidin **25**, Fig. **6**), and among this collection, delphinidin demonstrated to be the most potent angiogenesis inhibitor. In this study, delphinidin was able to inhibit VEGFR-2 leading to the inhibition of downstream signaling triggered by this tyrosine kinase. For instance, delphinidin inhibited VEGF-induced activation of ERK1/2 signaling pathway and the chemotactic motility and differentiation of human ECs into capillary-like tubular structures. *In vivo*, delphinidin was able to suppress angiogenesis formation related to its inhibitory effect on VEGFR-2 activity *via* bFGF and VEGF actions in the mouse Matrigel plug assay [90]. In 2017, a study also described that delphinidin inhibited VEGF transcriptional activity and tumor angiogenesis by decreasing the stimulated HIF-1α protein expression and considerably suppressing EGF-induced angiogenesis in the human lung adenocarcinoma A549 cells [91].

In 2005, Singh *et al.* found that silibinin **26** (Fig. **6**) was able to suppress tumor xenograft growth with an increase in apoptosis and reduction in tumor vasculature. Induction of G1 cell arrest accompanied by increased Kip1/p27, Cip, p21 and p53 seemed to be behind this growth inhibition [92]. In lung tumors, silibinin appears to strongly decrease both tumor number and size, an antitumor effect that correlates with reduced antiangiogenic activity by decreasing microvessels size. In this study, the therapeutic efficacy of silibinin in lung tumor growth inhibition and regression by antiangiogenic mechanisms appeared to be mediated by decreased tumor associated macrophages (TAMs) and cytokines, inhibition of HIF-1α, NF-κB and STAT3 activation, and up-regulation of the angiogenic inhibitors, Ang-2- and Tie-2 [93]. Furthermore, in experiments for colorectal carcinoma, silibinin was able to strongly decrease inducible nitric oxide synthase (NOS) and NOS3, cyclooxygenase-1 (COX-1) and COX-2, and HIF-1α and VEGF. Additionally, antiproliferative and proapoptotic effects were noticed through inhibition of ERK1/2 and AKT signaling [94].

Emerging research has shown that the bioflavonoid apigenin **15** (Fig. **6**) has antitumor properties *via* distinct pathways. In particular, Mirvoeva *et al.* demonstrated that apigenin inhibited hypoxia-induced elevation of VEGF at low oxygen conditions [95]. In 2013, these researchers investigated the inhibitory effect of apigenin on TGF-β-induced VEGF production and concluded that VEGF expression is induced by TGF-β1 in human prostate cancer cells. Treatment with apigenin markedly decreased VEGF production by modulating TGF-β-activated pathways linked to cancer progression and metastases, particularly the Smad2/3 and Src/FAK/AKT pathways [96].

Baicalein **16** (Fig. **6**), the main flavonoid extracted from the dried root of *Scutellaria baicalensis Georgi*, demonstrated many pharmacological effects. Along with these bioactivities, several studies found that baicalein inhibits tumor angiogenesis, disrupting tumor vasculature [97]. Miocinovic *et al.* reported that baicalein displays marked angiogenesis inhibition by decreasing the average number and length of sprouts formed by the endothelial cell aggregates of the treated group. Inspection of the signaling molecules altered by baicalein revealed the importance of p53/Rb signaling in the antiproliferative and antiangiogenic effects of this flavonoid [98]. Park *et al.* found by *in vivo* studies that baicalein reduced the tumor growth rate and volume in the early stages of tumor progression through reduction of CD31 expression (endothelial cell marker) and α-SMA (mural cell marker) in the tumors [99].

Another well-described flavonoid isolated from the root of *S. baicalensis* with antiangiogenic and antitumor properties is wogonin **17** (Fig. **6**). In 2014, Zhao *et al.* revealed that wogonin suppressed LPS-induced tumor angiogenesis *via* inhibiting PI3K/AKT/NF-κB signaling pathway. They found that wogonin not only downregulated the levels of PI3K and p-AKT, but also inhibited NF-κB nuclear accumulation [100]. In the same year, Zhou and co-workers reported that wogonin could also suppress PI3K/AKT and IKK/ NF-κB signaling pathways on H_2O_2-induced angiogenesis both *in vitro* and *in vivo* [101].

Imperatorin **27** (Fig. **6**) is a bioactive furocoumarin of *Angelica dahurica* used in traditional Chinese medicine for its anti-inflammatory, antitumoral, anticonvulsant, antihypertensive and vasodilator effects. In 2017, Mi *et al.* showed that imperatorin **27** not only downregulated HIF-1α by decreasing its protein expression without affecting mRNA levels, but also the expression of HIF target genes such as VEGF and erythropoietin (EPO) [102]. They also demonstrated that imperatorin inhibited HIF-1α protein synthesis by suppressing mTOR/ p70S6K/4E-BP1 and MAPK signaling pathways.

The flavone eupatorin **18** (Fig. **6**) has also shown to be a promising antiproliferative agent against several cancer cell lines, including human cervical adenocarcinoma (HeLa), human gastric adenocarcinoma (MK-1), murine melanoma (B16F10), murine colon carcinoma (26-L5), or human breast cancer cell line (MDA-MB-468), with no cytotoxic effects in non-neoplastic human breast cell line (MCF-10A) [103, 104]. In 2012, researchers found that eupatorin is a nonspecific kinase inhibitor with residual activities for RIPK2, VEGFR-1 and MLK3 in treated groups [105]. At the same time, Ahamed *et al.* described that eupatorin significantly inhibited the key aspects of angiogenesis in endothelial cells, such as migration and tube formation [103]. Additionally, it suppressed VEGF-induced phosphorylation of VEGFR-2 in HUVECs.

Deguelin **28** (Fig. **6**), a natural rotenoid extracted from *Derris trifoliata Lour.* and *Mundulea sericea*, has shown effective anti-tumorigenic, anti-angiogenic and anti-metastasis activities in several types of human cancer [106, 107]. In 2010, Lee et al. observed that deguelin inhibited angiogenesis in gastric cancer cells by VEGF mRNA downregulation and destabilization of HIF-1α protein. They hypothesized that deguelin bound to Hsp90 disrupting its function and triggering ubiquitin-mediated degradation of HIF-1α [108]. In 2018, a study described the inhibitory effect of deguelin on non-small cell lung cancer cell migration and invasion *in vitro* and metastasis *in vivo* through the suppression of the CtsZ/FAK/Src/Paxillin signaling pathway linked to cell proliferation, migration, as well as angiogenesis [109].

Ellagic acid **29** (Fig. **7**), a dimeric derivative of gallic acid, is a polyphenol found in several plants and fruits and has already proven its antiproliferative and antioxidant properties in cancer cell lines and animal models [110]. In 2013, Zhao *et al.* reported that ellagic acid inhibited the production of pro-angiogenic IL-6, IL-8 and VEGF in pancreatic tumor-induced Balb c nude mice [111]. Invasiveness-promoting Snail, MMP-2 and MMP-9 were also inhibited, suggesting suppression of cancer growth, angiogenesis and metastasis through the inhibition of AKT, Shh and Notch pathways. At the same time, Vanella *et al.* investigated the effect of ellagic acid in prostate cancer cells angiogenesis [112]. Ellagic acid treatment induced a significant decrease in hemeoxygenase-1 (HO-1), HO-2 and CYP2J2 expression, and in VEGF and OPG levels. These results suggest the ability of ellagic acid to modulate a new pathway *via* the decrease in eicosanoid synthesis and a down-regulation of the HO system in prostate cancer.

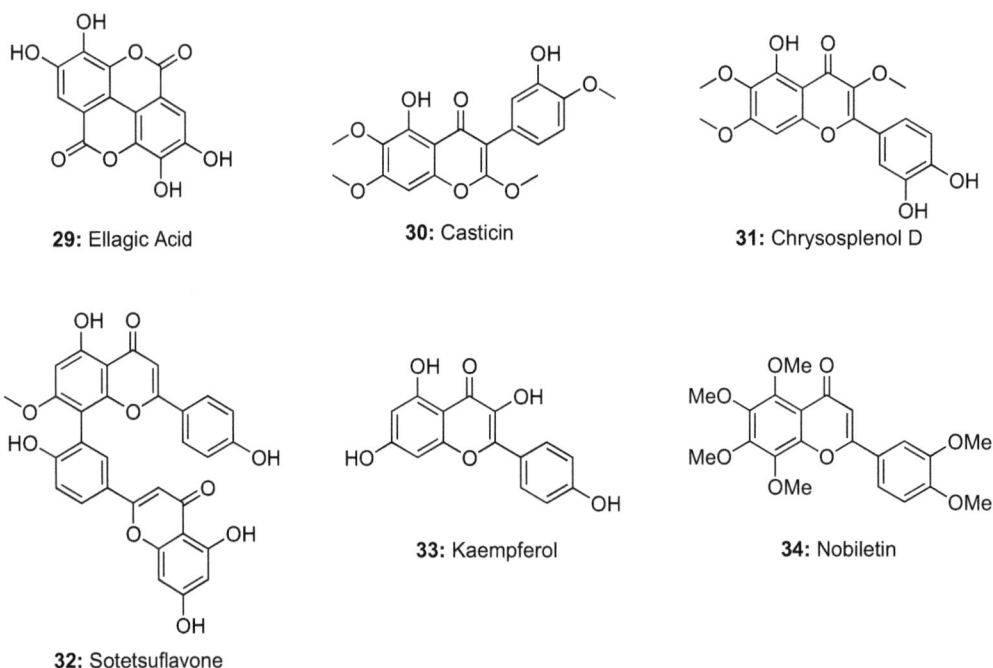

29: Ellagic Acid **30: Casticin** **31: Chrysosplenol D**

32: Sotetsuflavone **33: Kaempferol** **34: Nobiletin**

Fig. (7). Natural chromenes with antiangiogenic properties. Examples of 2*H*-chromen-2-one and several 4*H*-chromen-4-ones.

Two flavonoids, casticin **30** and chrysosplenol D **31** (Fig. **7**), were extracted from *Arteminisia annua L.* and studied for their antiangiogenic properties by Zhu *et al.* [113]. Both flavonoids were found to be involved in the suppression of several molecules related to the angiogenic process, including NO, PGE2, VEGF, IL-1β, IL-6 and TNF-α, both in rat peritoneal cells and human peripheral blood mononuclear cells.

Sotetsuflavone **32** (Fig. **7**) is a double flavonoid extracted from the stem and leaf of *Cycas revolute*. Recently, Wang *et al.* discovered that sotetsuflavone can inhibit the migration, invasion and epithelial-mesenchymal transition (EMT) of A549 cells (non-small-cell lung cancer) [114]. This inhibition was associated with the upregulation of E-cadherin, and down-regulation of N-cadherin, vimentin, and Snail. Sotetsuflavone also downregulated VEGF expression, upregulated angiostatin and concurrently affected the expression of MMPs and decreased MMP-9 and MMP-13 expression.

Extracted from *Dysosma versipellis*, a perennial herb that belongs to the *Berberidaceae* family, kaempferol **33** (Fig. **7**) is described as an effective angiogenesis inhibitor. The stem and radix of *D. versipellis* have been used to treat viral infections and solid tumors and reduce fever and pain. In 2009, Luo and co-workers found that kaempferol could inhibit angiogenesis and VEGF expression through both HIF-dependent (AKT/HIF) and HIF-independent (ESRRA) pathways in human ovarian cancer cells [115]. A few years later, Liang *et al.* demonstrated that kaempferol inhibited proliferation and migration of HUVECs through the suppression of VEGF and FGF signaling pathways [116]. Moreover, the growth of vascular intersegmental vessels was abrogated when zebrafish embryos were co-treated with sub-optimal concentrations of kaempferol and an FGFR inhibitor.

Nobiletin **34** (Fig. **7**) is a polymethoxy flavonoid compound isolated from citrus fruits such as *Citrus depressa* and *Citrus reticulate*. Over the years, nobiletin demonstrated a growth inhibition effect on numerous human cancer types showing suppression of PI3K/AKT pathway in human HepG2 cells, and the inhibition of invasion [117] and migration of human gastric adenocarcinoma AGS cells through FAK/PI3K/AKT pathway [118]. In 2015, Chen *et al.* assessed nobiletin *in vivo* properties finding that nobiletin could suppress tumor growth rates of CP-70 human ovarian cancer cells in the nude mouse model [119]. Furthermore, in the CAM model, nobiletin treatment significantly reduced not only the tumor size but also the number of tumor-associated blood vessels.

A wide range of flavonoids were isolated from *Scutellaria barbata* D. Don, an herb used in traditional Chinese medicine and widely distributed in China and Korea. *S. barbata* has already been recognized by its anti-inflammatory and antitumor effects on several cancer cell lines [120 - 122]. In 2013, Dai *et al.* found that total flavones of *S. barbata* could suppress the angiogenic process *in vitro* inhibiting endothelial cell proliferation, migration and tube formation in a dose dependent manner [120]. *In vivo*, the total number of blood vessels was significantly decreased in the CAM model.

Antiangiogenic and anti-inflammatory properties were also associated with flavonoids extracted from *Lycium barbarum* fruits [123]. Wu and co-workers reported that the flavonoids from *L. barbarum* could retard VEGF-induced proliferation, migration and angiogenesis (tube formation and aortic ring sprouting) in HUVECs in a dose-dependent manner partially through reduction of HUVECs adhesion [124]. The expression of intercellular adhesion molecule-1 (ICAM-1) and vascular cell adhesion molecule (VCAM-1) induced by TNF-α was inhibited in the same cell line. Moreover, the flavonoid extract inhibited TNF-α and H_2O_2-induced intracellular reactive oxygen species (ROS) production leading to the reduction of TNFα-induced IkB phosphorylation as well as NF-κB, p65 and p50 translocation from the cytosol to the nucleus.

Derivatives of Natural Chromenes as Angiogenesis Inhibitors

Increasing interest in resveratrol **35** (Fig. **8**) has shown that this stilbene holds antioxidant, anticancer, anti-aging, and anti-inflammatory properties. In particular, the cardioprotective effect of resveratrol has been intensively investigated. Examining the role of resveratrol in angiogenesis, Wang *et al.* observed that it could modulate angiogenesis in a biphasic pattern by the CAM assay [125]. These researchers found that low concentrations of resveratrol promoted angiogenesis in the HUVEC cell line, whereas high concentrations had an inhibitory effect by modulating GSK3β/β-catenin/TCF pathways, which is in turn regulated by the activation of PI3K/AKT and MEK/ERK signaling pathways.

Two phenolic acids have been studied by Kim *et al.* (2013) for their anti-angiogenic potential, caffeic **36** and rosmarinic **37** acids (Fig. **8**). In retinopathy of a premature mouse model, caffeic acid inhibited VEGF-induced proliferation, migration and tube formation in a concentration-dependent manner [126, 127]. On the other hand, in human retinal endothelial cells, rosmarinic acid inhibited cell proliferation associated with cell cycle arrest, with increased levels of p21[WAF1].

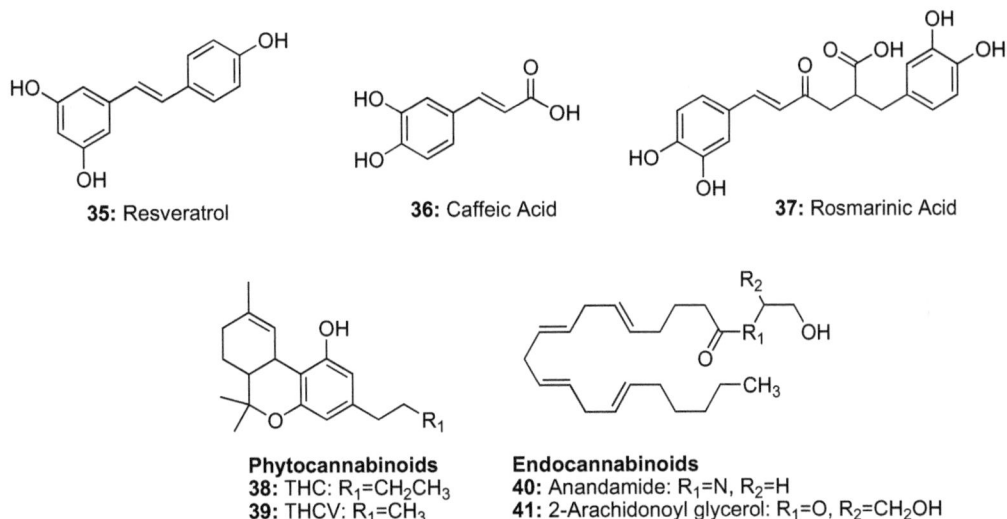

35: Resveratrol   **36:** Caffeic Acid   **37:** Rosmarinic Acid

Phytocannabinoids
38: THC: $R_1=CH_2CH_3$
39: THCV: $R_1=CH_3$

Endocannabinoids
40: Anandamide: $R_1=N$, $R_2=H$
41: 2-Arachidonoyl glycerol: $R_1=O$, $R_2=CH_2OH$

Fig. (8). Chromene derivatives with antiangiogenic properties. Chromene inspired compounds bearing interesting biological activity in angiogenic related pathways.

The hemp plant *Cannabis sativa* produces approximately 60 unique compounds known as cannabinoids **38-41** (examples in Fig. **8**). The antiproliferative properties of cannabis compounds were first reported in 1975 by Munson *et al.* [128]. Since then, promising results were found including growth inhibition of various tumor xenografts, including lung carcinomas, gliomas, thyroid epitheliomas, skin carcinomas and lymphomas. Immunohistochemical and functional studies in mouse models of glioma [129] and skin carcinoma [130] have shown that the administration of cannabinoids modifies vascular hyperplasia from actively growing tumors into a pattern of blood vessels characterized by small, differentiated and impermeable capillaries. These alterations are associated with reduced expression of VEGF, pro-angiogenic cytokines as well as VEGF receptors. Moreover, the administration of cannabinoids to tumor-bearing mice also decreased the activity and expression of MMP-2 [131].

Synthetic Chromenes as Angiogenesis Inhibitors

Hematoxylin analogue **42** (DW534, Fig. **9**) was synthetized and tested in different cell lines including HT-29 (human colorectal adenocarcinoma), K562 (human erythromyeloblastoid leukemia), T47D (human breast cancer), MCF-7 (human breast adenocarcinoma), PC-3 (prostate cancer), HCT-116 (human colon carcinoma), A549 (human lung adenocarcinoma) and MDAMB-231 (human breast cancer), by ELISA assay and Western blot [132]. According to the results DW532 inhibited cell growth, arrested cell cycle and induces apoptosis selectively in cancer cells. It was also demonstrated that compound **42** suppressed dose-dependently angiogenesis *in vitro* inhibiting EGFR and VEGFR-2 kinase activity and their downstream signaling.

Baicalein was reported to inhibit tumor angiogenesis through the disruption of the tumor vasculature but presented also serious disadvantages as poor oral bioavailability and low aqueous solubility. Thus, this molecule was used as inspiration for the synthesis of several derivatives **43** (Fig. 9) with an enhanced anticancer profile [97]. Qu *et al.*, used the phenotype-driven chemical genetic screen in transgenic zebrafish model to test 6-*O*-alkyl alcohol derivatives **43** of baicalein. The molecules were studied for their antiangiogenic and anticancer activities and the most promising candidate (R^1=Bn and R^2=piperazine) exhibited an IC_{50} value in the µM range for A549 cells and induced late apoptosis. Selectivity towards cancer cells was also tested using the human normal fibroblast L929 cells and lower cytotoxicity was demonstrated for this cell line. This compound demonstrated dose-dependent antiangiogenic effect by blocking new blood vessel formation and not by the destruction of existing vasculature when using the zebrafish model which was also confirmed using HUVECs proliferation, migration and tube formation *in vitro* mammalian assays.

Cheng and co-workers [133] focused their study on wogonin derivatives, since this naturally occurring flavonoid was reported to suppress proliferation, induce cell cycle arrest in human CRC cells and also inhibit tumor angiogenesis [100, 101, 134, 135]. The authors prepared 4'-hydroxywogonin **44** (Fig. 9) and used CRC model and SW620 cell line to investigate the potential of this compound. A decrease in cell viability was found in a concentration and time-dependent manner and reduced angiogenesis was also observed, which was associated with the downregulation of VEGF-A expression by disrupting the PI3K/AKT pathway.

Newly synthesized methoxy and 4-thio derivatives of naturally occurring quercetin **45** and luteolin **46** were identified as inhibitors of angiogenesis (Fig. **9**) [136]. Several synthetic derivatives and the corresponding natural products were tested by an established *in vitro* model using HUVECs and inhibition of VEGFR-stimulated migration was observed (scratch/wound healing assay). This inhibition was also confirmed by Western blot studies, where several compounds proved to suppress the VEGFR-2 activity. The antiproliferative activity of these compounds was also investigated in MCF-7 breast cancer cell line and underlined the importance of minimal structural modification in the antiproliferative and antiangiogenic properties of these compounds.

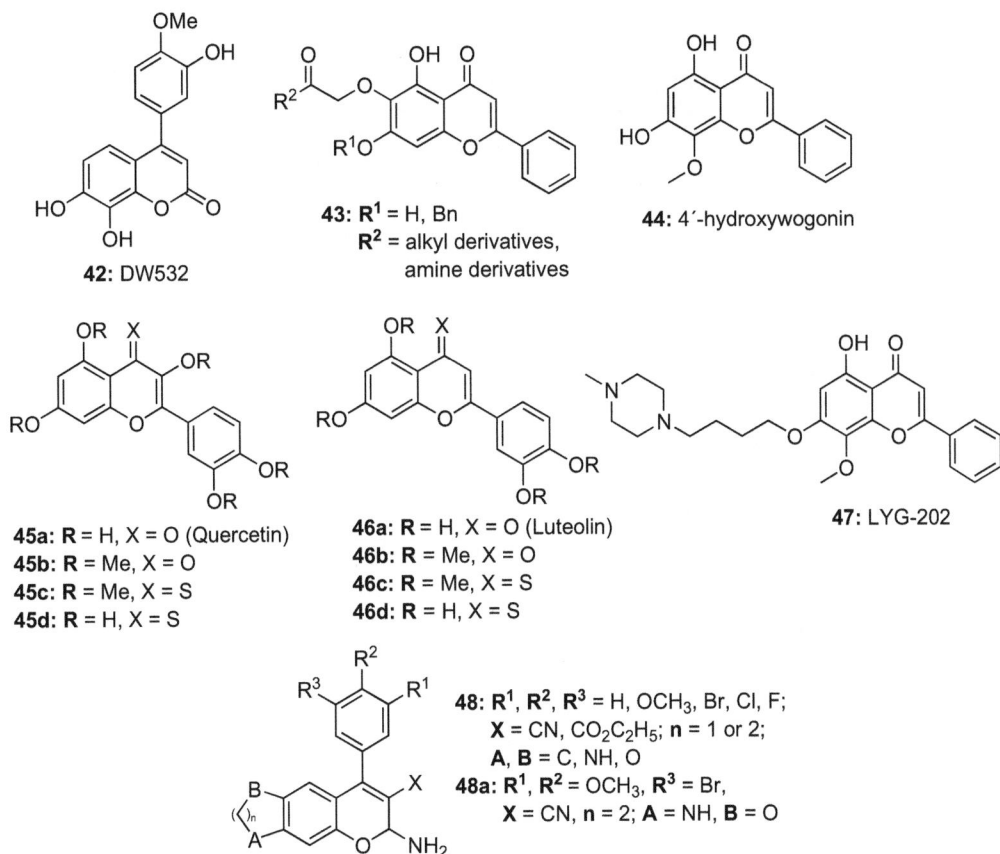

Fig. (9). Synthetic chromenes with antiangiogenic activity. Diverse chromene-based compounds developed using synthetic methodologies to target angiogenesis inhibition.

The anticancer properties of flavonoid derivative **47** LYG-202 (Fig. **9**) were studied to elucidate the mechanism of action, especially as an antiangiogenic agent [137]. LYG-202 proved to be a potent inhibitor using the HUVEC model for VEGF stimulated migration and tube formation. This flavonoid was also able to inhibit phosphorylation of VEGFR-2 and downstream signaling molecules, as AKT, ERK and p38 MAPK, by Western blot analysis. Also, the CAM assay proved that this compound suppressed neovascularization and the rat aortic ring model demonstrated microvessel outgrowth suppression.

Huang *et al.* synthesized a series of 4-aryl-4*H*-chromene-based compounds **48** (Fig. **9**) and studied their antiproliferative and antiangiogenic effect in A375 human melanoma cell line [138]. These compounds demonstrated a highly potent profile with IC_{50} values in the nM range, inhibited microtubule distribution, induced cell cycle arrest and apoptosis. Ultimately, they also inhibited HUVEC capillary tube formation at very low concentrations (nM range). Derivative **48a** demonstrated to be the most potent microtubule destabilizer and vascular disrupting agent, among all the other synthesized compounds. This compound showed also promising IC_{50} values for other cell lines (CHL-1, B16-F10, HeLa, A549, HT-29, HCT116, SW480, Jurkat) and excellent selectivity profile towards non-neoplastic cell lines (HUVECs and Peripheral Blood Mononuclear Cells).

4*H*-Chromene **49** (SP-6-27, Fig. **10**) was studied as a potential anticancer agent in ovarian cancer cells, with an especial focus on resistant cell lines [21]. The authors used cisplatin sensitive cell lines A2780, SKOV-3 and TOV112D and cisplatin-resistant cell lines OVCAR-3, cis-A2780 and cis- TOV112D, since chemo-resistance is a serious problem in this type of cancer. This chromene presented excellent IC_{50} values, for both sensitive and resistant cell lines (nM range values for 72h treatment). Cytotoxicity was also evaluated in normal ovarian epithelial cells (HOSEpiC) and no effect was observed at the studied concentrations. SP-6-27 was found to be a microtubule inhibitor, promoted cell cycle arrest at G2/M and enhanced intrinsic apoptosis was also detected (*via* upregulation of Bax, Apaf-1, Caspase-3, -6 and -9). A combination of this chromene with cisplatin led to enhanced cytotoxicity in both types of studied cell lines. Nonetheless, SP-6-27 was capable of affecting angiogenesis by inhibiting capillary tube formation in HUVECs. The compound inhibited endothelial cell tube formation and in the presence of ovarian tumor conditioned media completely prevented tube formation, which proved the potential of SP-6-27 as vascular disrupting agent leading therefore to suppressed angiogenesis.

Several naphtopyran analogues of chromene-based LY290181 (**50a**, Fig. **10**) were synthesized and their anticancer properties were evaluated [139]. Antiproliferative activity was measured and IC_{50} was determined for several cancer cell lines, 518A2, HT-29, A2780, A2780cis, DLD-1, Panc-1, HCT-116, KB-V1, MCF-7, and also in human endothelial hybrid cells Ea.Hy926, presenting low nM values (72 h treatment). These compounds led to cell cycle arrest in G2/M and tubulin dynamics disruption. The antiangiogenic potential was evaluated using the *in vitro* tube formation assay and 4 compounds were able to form only rudimentary cords or cells were simply in small colonies, proving the inhibition of tube formation. The vascular disrupting potential was assessed *in vivo* using the CAM assay and significant blood vessel reduction was observed for several tested compounds. Chromene **50b** (Fig. **10**) was able to reduce tumor growth *in vivo* in mice bearing cisplatin-resistant A2780cis xenograft.

A series of coumarin derivatives **51** (Fig. **10**) were synthesized using a multi-step synthetic approach and their antiproliferative activity was evaluated in EAC (Ehrlich ascites carcinoma) and DLA (Daltons lymphoma ascites) cell lines, and the IC$_{50}$ values were determined [140]. Compound **51a** was found to be the lead compound, with IC$_{50}$ values in low μM range. The coumarin induced cell shrinkage, condensed nucleus, formation of apoptotic bodies and DNA fragmentation, corroborate its anti-apoptotic potential. *In vivo* tests using murine ascites and solid tumor models confirmed the anticancer potential of this compound, with the prevention of tumor progression in both systems without any detected side effects (hematological and serum profile parameter analyses). Significant tumor size reduction was achieved and a three-fold increase in the life span of animals receiving treatment was observed. Coumarin **51a** treatment showed also a decrease in angiogenesis in a mice-bearing tumor model, when compared to the immense angiogenesis in the peritoneum lining of untreated tumor. Histological observation of H&E stained with formalin fixed peritoneum sections allowed the measurement of micro-vessel density and a significant decrease in the vessel number was detected. Angiogenesis was further studied using the CAM model, reducing rVEGF$_{165}$ neovascularisation, and the antiangiogenic profile of this chromene was also observed.

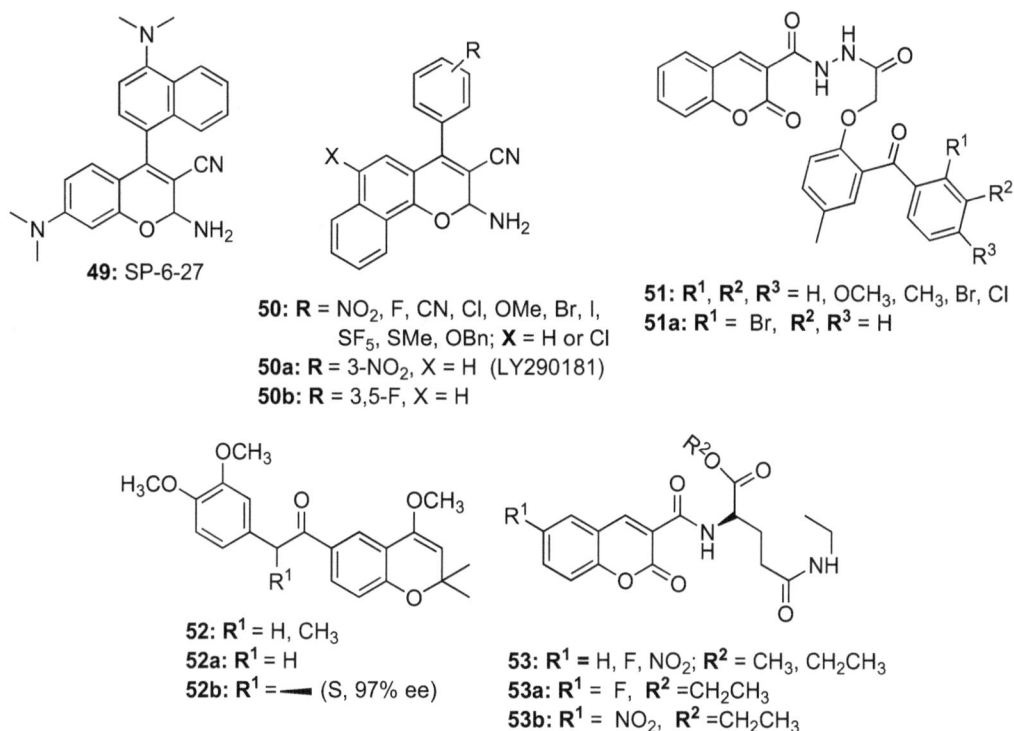

49: SP-6-27

50: R = NO$_2$, F, CN, Cl, OMe, Br, I,
    SF$_5$, SMe, OBn; **X** = H or Cl
50a: **R** = 3-NO$_2$, X = H (LY290181)
50b: **R** = 3,5-F, X = H

51: **R^1**, **R^2**, **R^3** = H, OCH$_3$, CH$_3$, Br, Cl
51a: **R^1** = Br, **R^2**, **R^3** = H

52: **R^1** = H, CH$_3$
52a: **R^1** = H
52b: **R^1** = ◄ (S, 97% ee)

53: **R^1** = H, F, NO$_2$; **R^2** = CH$_3$, CH$_2$CH$_3$
53a: **R^1** = F, **R^2** =CH$_2$CH$_3$
53b: **R^1** = NO$_2$, **R^2** =CH$_2$CH$_3$

Fig. (10). Chromene derivatives inhibiting VEGFR-2 signaling pathway. Synthetic chromenes exhibiting interesting antiangiogenic properties.

Suh *et al.* focused on the natural Deguelin (see Fig. **6**) and synthesized several analogues **52** (Fig. **10**) [141]. These compounds were assessed for their anticancer potential in the H1299 cell line and derivatives **52a** and **52b** demonstrated a high antiproliferative activity with IC_{50} values in the nM range. The HIF-1α inhibitory capacity was evaluated for these compounds, since it is a HSP90 client protein and also because of its role in the transcriptional activity of VEGF in terms of the regulation of angiogenesis. Inhibition of HIF-1α was achieved by both compounds and through HSP90, confirmed by immunoprecipitation and immunoblotting assays. The interruption of the interaction between HIF-1α and HSP90 was confirmed and this profile was favourable for angiogenesis inhibition. The authors performed further experiments to prove the antiangiogenic effect of the compounds using a transgenic zebrafish line. The depletion of sub-intestinal veins was detected for **52a**, whereas the antiangiogenic activity of **52b**, although higher than **52a**, was not revealed by the authors.

Novel fluorescent coumarins linked to a theanine moiety **53** (Fig. **10**) were explored as anticancer agents in NSCLC cells and leukemia model [142]. Studies included *in vitro*, *ex vivo* and *in vivo* experiments of human and mouse cancer models. *In vitro* results showed the cell migration inhibition capacity of the compound in Lewis lung cancer (LLC) and A549 cells and the most promising compounds also inhibited cell growth in different cancer models (LLC, A549, H460 and K562 cells) with IC_{50} values in the µM range (72h treatment). Selectivity towards cancer cell lines was also tested for compounds **53a** and **53b** and at the used concentrations no inhibition of cell growth was detected for normal human embryonic lung fibroblasts (MRC-5) and human peripheral blood lymphocytes (PBL). *In vivo* experiments with A549 cells in mice, using these two coumarins, demonstrated inhibition of cell growth after a few hours of oral administration, especially in combination with the known drugs cytarabine, vincristine and methotrexate. Both **53a** and **53b** compounds were able to inhibit tumor growth in tumor-bearing mice (LLC and A549 cell lines). To determine their mechanism of action the authors used A549 and LLC cell lines and both compounds demonstrated anti-apoptotic activity (Annexin V-FITC/PI double-staining), downregulated Bcl-2 and cyclin D1 protein levels and, on the contrary, up-regulated Bax protein levels, cytosolic cytochrome c, caspase-3, PARP-1, p53, and p21 in LLC cells (analysed by Western blotting). Coumarins diminished the expressions of VEGFR-1, VEGFR-2, the phosphorylation and expression of EGFR and AKT in LLC cells.

Another coumarin-based approach for anticancer agents with VEGFR-2 inhibition potential, as a marker for angiogenesis inhibition, led to the synthesis of compounds **54** (Fig. **11**) [143]. The anticancer activity of these chromenes was tested using the breast cancer cell line MCF-7 and µM range IC_{50} values were obtained, with compounds 54a, b and 54c displaying the most promising results. The VEGFR-2 kinase inhibitory activity (% inhibition) was determined for all the synthesized compounds and 54a, b and 54c demonstrated an equal 94% capacity to inhibit this kinase comparable with the commercial drug Tamoxifen (95% inhibition).

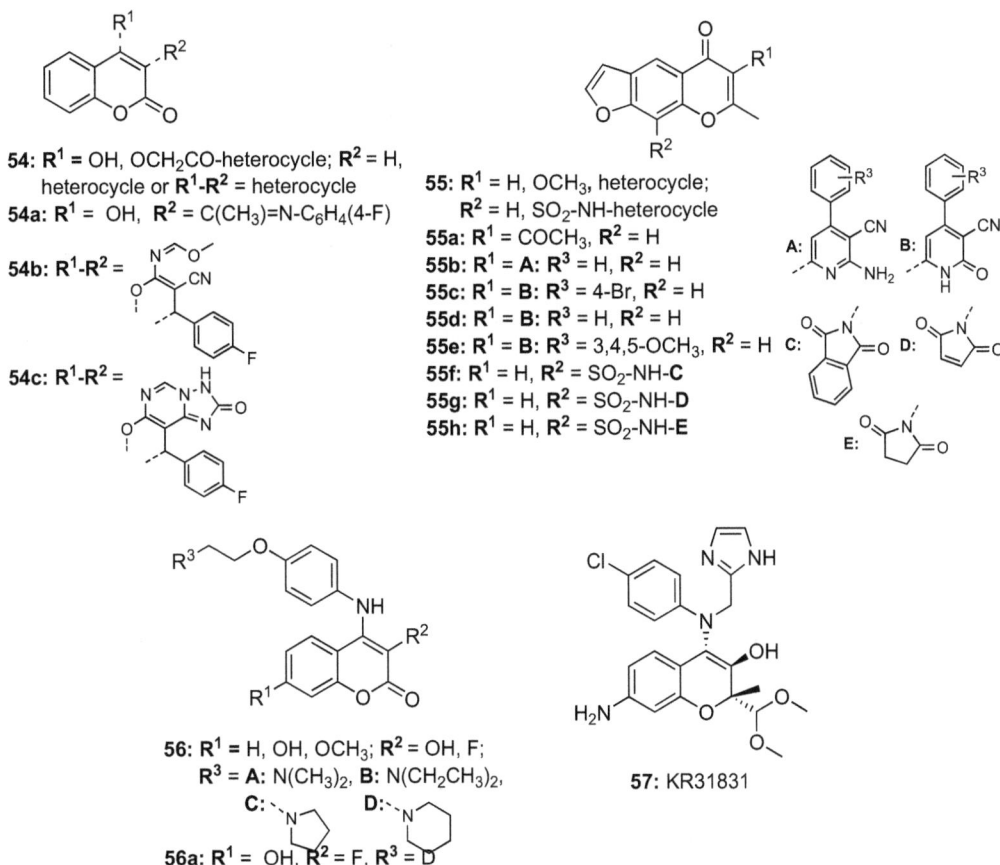

54: R^1 = OH, OCH$_2$CO-heterocycle; R^2 = H, heterocycle or R^1-R^2 = heterocycle
54a: R^1 = OH, R^2 = C(CH$_3$)=N-C$_6$H$_4$(4-F)
54b: R^1-R^2 =
54c: R^1-R^2 =

55: R^1 = H, OCH$_3$, heterocycle; R^2 = H, SO$_2$-NH-heterocycle
55a: R^1 = COCH$_3$, R^2 = H
55b: R^1 = A: R^3 = H, R^2 = H
55c: R^1 = B: R^3 = 4-Br, R^2 = H
55d: R^1 = B: R^3 = H, R^2 = H
55e: R^1 = B: R^3 = 3,4,5-OCH$_3$, R^2 = H
55f: R^1 = H, R^2 = SO$_2$-NH-**C**
55g: R^1 = H, R^2 = SO$_2$-NH-**D**
55h: R^1 = H, R^2 = SO$_2$-NH-**E**

56: R^1 = H, OH, OCH$_3$; R^2 = OH, F; R^3 = A: N(CH$_3$)$_2$, B: N(CH$_2$CH$_3$)$_2$, **C:**   **D:**
56a: R^1 = OH, R^2 = F, R^3 = D

57: KR31831

Fig. (11). Chromene-based compounds as anticancer agents. Compilation of a series of synthesized compounds reported as biologically active structures.

Amhed *et al.* reported the synthesis of several furochromones and benzofuran derivatives **55** (Fig. **11**) [144]. These chromene derivatives were evaluated for their anticancer potential in fifteen human cancer cell lines (KB, SK OV-3, SF-268, NCI H 460, RKOP27, HL60, U937, K561, G361, SK-MEL-28, GOTO, NB-1, PC-3, HT1080, HepG2). In general, compounds exhibited low IC$_{50}$ values, in the μM range, in most of the cell lines. Chromenes **55a-h** demonstrated the most promising activity profile. All the synthesized compounds were evaluated for their ability to inhibit VEGFR-2 activity (using VEGFR-2 kinase activity assays by ELISA) and although all presented inhibition, chromene **55a** displayed the most promising result, with the same IC_{50} value as the reference drug sorafenib. *In vivo* anti-prostate cancer activity was also evaluated in rats and the anticancer activity was accessed as a percentage of inhibition of the testosterone propionate effect. Imide substituted chromenes **55f, 55g** and **55h** showed the most significant *in vivo* anti-prostate cancer activity, with ED_{50} (effective dose) values in the low µM range, lower than the control drug flutamide.

Coumarin derivatives **56** were designed, synthesized and projected to be dual ERα /VEGFR-2 ligands for breast cancer treatment (Fig. **11**) [145]. A series of coumarins were examined for their anticancer activity, inhibiting proliferation in MCF-7 breast cancer cells (ERα positive) and in Ishikawa human endometrial cancers (Tamoxifen-induced endometrial cancer model). In general, the compounds exhibited IC_{50} values in MCF-7 cell line in the low µM range, good anti-endometrial hyperplasia activity against Ishikawa cells and some presented excellent binding affinity in ERα assay. Based on these two results the best compounds were selected for antiangiogenic activity determination and screened for their potency to inhibit overexpressed VEGFR-2 in HUVECs. Several chromenes exhibited inhibition of VEGFR-2 (83-88% inhibition) when compared to the control (Vandetanib, 96% inhibition). Compound **56a** presented the best combination of ERα binding affinity, cytotoxicity against MCF-7 and Ishikawa cells and was considered a promising candidate in terms of antiangiogenic activity. This chromene was selected for further studies in order to understand the multifunctional effect of this family of compounds. Using MCF-7 cells, **56a** proved to inhibit cell migration, arrested cell cycle at G0/G1 phase and was able to inhibit the activation of VEGFR-2 and the signalling transduction of Raf-1/MAPK/ERK pathway (detected by Western blot).

Kim *et al.* reported chromene-based compound **57** (KR31831, Fig. **11**) as an antiangiogenic agent and studied its inhibitory mechanism, especially for VEGF-signalling pathway in HUVECs [146]. This chromene was capable to inhibit VEGF-induced tube formation and proliferation *via* the release of intracellular Ca^{2+} and phosphorylation of ERK1/2 (activation was significantly inhibited) in HUVECs (Western blot). Next, VEGFR-2 levels were investigated in order to see if the inhibition of both Ca^{2+} release and ERK1/2 activation was due to its downregulation. In fact, compound **57** was able to reduce the expression of VEGFR-2 in a dose-dependent manner (RT-PCR and Western blot analysis) and may have inhibitory effects on tumor angiogenesis.

CONCLUSION

Tumor vascularization is associated with tumor aggressiveness and progression. New vessel formation is essential to sustain tumor growth, by providing the necessary oxygen and nutrients, but also for tumor metastization. Thus, angiogenesis constitutes an important hallmark of cancer and it is a rational target for cancer therapy. In this context, different inhibitors, from antibodies to small inhibitors, reached clinical approval. However, despite initial encouraging results in terms of survival rates, it soon became evident that there was no major benefit in patient global survival. Despite this limitation, antiangiogenic agents are still being used but mainly in combination with classical chemotherapy, in cancers where they demonstrated benefit. Therefore, targeting angiogenesis in cancer therapy still requires optimization and there is the need to search for more effective agents.

In this line of thought, several families of naturally occurring compounds have been explored as antiangiogenic agents, aiming to improve the efficacy of this therapeutic approach. These include plant polyphenols, chromenes and coumarins, which due to their structure variety, hold great potential. There is already a comprehensive number of studies exploring these polyphenols as vascular-disrupting agents, with demonstrated antiangiogenic properties in different cancer models and, importantly, with very low toxicity. However, so far, very few of these compounds reached clinical use. Most of the available studies on the activities of these compounds are performed in *in vitro*, *ex vivo* or *in vivo* immunocompromised cancer models. Also, *in vivo* bioavailability studies are lacking. Thus, clinical translation is still quite far away for most of the compounds. Nevertheless, based on the available pre-clinical data, these compounds hold promise as anti-cancer agents and the clinical trial promoters should make a bigger effort to take them to the next level.

CONSENT FOR PUBLICATION

Not applicable.

CONFLICT OF INTEREST

The author confirms that this chapter contents have no conflict of interest.

ACKNOWLEDGEMENTS

This study was partially developed under the scope of the projects NORTE-01-0145-FEDER-000013 and NORTE-01-0145-FEDER-000023, supported by the Northern Portugal Regional Operational Programme (NORTE 2020), under the

Portugal 2020 Partnership Agreement, through the European Regional Development Fund (FEDER). Olívia Pontes is recipient of a PhD fellowship (SFRH/BD/128850/2017) and Ana Raquel-Cunha is also recipients of a PhD fellowship (SFRH/BD/148199/2019) from Fundação para a Ciência e Tecnologia (FCT), Portugal. Olga Martinho is an auxiliary researcher from the above cited project: NORTE-01-0145-FEDER-000023.

REFERENCES

[1]   Carmeliet P. Angiogenesis in health and disease. Nat Med 2003; 9(6): 653-60.
        [http://dx.doi.org/10.1038/nm0603-653] [PMID: 12778163]

[2]   Pluda JM. Tumor-associated angiogenesis: mechanisms, clinical implications, and therapeutic strategies. Semin Oncol 1997; 24(2): 203-18.
        [PMID: 9129690]

[3]   Hunter J. A treatise on the blood, inflammation, and gun-shot wounds. 1794. Clin Orthop Relat Res 2007; 458(458): 27-34.
        [http://dx.doi.org/10.1097/BLO.0b013e31803dd01c] [PMID: 17473595]

[4]   Folkman J. Tumor angiogenesis: therapeutic implications. N Engl J Med 1971; 285(21): 1182-6.
        [http://dx.doi.org/10.1056/NEJM197111182852108] [PMID: 4938153]

[5]   Gupta K, Zhang J. Angiogenesis: a curse or cure? Postgrad Med J 2005; 81(954): 236-42.
        [http://dx.doi.org/10.1136/pgmj.2004.023309] [PMID: 15811887]

[6]   Veith AP, Henderson K, Spencer A, Sligar AD, Baker AB. Therapeutic strategies for enhancing angiogenesis in wound healing 2018.
        [http://dx.doi.org/10.1016/j.addr.2018.09.010]

[7]   Pandya NM, Dhalla NS, Santani DD. Angiogenesis--a new target for future therapy. Vascul Pharmacol 2006; 44(5): 265-74.
        [http://dx.doi.org/10.1016/j.vph.2006.01.005] [PMID: 16545987]

[8]   Saharinen P, Bry M, Alitalo K. How do angiopoietins Tie in with vascular endothelial growth factors? Curr Opin Hematol 2010; 17(3): 198-205.
        [http://dx.doi.org/10.1097/MOH.0b013e3283386673] [PMID: 20375888]

[9]   Andrae J, Gallini R, Betsholtz C. Role of platelet-derived growth factors in physiology and medicine. Genes Dev 2008; 22(10): 1276-312.
        [http://dx.doi.org/10.1101/gad.1653708] [PMID: 18483217]

[10]   Yun YR, Won JE, Jeon E, et al. Fibroblast growth factors: biology, function, and application for tissue regeneration. J Tissue Eng 2010; 2010(7)218142
        [http://dx.doi.org/10.4061/2010/218142] [PMID: 21350642]

[11]   Nishida N, Yano H, Nishida T, Kamura T, Kojiro M. Angiogenesis in cancer. Vasc Health Risk Manag 2006; 2(3): 213-9.
        [http://dx.doi.org/10.2147/vhrm.2006.2.3.213] [PMID: 17326328]

[12]   Eales KL, Hollinshead KE, Tennant DA. Hypoxia and metabolic adaptation of cancer cells. Oncogenesis 2016; 5e190
        [http://dx.doi.org/10.1038/oncsis.2015.50] [PMID: 26807645]

[13]   Pugh CW, Ratcliffe PJ. Regulation of angiogenesis by hypoxia: role of the HIF system. Nat Med 2003; 9(6): 677-84.
        [http://dx.doi.org/10.1038/nm0603-677] [PMID: 12778166]

[14]   Hanahan D, Weinberg RA. Hallmarks of cancer: the next generation. Cell 2011; 144(5): 646-74.
        [http://dx.doi.org/10.1016/j.cell.2011.02.013] [PMID: 21376230]

[15]   Ribatti D, Nico B, Crivellato E, Roccaro AM, Vacca A. The history of the angiogenic switch concept. Leukemia 2007; 21(1): 44-52.
[http://dx.doi.org/10.1038/sj.leu.2404402] [PMID: 16990761]

[16]   Yehya AHS, Asif M, Petersen SH, *et al.* Angiogenesis: Managing the Culprits behind Tumorigenesis and Metastasis. Medicina (Kaunas) 2018; 54(1): 8-28.
[http://dx.doi.org/10.3390/medicina54010008] [PMID: 30344239]

[17]   Eckardt KU, Bernhardt W, Willam C, Wiesener M. Hypoxia-inducible transcription factors and their role in renal disease. Semin Nephrol 2007; 27(3): 363-72.
[http://dx.doi.org/10.1016/j.semnephrol.2007.02.007] [PMID: 17533012]

[18]   Viallard C, Larrivée B. Tumor angiogenesis and vascular normalization: alternative therapeutic targets. Angiogenesis 2017; 20(4): 409-26.
[http://dx.doi.org/10.1007/s10456-017-9562-9] [PMID: 28660302]

[19]   Giaccia AJ, Simon MC, Johnson R. The biology of hypoxia: the role of oxygen sensing in development, normal function, and disease. Genes Dev 2004; 18(18): 2183-94.
[http://dx.doi.org/10.1101/gad.1243304] [PMID: 15371333]

[20]   Meneses AM, Wielockx B. PHD2: from hypoxia regulation to disease progression. Hypoxia (Auckl) 2016; 4: 53-67.
[PMID: 27800508]

[21]   Wang GL, Jiang BH, Rue EA, Semenza GL. Hypoxia-inducible factor 1 is a basic-helix-loop-helix-PAS heterodimer regulated by cellular O_2 tension. Proc Natl Acad Sci USA 1995; 92(12): 5510-4.
[http://dx.doi.org/10.1073/pnas.92.12.5510] [PMID: 7539918]

[22]   Chan MC, Holt-Martyn JP, Schofield CJ, Ratcliffe PJ. Pharmacological targeting of the HIF hydroxylases--A new field in medicine development. Mol Aspects Med 2016; 47-48: 54-75.
[http://dx.doi.org/10.1016/j.mam.2016.01.001] [PMID: 26791432]

[23]   Masoud GN, Li W. HIF-1α pathway: role, regulation and intervention for cancer therapy. Acta Pharm Sin B 2015; 5(5): 378-89.
[http://dx.doi.org/10.1016/j.apsb.2015.05.007] [PMID: 26579469]

[24]   Marín-Hernández A, Gallardo-Pérez JC, Ralph SJ, Rodríguez-Enríquez S, Moreno-Sánchez R. HIF-1alpha modulates energy metabolism in cancer cells by inducing over-expression of specific glycolytic isoforms. Mini Rev Med Chem 2009; 9(9): 1084-101.
[http://dx.doi.org/10.2174/138955709788922610] [PMID: 19689405]

[25]   Darby IA, Hewitson TD. Hypoxia in tissue repair and fibrosis. Cell Tissue Res 2016; 365(3): 553-62.
[http://dx.doi.org/10.1007/s00441-016-2461-3] [PMID: 27423661]

[26]   Neufeld G, Cohen T, Gengrinovitch S, Poltorak Z. Vascular endothelial growth factor (VEGF) and its receptors. FASEB J 1999; 13(1): 9-22.
[http://dx.doi.org/10.1096/fasebj.13.1.9] [PMID: 9872925]

[27]   Baeriswyl V, Christofori G. The angiogenic switch in carcinogenesis. Semin Cancer Biol 2009; 19(5): 329-37.
[http://dx.doi.org/10.1016/j.semcancer.2009.05.003] [PMID: 19482086]

[28]   Goel HL, Mercurio AM. VEGF targets the tumour cell. Nat Rev Cancer 2013; 13(12): 871-82.
[http://dx.doi.org/10.1038/nrc3627] [PMID: 24263190]

[29]   Shalaby F, Rossant J, Yamaguchi TP, *et al.* Failure of blood-island formation and vasculogenesis in Flk-1-deficient mice. Nature 1995; 376(6535): 62-6.
[http://dx.doi.org/10.1038/376062a0] [PMID: 7596435]

[30]   Olofsson B, Korpelainen E, Pepper MS, *et al.* Vascular endothelial growth factor B (VEGF-B) binds to VEGF receptor-1 and regulates plasminogen activator activity in endothelial cells. Proc Natl Acad Sci USA 1998; 95(20): 11709-14.

[http://dx.doi.org/10.1073/pnas.95.20.11709] [PMID: 9751730]

[31]   Alitalo K, Tammela T, Petrova TV. Lymphangiogenesis in development and human disease. Nature 2005; 438(7070): 946-53.
[http://dx.doi.org/10.1038/nature04480] [PMID: 16355212]

[32]   Tammela T, Zarkada G, Wallgard E, *et al.* Blocking VEGFR-3 suppresses angiogenic sprouting and vascular network formation. Nature 2008; 454(7204): 656-60.
[http://dx.doi.org/10.1038/nature07083] [PMID: 18594512]

[33]   Hamada K, Oike Y, Takakura N, *et al.* VEGF-C signaling pathways through VEGFR-2 and VEGFR-3 in vasculoangiogenesis and hematopoiesis. Blood 2000; 96(12): 3793-800.
[http://dx.doi.org/10.1182/blood.V96.12.3793] [PMID: 11090062]

[34]   Lyttle DJ, Fraser KM, Fleming SB, Mercer AA, Robinson AJ. Homologs of vascular endothelial growth factor are encoded by the poxvirus orf virus. J Virol 1994; 68(1): 84-92.
[PMID: 8254780]

[35]   Yadav L, Puri N, Rastogi V, Satpute P, Sharma V. Tumour Angiogenesis and Angiogenic Inhibitors: A Review. J Clin Diagn Res 2015; 9(6): XE01-5.
[http://dx.doi.org/10.7860/JCDR/2015/12016.6135] [PMID: 26266204]

[36]   Borrello MG, Degl'Innocenti D, Pierotti MA. Inflammation and cancer: the oncogene-driven connection. Cancer Lett 2008; 267(2): 262-70.
[http://dx.doi.org/10.1016/j.canlet.2008.03.060] [PMID: 18502035]

[37]   Díaz-Rubio E, Schmoll HJ. Introduction. Critical role of anti-angiogenesis and VEGF inhibition in colorectal cancer. Oncology 2005; 69 (Suppl. 3): 1-3.
[PMID: 16301829]

[38]   Zirlik K, Duyster J. Anti-Angiogenics: Current Situation and Future Perspectives. Oncol Res Treat 2018; 41(4): 166-71.
[http://dx.doi.org/10.1159/000488087] [PMID: 29562226]

[39]   Ferrara N. VEGF and the quest for tumour angiogenesis factors. Nat Rev Cancer 2002; 2(10): 795-803.
[http://dx.doi.org/10.1038/nrc909] [PMID: 12360282]

[40]   Ferrara N, Hillan KJ, Novotny W. Bevacizumab (Avastin), a humanized anti-VEGF monoclonal antibody for cancer therapy. Biochem Biophys Res Commun 2005; 333(2): 328-35.
[http://dx.doi.org/10.1016/j.bbrc.2005.05.132] [PMID: 15961063]

[41]   Giantonio BJ, Catalano PJ, Meropol NJ, *et al.* Bevacizumab in combination with oxaliplatin, fluorouracil, and leucovorin (FOLFOX4) for previously treated metastatic colorectal cancer: results from the Eastern Cooperative Oncology Group Study E3200. J Clin Oncol 2007; 25(12): 1539-44.
[http://dx.doi.org/10.1200/JCO.2006.09.6305] [PMID: 17442997]

[42]   Hurwitz H, Fehrenbacher L, Novotny W, *et al.* Bevacizumab plus irinotecan, fluorouracil, and leucovorin for metastatic colorectal cancer. N Engl J Med 2004; 350(23): 2335-42.
[http://dx.doi.org/10.1056/NEJMoa032691] [PMID: 15175435]

[43]   Saltz LB, Clarke S, Díaz-Rubio E, *et al.* Bevacizumab in combination with oxaliplatin-based chemotherapy as first-line therapy in metastatic colorectal cancer: a randomized phase III study. J Clin Oncol 2008; 26(12): 2013-9.
[http://dx.doi.org/10.1200/JCO.2007.14.9930] [PMID: 18421054]

[44]   Burger RA, Brady MF, Bookman MA, *et al.* Incorporation of bevacizumab in the primary treatment of ovarian cancer. N Engl J Med 2011; 365(26): 2473-83.
[http://dx.doi.org/10.1056/NEJMoa1104390] [PMID: 22204724]

[45]   Perren TJ, Swart AM, Pfisterer J, *et al.* A phase 3 trial of bevacizumab in ovarian cancer. N Engl J Med 2011; 365(26): 2484-96.
[http://dx.doi.org/10.1056/NEJMoa1103799] [PMID: 22204725]

[46] Pujade-Lauraine E, Hilpert F, Weber B, *et al.* Bevacizumab combined with chemotherapy for platinum-resistant recurrent ovarian cancer: The AURELIA open-label randomized phase III trial. J Clin Oncol 2014; 32(13): 1302-8.
[http://dx.doi.org/10.1200/JCO.2013.51.4489] [PMID: 24637997]

[47] Sandler A, Gray R, Perry MC, *et al.* Paclitaxel-carboplatin alone or with bevacizumab for non-smal--cell lung cancer. N Engl J Med 2006; 355(24): 2542-50.
[http://dx.doi.org/10.1056/NEJMoa061884] [PMID: 17167137]

[48] Tewari KS, Sill MW, Long HJ III, *et al.* Improved survival with bevacizumab in advanced cervical cancer. N Engl J Med 2014; 370(8): 734-43.
[http://dx.doi.org/10.1056/NEJMoa1309748] [PMID: 24552320]

[49] Zalcman G, Mazieres J, Margery J, *et al.* Bevacizumab for newly diagnosed pleural mesothelioma in the Mesothelioma Avastin Cisplatin Pemetrexed Study (MAPS): a randomised, controlled, open-label, phase 3 trial. Lancet 2016; 387(10026): 1405-14.
[http://dx.doi.org/10.1016/S0140-6736(15)01238-6] [PMID: 26719230]

[50] de Gramont A, Van Cutsem E, Schmoll HJ, *et al.* Bevacizumab plus oxaliplatin-based chemotherapy as adjuvant treatment for colon cancer (AVANT): a phase 3 randomised controlled trial. Lancet Oncol 2012; 13(12): 1225-33.
[http://dx.doi.org/10.1016/S1470-2045(12)70509-0] [PMID: 23168362]

[51] Rini BI, Bellmunt J, Clancy J, *et al.* Randomized phase III trial of temsirolimus and bevacizumab *versus* interferon alfa and bevacizumab in metastatic renal cell carcinoma: INTORACT trial. J Clin Oncol 2014; 32(8): 752-9.
[http://dx.doi.org/10.1200/JCO.2013.50.5305] [PMID: 24297945]

[52] Jayson GC, Kerbel R, Ellis LM, Harris AL. Antiangiogenic therapy in oncology: current status and future directions. Lancet 2016; 388(10043): 518-29.
[http://dx.doi.org/10.1016/S0140-6736(15)01088-0] [PMID: 26853587]

[53] Al-Halafi AM. Vascular endothelial growth factor trap-eye and trap technology: Aflibercept from bench to bedside. Oman J Ophthalmol 2014; 7(3): 112-5.
[http://dx.doi.org/10.4103/0974-620X.142591] [PMID: 25378873]

[54] Van Cutsem E, Tabernero J, Lakomy R, *et al.* Addition of aflibercept to fluorouracil, leucovorin, and irinotecan improves survival in a phase III randomized trial in patients with metastatic colorectal cancer previously treated with an oxaliplatin-based regimen. J Clin Oncol 2012; 30(28): 3499-506.
[http://dx.doi.org/10.1200/JCO.2012.42.8201] [PMID: 22949147]

[55] Zaltrap ACM. Synthèse de mise sur le marché dans le cancer colorectal métastatique. Bull Cancer 2013; 100: 1023-5.

[56] Torimura T, Iwamoto H, Nakamura T, *et al.* Antiangiogenic and Antitumor Activities of Aflibercept, a Soluble VEGF Receptor-1 and -2, in a Mouse Model of Hepatocellular Carcinoma. Neoplasia 2016; 18(7): 413-24.
[http://dx.doi.org/10.1016/j.neo.2016.05.001] [PMID: 27435924]

[57] Spratlin JL, Mulder KE, Mackey JR. Ramucirumab (IMC-1121B): a novel attack on angiogenesis. Future Oncol 2010; 6(7): 1085-94.
[http://dx.doi.org/10.2217/fon.10.75] [PMID: 20624120]

[58] Takeda K, Daga H. Ramucirumab for the treatment of advanced or metastatic non-small cell lung cancer. Expert Opin Biol Ther 2016; 16(12): 1541-7.
[http://dx.doi.org/10.1080/14712598.2016.1248397] [PMID: 27737562]

[59] Arrieta O, Zatarain-Barrón ZL, Cardona AF, Carmona A, Lopez-Mejia M. Ramucirumab in the treatment of non-small cell lung cancer. Expert Opin Drug Saf 2017; 16(5): 637-44.
[http://dx.doi.org/10.1080/14740338.2017.1313226] [PMID: 28395526]

[60] Poole RM, Vaidya A. Ramucirumab: first global approval. Drugs 2014; 74(9): 1047-58.

[http://dx.doi.org/10.1007/s40265-014-0244-2] [PMID: 24916147]

[61] Escudier B, Eisen T, Stadler WM, *et al.* Sorafenib in advanced clear-cell renal-cell carcinoma. N Engl J Med 2007; 356(2): 125-34.
[http://dx.doi.org/10.1056/NEJMoa060655] [PMID: 17215530]

[62] Bruix J, Cheng AL, Meinhardt G, Nakajima K, De Sanctis Y, Llovet J. Prognostic factors and predictors of sorafenib benefit in patients with hepatocellular carcinoma: Analysis of two phase III studies. J Hepatol 2017; 67(5): 999-1008.
[http://dx.doi.org/10.1016/j.jhep.2017.06.026] [PMID: 28687477]

[63] Escudier B, Worden F, Kudo M. Sorafenib: key lessons from over 10 years of experience. Expert Rev Anticancer Ther 2018; •••: 1-13.
[PMID: 30575405]

[64] Pasqualetti G, Ricciardi S, Mey V, Del Tacca M, Danesi R. Synergistic cytotoxicity, inhibition of signal transduction pathways and pharmacogenetics of sorafenib and gemcitabine in human NSCLC cell lines. Lung Cancer 2011; 74(2): 197-205.
[http://dx.doi.org/10.1016/j.lungcan.2011.03.003] [PMID: 21529991]

[65] Ferrari SM, Centanni M, Virili C, *et al.* Sunitinib in the treatment of thyroid cancer. Curr Med Chem 2019; 26(6): 963-72.
[http://dx.doi.org/10.2174/0929867324666171006165942] [PMID: 28990511]

[66] Martens UM. Small Molecules in Oncology. 2018.
[http://dx.doi.org/10.1007/978-3-319-91442-8]

[67] Comunanza V, Bussolino F. Therapy for Cancer: Strategy of Combining Anti-Angiogenic and Target Therapies. Front Cell Dev Biol 2017; 5: 101-12.
[http://dx.doi.org/10.3389/fcell.2017.00101] [PMID: 29270405]

[68] Sitohy B, Nagy JA, Dvorak HF. Anti-VEGF/VEGFR therapy for cancer: reassessing the target. Cancer Res 2012; 72(8): 1909-14.
[http://dx.doi.org/10.1158/0008-5472.CAN-11-3406] [PMID: 22508695]

[69] Lewandowska U, Gorlach S, Owczarek K, Hrabec E, Szewczyk K. Synergistic interactions between anticancer chemotherapeutics and phenolic compounds and anticancer synergy between polyphenols. Postepy Hig Med Dosw 2014; 68: 528-40.
[http://dx.doi.org/10.5604/17322693.1102278] [PMID: 24864104]

[70] Ribeiro A, Abreu RMV, Dias MM, Barreiro MF, Ferreira ICFR. Antiangiogenic compounds: well-established drugs *versus* emerging natural molecules. Cancer Lett 2018; 415: 86-105.
[http://dx.doi.org/10.1016/j.canlet.2017.12.006] [PMID: 29222042]

[71] Pratap R, Ram VJ. Natural and synthetic chromenes, fused chromenes, and versatility of dihydrobenzo[h]chromenes in organic synthesis. Chem Rev 2014; 114(20): 10476-526.
[http://dx.doi.org/10.1021/cr500075s] [PMID: 25303539]

[72] Ellis GP. Chromenes, chromanones, and chromones. 1977.
[http://dx.doi.org/10.1002/9780470187012]

[73] Borges F, Roleira F, Milhazes N, Santana L, Uriarte E. Simple coumarins and analogues in medicinal chemistry: occurrence, synthesis and biological activity. Curr Med Chem 2005; 12(8): 887-916.
[http://dx.doi.org/10.2174/0929867053507315] [PMID: 15853704]

[74] Costa M, Dias TA, Brito A, Proença F. Biological importance of structurally diversified chromenes. Eur J Med Chem 2016; 123: 487-507.
[http://dx.doi.org/10.1016/j.ejmech.2016.07.057] [PMID: 27494166]

[75] Kostova I. Synthetic and natural coumarins as antioxidants. Mini Rev Med Chem 2006; 6(4): 365-74.
[http://dx.doi.org/10.2174/138955706776361457] [PMID: 16613573]

[76] Ravishankar D, Rajora AK, Greco F, Osborn HM. Flavonoids as prospective compounds for anti-

cancer therapy. Int J Biochem Cell Biol 2013; 45(12): 2821-31.
[http://dx.doi.org/10.1016/j.biocel.2013.10.004] [PMID: 24128857]

[77]   Patil SA, Patil R, Pfeffer LM, Miller DD. Chromenes: potential new chemotherapeutic agents for cancer. Future Med Chem 2013; 5(14): 1647-60.
[http://dx.doi.org/10.4155/fmc.13.126] [PMID: 24047270]

[78]   A Phase I/II Trial of Crolibulin (EPC2407) Plus Cisplatin in Adults With Solid Tumors With a Focus on Anaplastic Thyroid Cancer (ATC). Retrieved from: https://clinicaltrials.gov/ct2/show/NCT01240590, in November 2, 2018.

[79]   Reis J, Gaspar A, Milhazes N, Borges F. Chromone as a Privileged Scaffold in Drug Discovery: Recent Advances. J Med Chem 2017; 60(19): 7941-57.
[http://dx.doi.org/10.1021/acs.jmedchem.6b01720] [PMID: 28537720]

[80]   Delost MD, Smith DT, Anderson BJ, Njardarson JT. From Oxiranes to Oligomers: Architectures of U.S. FDA Approved Pharmaceuticals Containing Oxygen Heterocycles. J Med Chem 2018; 61(24): 10996-1020.
[http://dx.doi.org/10.1021/acs.jmedchem.8b00876] [PMID: 30024747]

[81]   Lin LG, Xie H, Li HL, *et al.* Naturally occurring homoisoflavonoids function as potent protein tyrosine kinase inhibitors by c-Src-based high-throughput screening. J Med Chem 2008; 51(15): 4419-29.
[http://dx.doi.org/10.1021/jm701501x] [PMID: 18610999]

[82]   Pan R, Dai Y, Gao XH, Lu D, Xia YF. Inhibition of vascular endothelial growth factor-induced angiogenesis by scopoletin through interrupting the autophosphorylation of VEGF receptor 2 and its downstream signaling pathways. Vascul Pharmacol 2011; 54(1-2): 18-28.
[http://dx.doi.org/10.1016/j.vph.2010.11.001] [PMID: 21078410]

[83]   Pratheeshkumar P, Son YO, Budhraja A, *et al.* Luteolin inhibits human prostate tumor growth by suppressing vascular endothelial growth factor receptor 2-mediated angiogenesis. PLoS One 2012; 7(12)e52279
[http://dx.doi.org/10.1371/journal.pone.0052279] [PMID: 23300633]

[84]   Pratheeshkumar P, Budhraja A, Son YO, *et al.* Quercetin inhibits angiogenesis mediated human prostate tumor growth by targeting VEGFR- 2 regulated AKT/mTOR/P70S6K signaling pathways. PLoS One 2012; 7(10)e47516
[http://dx.doi.org/10.1371/journal.pone.0047516] [PMID: 23094058]

[85]   Vivek Sagayaraj Rathinasamy NP. Malathi Ragunathan. Effect of genistein on regenerative angiogenesis using zebrafish as model organism. Biomedicine & Preventive Nutrition 2014; 4(4): 469-74.
[http://dx.doi.org/10.1016/j.bionut.2014.07.002]

[86]   Piao M, Mori D, Satoh T, Sugita Y, Tokunaga O. Inhibition of endothelial cell proliferation, *in vitro* angiogenesis, and the down-regulation of cell adhesion-related genes by genistein 2006.

[87]   Ruiz PA, Haller D. Functional diversity of flavonoids in the inhibition of the proinflammatory NF-kappaB, IRF, and Akt signaling pathways in murine intestinal epithelial cells. J Nutr 2006; 136(3): 664-71.
[http://dx.doi.org/10.1093/jn/136.3.664] [PMID: 16484540]

[88]   Wang B, Zou Y, Li H, Yan H, Pan JS, Yuan ZL. Genistein inhibited retinal neovascularization and expression of vascular endothelial growth factor and hypoxia inducible factor 1alpha in a mouse model of oxygen-induced retinopathy. J Ocul Pharmacol Ther 2005; 21(2): 107-13.
[http://dx.doi.org/10.1089/jop.2005.21.107] [PMID: 15857276]

[89]   Berndt S, Issa ME, Carpentier G, Cuendet M. A Bivalent Role of Genistein in Sprouting Angiogenesis. Planta Med 2018; 84(9-10): 653-61.
[http://dx.doi.org/10.1055/a-0587-5991] [PMID: 29539645]

[90] Lamy S, Blanchette M, Michaud-Levesque J, *et al.* Delphinidin, a dietary anthocyanidin, inhibits vascular endothelial growth factor receptor-2 phosphorylation. Carcinogenesis 2006; 27(5): 989-96.
[http://dx.doi.org/10.1093/carcin/bgi279] [PMID: 16308314]

[91] Kim MH, Jeong YJ, Cho HJ, *et al.* Delphinidin inhibits angiogenesis through the suppression of HIF-1α and VEGF expression in A549 lung cancer cells. Oncol Rep 2017; 37(2): 777-84.
[http://dx.doi.org/10.3892/or.2016.5296] [PMID: 27959445]

[92] Singh RP, Dhanalakshmi S, Agarwal C, Agarwal R. Silibinin strongly inhibits growth and survival of human endothelial cells *via* cell cycle arrest and downregulation of survivin, Akt and NF-kappaB: implications for angioprevention and antiangiogenic therapy. Oncogene 2005; 24(7): 1188-202.
[http://dx.doi.org/10.1038/sj.onc.1208276] [PMID: 15558015]

[93] Tyagi A, Singh RP, Ramasamy K, *et al.* Growth inhibition and regression of lung tumors by silibinin: modulation of angiogenesis by macrophage-associated cytokines and nuclear factor-kappaB and signal transducers and activators of transcription 3. Cancer Prev Res (Phila) 2009; 2(1): 74-83.
[http://dx.doi.org/10.1158/1940-6207.CAPR-08-0095] [PMID: 19139021]

[94] Singh RP, Gu M, Agarwal R. Silibinin inhibits colorectal cancer growth by inhibiting tumor cell proliferation and angiogenesis. Cancer Res 2008; 68(6): 2043-50.
[http://dx.doi.org/10.1158/0008-5472.CAN-07-6247] [PMID: 18339887]

[95] Mirzoeva S, Kim ND, Chiu K, Franzen CA, Bergan RC, Pelling JC. Inhibition of HIF-1 alpha and VEGF expression by the chemopreventive bioflavonoid apigenin is accompanied by Akt inhibition in human prostate carcinoma PC3-M cells. Mol Carcinog 2008; 47(9): 686-700.
[http://dx.doi.org/10.1002/mc.20421] [PMID: 18240292]

[96] Mirzoeva S, Franzen CA, Pelling JC. Apigenin inhibits TGF-β-induced VEGF expression in human prostate carcinoma cells *via* a Smad2/3- and Src-dependent mechanism. Mol Carcinog 2014; 53(8): 598-609.
[PMID: 23359392]

[97] Jiang X, Zhou J, Lin Q, *et al.* Anti-angiogenic and anticancer effects of baicalein derivatives based on transgenic zebrafish model. Bioorg Med Chem 2018; 26(15): 4481-92.
[http://dx.doi.org/10.1016/j.bmc.2018.07.037] [PMID: 30098912]

[98] Ling Y, Chen Y, Chen P, *et al.* Baicalein potently suppresses angiogenesis induced by vascular endothelial growth factor through the p53/Rb signaling pathway leading to G_1/S cell cycle arrest. Exp Biol Med (Maywood) 2011; 236(7): 851-8.
[http://dx.doi.org/10.1258/ebm.2011.010395] [PMID: 21659383]

[99] Park YG, Choi J, Jung HK, *et al.* Baicalein inhibits tumor progression by inhibiting tumor cell growth and tumor angiogenesis. Oncol Rep 2017; 38(5): 3011-8.
[http://dx.doi.org/10.3892/or.2017.6007] [PMID: 29048641]

[100] Zhao K, Song X, Huang Y, *et al.* Wogonin inhibits LPS-induced tumor angiogenesis *via* suppressing PI3K/Akt/NF-κB signaling. Eur J Pharmacol 2014; 737: 57-69.
[http://dx.doi.org/10.1016/j.ejphar.2014.05.011] [PMID: 24858369]

[101] Zhou M, Song X, Huang Y, *et al.* Wogonin inhibits H2O2-induced angiogenesis *via* suppressing PI3K/Akt/NF-κB signaling pathway. Vascul Pharmacol 2014; 60(3): 110-9.
[http://dx.doi.org/10.1016/j.vph.2014.01.010] [PMID: 24534483]

[102] Mi C, Ma J, Wang KS, *et al.* Imperatorin suppresses proliferation and angiogenesis of human colon cancer cell by targeting HIF-1α *via* the mTOR/p70S6K/4E-BP1 and MAPK pathways. J Ethnopharmacol 2017; 203: 27-38.
[http://dx.doi.org/10.1016/j.jep.2017.03.033] [PMID: 28341244]

[103] Ahamed MB, Aisha AF, Nassar ZD, *et al.* Cat's whiskers tea (*Orthosiphon stamineus*) extract inhibits growth of colon tumor in nude mice and angiogenesis in endothelial cells *via* suppressing VEGFR phosphorylation. Nutr Cancer 2012; 64(1): 89-99.

[http://dx.doi.org/10.1080/01635581.2012.630160] [PMID: 22136553]

[104] Salmela AL, Pouwels J, Kukkonen-Macchi A, *et al.* The flavonoid eupatorin inactivates the mitotic checkpoint leading to polyploidy and apoptosis. Exp Cell Res 2012; 318(5): 578-92.
[http://dx.doi.org/10.1016/j.yexcr.2011.12.014] [PMID: 22227008]

[105] Dolečková I, Rárová L, Grúz J, Vondrusová M, Strnad M, Kryštof V. Antiproliferative and antiangiogenic effects of flavone eupatorin, an active constituent of chloroform extract of *Orthosiphon stamineus* leaves. Fitoterapia 2012; 83(6): 1000-7.
[http://dx.doi.org/10.1016/j.fitote.2012.06.002] [PMID: 22698713]

[106] Boreddy SR, Srivastava SK. Deguelin suppresses pancreatic tumor growth and metastasis by inhibiting epithelial-to-mesenchymal transition in an orthotopic model. Oncogene 2013; 32(34): 3980-91.
[http://dx.doi.org/10.1038/onc.2012.413] [PMID: 22986522]

[107] Murillo G, Salti GI, Kosmeder JW II, Pezzuto JM, Mehta RG. Deguelin inhibits the growth of colon cancer cells through the induction of apoptosis and cell cycle arrest. Eur J Cancer 2002; 38(18): 2446-54.
[http://dx.doi.org/10.1016/S0959-8049(02)00192-2] [PMID: 12460790]

[108] Lee H, Lee JH, Jung KH, Hong SS. Deguelin promotes apoptosis and inhibits angiogenesis of gastric cancer. Oncol Rep 2010; 24(4): 957-63.
[PMID: 20811676]

[109] Li W, Yu X, Ma X, *et al.* Deguelin attenuates non-small cell lung cancer cell metastasis through inhibiting the CtsZ/FAK signaling pathway. Cell Signal 2018; 50: 131-41.
[http://dx.doi.org/10.1016/j.cellsig.2018.07.001] [PMID: 30018008]

[110] Gulzar M, Syed SB, Khan FI, *et al.* Elucidation of interaction mechanism of ellagic acid to the integrin linked kinase. Int J Biol Macromol 2019; 122: 1297-304.
[http://dx.doi.org/10.1016/j.ijbiomac.2018.09.089] [PMID: 30227205]

[111] Zhao M, Tang SN, Marsh JL, Shankar S, Srivastava RK. Ellagic acid inhibits human pancreatic cancer growth in Balb c nude mice. Cancer Lett 2013; 337(2): 210-7.
[http://dx.doi.org/10.1016/j.canlet.2013.05.009] [PMID: 23684930]

[112] Vanella L, Di Giacomo C, Acquaviva R, *et al.* Effects of ellagic Acid on angiogenic factors in prostate cancer cells. Cancers (Basel) 2013; 5(2): 726-38.
[http://dx.doi.org/10.3390/cancers5020726] [PMID: 24216999]

[113] Zhu XX, Yang L, Li YJ, *et al.* Effects of sesquiterpene, flavonoid and coumarin types of compounds from *Artemisia annua L.* on production of mediators of angiogenesis. Pharmacol Rep 2013; 65(2): 410-20.
[http://dx.doi.org/10.1016/S1734-1140(13)71016-8] [PMID: 23744425]

[114] Wang S, Yan Y, Cheng Z, Hu Y, Liu T. Sotetsuflavone suppresses invasion and metastasis in non-small-cell lung cancer A549 cells by reversing EMT *via* the TNF-α/NF-κB and PI3K/AKT signaling pathway. Cell Death Discov 2018; 4: 26-37.
[http://dx.doi.org/10.1038/s41420-018-0026-9] [PMID: 29531823]

[115] Luo H, Rankin GO, Liu L, Daddysman MK, Jiang BH, Chen YC. Kaempferol inhibits angiogenesis and VEGF expression through both HIF dependent and independent pathways in human ovarian cancer cells. Nutr Cancer 2009; 61(4): 554-63.
[http://dx.doi.org/10.1080/01635580802666281] [PMID: 19838928]

[116] Liang F, Han Y, Gao H, *et al.* Kaempferol Identified by Zebrafish Assay and Fine Fractionations Strategy from Dysosma versipellis Inhibits Angiogenesis through VEGF and FGF Pathways. Sci Rep 2015; 5: 14468.
[http://dx.doi.org/10.1038/srep14468] [PMID: 26446489]

[117] Shi MD, Liao YC, Shih YW, Tsai LY. Nobiletin attenuates metastasis *via* both ERK and PI3K/Akt

pathways in HGF-treated liver cancer HepG2 cells. Phytomedicine: international journal of phytotherapy and phytopharmacology. 2013;20(8-9):743-52.

[118] Lee YC, Cheng TH, Lee JS, *et al.* Nobiletin, a citrus flavonoid, suppresses invasion and migration involving FAK/PI3K/Akt and small GTPase signals in human gastric adenocarcinoma AGS cells. Mol Cell Biochem 2011; 347(1-2): 103-15.
[http://dx.doi.org/10.1007/s11010-010-0618-z] [PMID: 20963626]

[119] Chen J, Chen AY, Huang H, *et al.* The flavonoid nobiletin inhibits tumor growth and angiogenesis of ovarian cancers *via* the Akt pathway. Int J Oncol 2015; 46(6): 2629-38.
[http://dx.doi.org/10.3892/ijo.2015.2946] [PMID: 25845666]

[120] Dai ZJ, Lu WF, Gao J, *et al.* Anti-angiogenic effect of the total flavonoids in *Scutellaria barbata* D. Don. BMC Complement Altern Med 2013; 13: 150.
[http://dx.doi.org/10.1186/1472-6882-13-150] [PMID: 23815868]

[121] Tang PM, Chan JY, Zhang DM, *et al.* Pheophorbide a, an active component in *Scutellaria barbata*, reverses P-glycoprotein-mediated multidrug resistance on a human hepatoma cell line R-HepG2. Cancer Biol Ther 2007; 6(4): 504-9.
[http://dx.doi.org/10.4161/cbt.6.4.3814] [PMID: 17457045]

[122] Dai ZJ, Gao J, Li ZF, *et al. In vitro* and *in vivo* antitumor activity of *Scutellaria barbate* extract on murine liver cancer. Molecules 2011; 16(6): 4389-400.
[http://dx.doi.org/10.3390/molecules16064389] [PMID: 21623310]

[123] Pan MH, Lai CS, Ho CT. Anti-inflammatory activity of natural dietary flavonoids. Food Funct 2010; 1(1): 15-31.
[http://dx.doi.org/10.1039/c0fo00103a] [PMID: 21776454]

[124] Wu WB, Hung DK, Chang FW, Ong ET, Chen BH. Anti-inflammatory and anti-angiogenic effects of flavonoids isolated from *Lycium barbarum Linnaeus* on human umbilical vein endothelial cells. Food Funct 2012; 3(10): 1068-81.
[http://dx.doi.org/10.1039/c2fo30051f] [PMID: 22751795]

[125] Wang H, Zhou H, Zou Y, *et al.* Resveratrol modulates angiogenesis through the GSK3β/β-catenin/TCF-dependent pathway in human endothelial cells. Biochem Pharmacol 2010; 80(9): 1386-95.
[http://dx.doi.org/10.1016/j.bcp.2010.07.034] [PMID: 20696143]

[126] Kim JH, Lee BJ, Kim JH, Yu YS, Kim MY, Kim KW. Rosmarinic acid suppresses retinal neovascularization *via* cell cycle arrest with increase of p21(WAF1) expression. Eur J Pharmacol 2009; 615(1-3): 150-4.
[http://dx.doi.org/10.1016/j.ejphar.2009.05.015] [PMID: 19470386]

[127] Kim JH, Lee BJ, Kim JH, Yu YS, Kim KW. Anti-angiogenic effect of caffeic acid on retinal neovascularization. Vascul Pharmacol 2009; 51(4): 262-7.
[http://dx.doi.org/10.1016/j.vph.2009.06.010] [PMID: 19589397]

[128] Munson AE, Harris LS, Friedman MA, Dewey WL, Carchman RA. Antineoplastic activity of cannabinoids. J Natl Cancer Inst 1975; 55(3): 597-602.
[http://dx.doi.org/10.1093/jnci/55.3.597] [PMID: 1159836]

[129] Blázquez C, Casanova ML, Planas A, *et al.* Inhibition of tumor angiogenesis by cannabinoids. FASEB J 2003; 17(3): 529-31.
[http://dx.doi.org/10.1096/fj.02-0795fje] [PMID: 12514108]

[130] Casanova ML, Blázquez C, Martínez-Palacio J, *et al.* Inhibition of skin tumor growth and angiogenesis *in vivo* by activation of cannabinoid receptors. J Clin Invest 2003; 111(1): 43-50.
[http://dx.doi.org/10.1172/JCI200316116] [PMID: 12511587]

[131] Guzmán M. Cannabinoids: potential anticancer agents. Nat Rev Cancer 2003; 3(10): 745-55.
[http://dx.doi.org/10.1038/nrc1188] [PMID: 14570037]

[132] Peng T, Wu JR, Tong LJ, *et al.* Identification of DW532 as a novel anti-tumor agent targeting both kinases and tubulin. Acta Pharmacol Sin 2014; 35(7): 916-28.
[http://dx.doi.org/10.1038/aps.2014.33] [PMID: 24858311]

[133] Sun D, Zhang F, Qian J, *et al.* 4′-hydroxywogonin inhibits colorectal cancer angiogenesis by disrupting PI3K/AKT signaling. Chem Biol Interact 2018; 296: 26-33.
[http://dx.doi.org/10.1016/j.cbi.2018.09.003] [PMID: 30217479]

[134] He L, Lu N, Dai Q, *et al.* Wogonin induced G1 cell cycle arrest by regulating Wnt/β-catenin signaling pathway and inactivating CDK8 in human colorectal cancer carcinoma cells. Toxicology 2013; 312: 36-47.
[http://dx.doi.org/10.1016/j.tox.2013.07.013] [PMID: 23907061]

[135] Song X, Yao J, Wang F, *et al.* Wogonin inhibits tumor angiogenesis *via* degradation of HIF-1α protein. Toxicol Appl Pharmacol 2013; 271(2): 144-55.
[http://dx.doi.org/10.1016/j.taap.2013.04.031] [PMID: 23707765]

[136] Ravishankar D, Watson KA, Boateng SY, Green RJ, Greco F, Osborn HM. Exploring quercetin and luteolin derivatives as antiangiogenic agents. Eur J Med Chem 2015; 97: 259-74.
[http://dx.doi.org/10.1016/j.ejmech.2015.04.056] [PMID: 25984842]

[137] Chen Y, Lu N, Ling Y, *et al.* LYG-202, a newly synthesized flavonoid, exhibits potent anti-angiogenic activity *in vitro* and *in vivo*. J Pharmacol Sci 2010; 112(1): 37-45.
[http://dx.doi.org/10.1254/jphs.09213FP] [PMID: 20093787]

[138] Zhang H, Fang X, Meng Q, *et al.* Design, synthesis and characterization of potent microtubule inhibitors with dual anti-proliferative and anti-angiogenic activities. Eur J Med Chem 2018; 157: 380-96.
[http://dx.doi.org/10.1016/j.ejmech.2018.07.043] [PMID: 30099258]

[139] Kulshrestha A, Katara GK, Ibrahim SA, Patil R, Patil SA, Beaman KD. Microtubule inhibitor, SP--27 inhibits angiogenesis and induces apoptosis in ovarian cancer cells. Oncotarget 2017; 8(40): 67017-28.
[http://dx.doi.org/10.18632/oncotarget.17549] [PMID: 28978013]

[140] Schmitt F, Gold M, Rothemund M, *et al.* New naphthopyran analogues of LY290181 as potential tumor vascular-disrupting agents. Eur J Med Chem 2019; 163: 160-8.
[http://dx.doi.org/10.1016/j.ejmech.2018.11.055] [PMID: 30503940]

[141] Vijay Avin BR, Thirusangu P, Lakshmi Ranganatha V, Firdouse A, Prabhakar BT, Khanum SA. Synthesis and tumor inhibitory activity of novel coumarin analogs targeting angiogenesis and apoptosis. Eur J Med Chem 2014; 75(21): 211-21.
[http://dx.doi.org/10.1016/j.ejmech.2014.01.050] [PMID: 24534537]

[142] Chang DJ, An H, Kim KS, *et al.* Design, synthesis, and biological evaluation of novel deguelin-based heat shock protein 90 (HSP90) inhibitors targeting proliferation and angiogenesis. J Med Chem 2012; 55(24): 10863-84.
[http://dx.doi.org/10.1021/jm301488q] [PMID: 23186287]

[143] Zhang G, Ye X, Ji D, *et al.* Inhibition of lung tumor growth by targeting EGFR/VEGFR-Akt/NF-κB pathways with novel theanine derivatives. Oncotarget 2014; 5(18): 8528-43.
[http://dx.doi.org/10.18632/oncotarget.2336] [PMID: 25138052]

[144] Batran RZ, Dawood DH, El-Seginy SA, *et al.* New Coumarin Derivatives as Anti-Breast and Anti-Cervical Cancer Agents Targeting VEGFR-2 and p38α MAPK. Arch Pharm (Weinheim) 2017; 350(9)
[http://dx.doi.org/10.1002/ardp.201700064] [PMID: 28787092]

[145] Abdelhafez OM, Ali HI, Amin KM, Abdalla MM, Ahmed EY. Design, synthesis and anticancer activity of furochromone and benzofuran derivatives targeting VEGFR-2 tyrosine kinase. RSC Advances 2015; 5(32): 25312-24.
[http://dx.doi.org/10.1039/C4RA16228E]

[146] Luo G, Li X, Zhang G, *et al.* Novel SERMs based on 3-aryl-4-aryloxy-2H-chromen-2-one skeleton - A possible way to dual ERα/VEGFR-2 ligands for treatment of breast cancer. Eur J Med Chem 2017; 140: 252-73.
[http://dx.doi.org/10.1016/j.ejmech.2017.09.015] [PMID: 28942113]

[147] Park SY, Seo EH, Song HS, *et al.* KR-31831, benzopyran derivative, inhibits VEGF-induced angiogenesis of HUVECs through suppressing KDR expression. Int J Oncol 2008; 32(6): 1311-5.
[http://dx.doi.org/10.3892/ijo.32.6.1311] [PMID: 18497993]

SUBJECT INDEX

A

Acids 135, 168
  nucleic 135
  phenolic 168
  saturated fatty 135
Activated HIF proteins 156
Activation 4, 9, 18, 20, 37, 39, 40, 60, 61, 105, 155, 156, 163, 176
  immune 105
  inhibited VEGF-induced 163
  thrombin-induced platelets 60
Acute medical illnesses 61
Agents 42, 55, 60, 62, 100, 128 138, 151, 156, 157, 165, 172, 177
  immuno-oncology reoviral 138
  innovative mediating 60
  ligand binding 156, 157
  natural anti-angiogentic 42
  pro-angiogenesis 128
  promising antiproliferative 165
  standard first-line anti-cancer 62
  tumoricidal 100
  undertrial chemical/biochemical 55
  vascular disrupting 151, 172
  vascular-disrupting 177
Age-related neovascular macular degeneration 47
Aggressive 8, 61
  growth 8
  tumor behavior 61
AGT technique 106
AI-immunotherapy combination approaches 19
Alternative gene therapy (AGT) 103, 106, 107
Angiogenesis 2, 6, 8, 9, 11, 15, 16, 31, 32, 33, 38, 39, 40, 42, 43, 58, 60, 86, 87, 88, 89, 94, 101, 105, 108, 125, 126, 128, 130, 133, 136, 152, 153, 156, 162, 164, 165, 166, 168, 172, 177
  activating 153
  blocking tumor 86, 101
  direct tumor 88

  embryonic 40
  inhibiting 6, 16
  inhibiting tumor 8
  intussusceptive 32
  modulate 168
  pathological 156
  physiological 2
  prostate cancer cells 166
  reduced tumor 108
  suppress 125, 136
  suppressed 162, 172
  suppressed LPS-induced tumor 165
  suppressing EGF-induced 164
  target 15
  targeting 130, 156, 177
  therapeutic 11
  tumor-induced 33, 42, 43
Angiogenesis inhibitors (AIs) 1, 3, 5, 6, 11, 13, 15, 16, 17, 18, 19, 20, 21, 92, 93, 130, 152
  endogenous 130, 152
Angiogenic 3, 19, 30, 32, 34, 36, 41, 45, 90, 94, 126, 128, 129, 136, 152, 154, 164, 166, 167
  biomechanisms 32
  genes 136, 154
  growth factors 3, 30, 32, 152, 154
  inducers 126, 154
  inhibitor 41, 45, 90, 128, 129, 154, 164
  processes 19, 30, 34, 36, 94, 166, 167
  promoters 36
Anthracycline antibiotics 46
Anti-angiogenesis gene therapy 93
Antiangiogenesis metargidin peptide (AMEP) 98
Anti-angiogenesis therapy 61, 67, 86, 90, 94, 125, 130
  microbial-based 86
  treatments 61, 67
Antiangiogenic 34, 62, 64, 90, 91, 94, 96, 100, 103, 138, 151, 152, 171, 176, 177
  agents 64, 91, 94, 96, 100, 103, 151, 152, 171, 176, 177
  polypeptide 138

www.ingramcontent.com/pod-product-compliance
Lightning Source LLC
Chambersburg PA
CBHW050846220326
41598CB00006B/446

* 9 7 8 9 8 1 1 4 3 2 8 6 6 *